Pain Care Essentials

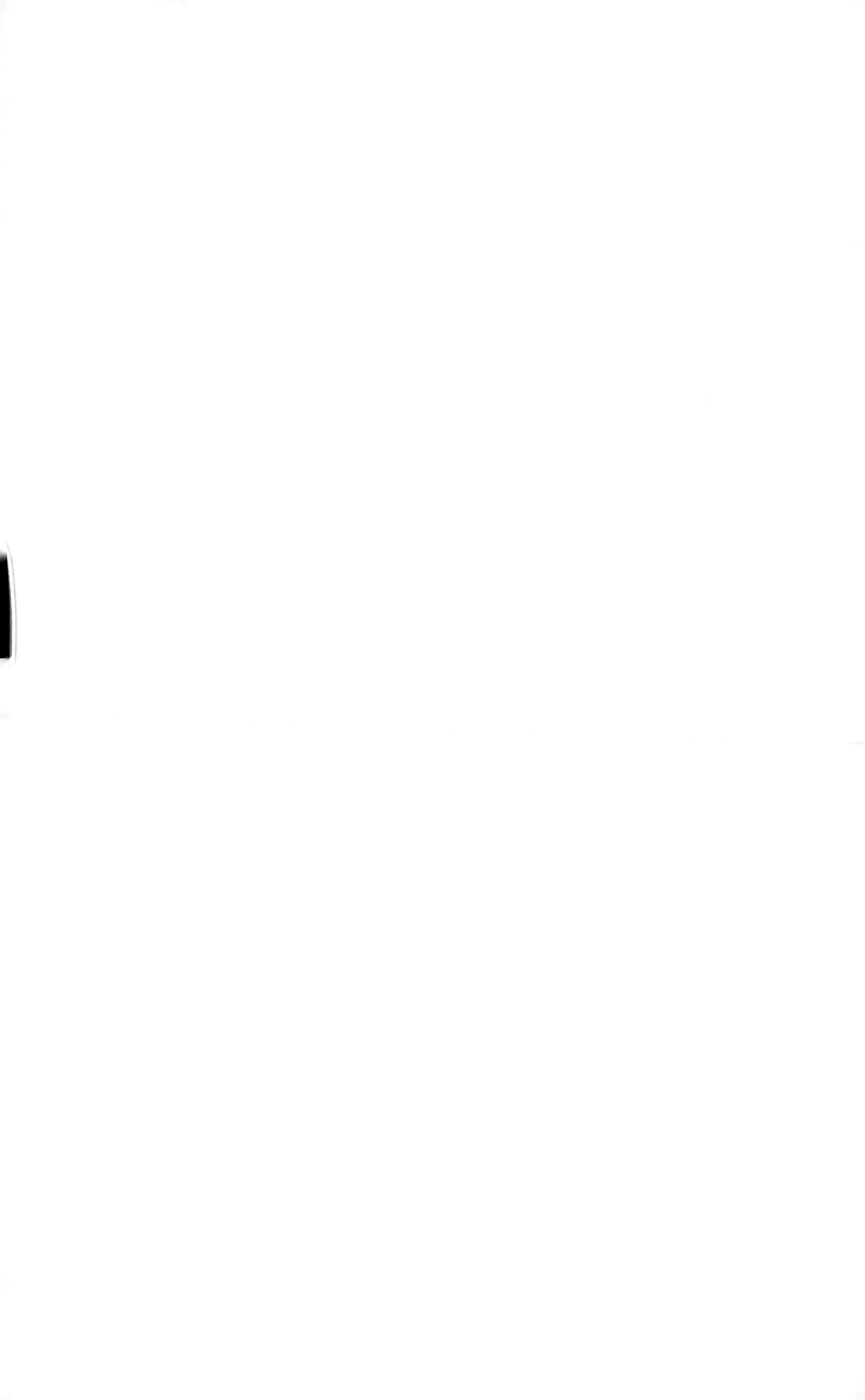

PAIN CARE ESSENTIALS

Edited by
Beth B. Hogans, MS, MD, PhD

Associate Professor and Director of Pain Education
Department of Neurology
Johns Hopkins School of Medicine
Associate Director for Education and Evaluation
Geriatric Research, Education, and Clinical Center
VA Maryland Health Care System
Baltimore, MD

Antje M. Barreveld, MD

Medical Director, Pain Management Service
Department of Anesthesiology
Newton-Wellesley Hospital
Newton, MA

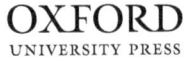

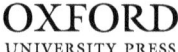

Oxford University Press is a department of the University of Oxford. It furthers
the University's objective of excellence in research, scholarship, and education
by publishing worldwide. Oxford is a registered trade mark of Oxford University
Press in the UK and certain other countries.

Published in the United States of America by Oxford University Press
198 Madison Avenue, New York, NY 10016, United States of America.

© Oxford University Press 2020

All rights reserved. No part of this publication may be reproduced, stored in
a retrieval system, or transmitted, in any form or by any means, without the
prior permission in writing of Oxford University Press, or as expressly permitted
by law, by license, or under terms agreed with the appropriate reproduction
rights organization. Inquiries concerning reproduction outside the scope of the
above should be sent to the Rights Department, Oxford University Press, at the
address above.

You must not circulate this work in any other form
and you must impose this same condition on any acquirer.

CIP data is on file at the Library of Congress
ISBN 978–0–19–976891–2

This material is not intended to be, and should not be considered, a substitute for medical or other
professional advice. Treatment for the conditions described in this material is highly dependent on
the individual circumstances. And, while this material is designed to offer accurate information
with respect to the subject matter covered and to be current as of the time it was written, research
and knowledge about medical and health issues is constantly evolving and dose schedules for
medications are being revised continually, with new side effects recognized and accounted for
regularly. Readers must therefore always check the product information and clinical procedures
with the most up-to-date published product information and data sheets provided by the
manufacturers and the most recent codes of conduct and safety regulation. The publisher and the
authors make no representations or warranties to readers, express or implied, as to the accuracy or
completeness of this material. Without limiting the foregoing, the publisher and the authors make
no representations or warranties as to the accuracy or efficacy of the drug dosages mentioned in the
material. The authors and the publisher do not accept, and expressly disclaim, any responsibility
for any liability, loss or risk that may be claimed or incurred as a consequence of the use and/or
application of any of the contents of this material.

To Eitan, Rachel, and Donnie, for their courage, kindness, and grace.
BBH

To Dorothee, Meenhard, Bernie, Sebastian, Annika and Julian—I like you a lot.
AMB

To our patients, for their hope and resilience.

[T]here's so much more to be learnt about pain, and you will only be frustrated if you don't do it properly. . . .

—Surgeon Norman Barrett speaking to Cicely Saunders in 1948

Cicely Saunders (1918–2005) trained first as a nurse, then as a medical social worker, and later as a physician. She established modern hospice care in the United Kingdom and influenced others globally. Saunders' work was lauded during her lifetime, and she was named Dame Commander of the Order of the British Empire (knighted) in 1979. Saunders advanced the concept of "total pain" encompassing physical, emotional, social, and spiritual distress and created an environment where care could address the comprehensive needs of patients.* Pain care is sometimes confused or incorrectly conflated with palliative care. Nonetheless, pain is present across the life span and should be addressed diligently even in the absence of life-limiting illness. We gratefully acknowledge Saunders' leadership in building bridges between the health professions, putting patients at the center, and promoting comprehensive "thinking and doing" to meet the needs of patients and caregivers.

---

* Dame Cicely Saunders (Obituary). C. Richmond. BMJ. 2005;331(7510):238.

Contents

xi Foreword; *by Judy Watt-Watson*
xv Preface; *by Beth B. Hogans and Antje M. Barreveld*
xix Contributors
xxiii About the Cover

1 Introduction
   Antje M. Barreveld and Beth B. Hogans

Part I The Multi-dimensionality of Pain: Neurobiology, Scope, and Impact

7 1. Pain Pathways: Anatomic Organization and Development
   Mark Schumacher and Beth B. Hogans

26 2. Nociceptive Processing: Neurochemistry and Neurophysiology
   Cynthia L. Renn and Susan G. Dorsey

41 3. Impact of Pain on the Individual and Others: Implications for Healthcare Professionals
   Paul Arnstein and Megan Keating

52 4. Pain Appraisal: Classification, Measurement, and Nomenclature
   Chris R. Abrecht, Beth B. Hogans, and Antje M. Barreveld

75 5. Pain Psychology: An Overview of Concepts and Methods
   Valerie Jackson

Part II Clinical Skills in the Assessment and Care of Pain

89 6. Clinical Assessment of Pain: History, Examination, and Clinical Reasoning
   Beth B. Hogans

103 7. Diagnostic Reasoning in the Pain-Focused Encounter
   Beth B. Hogans

117 8. Professionalism in Pain Care
   Beth B. Hogans

Part III Pain Treatments and Approaches to Management

133   9. Standard Systemic Analgesic Agents: Acetaminophen, Nonsteroidal Anti-Inflammatory Drugs, and Opioids
Michele L. Matthews and Benjamin S. Kematick

158 10. Neuromodulating Agents
Beth B. Hogans

176 11. Interventional Techniques and Surgical Management of Pain
Mark Young, Andrew Rubens, and Antje M. Barreveld

199 12. Rehabilitation Approaches to Pain and Applications in Outpatient Practice
Marlis Gonzalez-Fernandez, Katherine S. Wright, Bernard Abrams, Ada L. Yao, Amira Noles, and Beth B. Hogans

Part IV Pain Care in Clinical Context

221 13. Pain Emergencies and Complications of Pain Treatment
Isaac Tong, R. Jason Yong, and Beth B. Hogans

241 14. Acute Pain: Postoperative, Trauma-Related, and Obstetric Pain
Nantthasorn Zinboonyahgoon and Kristin Schreiber

259 15. Urgent Pain Problems
Beth B. Hogans

273 16. Common Chronic Pain Problems
Beth B. Hogans

291 17. Extremes of Pain
Beth B. Hogans

306 18. Basics of Pediatric Pain Management
Tommy Rappold, Matthew Digiusto, and M-Irfan Suleman

319 19. Pain in Older Patients
Staja Q. Booker and Keela A. Herr

339 20. Opioid Misuse and Addiction Among Patients With Chronic Pain: From Risk Factors to Risk Reduction
Marc O. Martel and Robert N. Jamison

     Appendices
355   I. Examination Template
359 II. Chemical Structure of Commonly Used Pain Medications
363 III. Comparison of Pain Treatments According to Pain Type

365   IV. Adjustments in Treatment for Liver and Renal Failure
369   V. Back Pain Diagnosis Flow Diagram
373   VI. Evidence-Based Basic Recommendations to Prevent or Reduce Chronic Pain
375   Index

Foreword

This book, *Pain Care Essentials*, is an excellent resource for newly graduated health professionals, including those without prior pain education, and experienced educators to recommend to their trainees. Acute and persistent (chronic) pain affects millions of people worldwide across the life span, and persistent pain is a global cause of morbidity and disability in both developed and developing countries (2016 Global Burden of Disease Study). The widespread prevalence of pain ensures that pain is a common concern of patients seeking help from all health professionals, and this book is relevant across these professions. Pain is a public health crisis that requires a more complex approach than many other health conditions. But are we sufficiently prepared to help people with pain manage their care?

The material in this book is important because pain content has not necessarily been recognized as essential and a key priority at all levels of professional education. Despite available curriculum resources, such as those from the International Association for the Study of Pain (IASP), surveys continue to demonstrate minimal or no pain content in health science curricula, particularly at the entry-to-practice level. It was concerning to find that graduates from veterinary colleges, who care for our pets, received more pain content and related clinical practice hours than the rest of us (Watt-Watson et al., 2009).[†] It is not surprising, therefore, that health professionals don't feel competent to manage pain, particularly with complex pain issues that require comprehensive treatment. Until now, many health professionals have learned pain management only on the job through the "informal curriculum" in clinical settings that perpetuate a culture of misbeliefs and inadequate pain care practices. As a result, health sciences schools and universities, education-accrediting bodies, and faculty across the globe are being asked to incorporate essential pain content into curricula. However, their aim of producing graduates with the knowledge and skills that are necessary to be competent in contemporary pain management will take time, and many clinicians have graduated without foundational understanding of pain care.

Pain Care Essentials is an important source of foundational information for newly graduated clinicians, trainees, and those wishing to update their pain knowledge. This book is unique in that the content is framed within the IASP Curriculum Domains, reflecting in particular the Interprofessional Pain Curriculum components. Effective pain management can be complex, requiring interprofessional, collaborative

---

[†] Watt-Watson J, McGillion M, Hunter J, Choiniere M, Clark AJ, Dewar A, Johnston C, Lynch M, Morley-Forster P, Moulin D, Thie N, von Baeyer CL, Webber K. A survey of prelicensure pain curricula in health science faculties in Canadian universities. Pain Res Manag. 2009 Nov-Dec;14(6):439–444.

approaches that exceed the expertise of any one profession, and this book provides knowledge and approaches relevant to all professions. The World Health Organization and National Academy of Medicine have both emphasized that interprofessional education is an important step in developing collaborative practice, which has demonstrated benefits for health service, delivery, and outcomes. Contributors represent the major health science professions, and many chapters provide integrated views despite their different disciplines.

The format of the book allows the reader to proceed sequentially through the chapters or to select a stand-alone section, depending on his or her needs. The chapters are organized in four parts, which take the reader through the key components of the multidimensional nature of pain, assessment, and management, and pain care in specific clinical contexts. While all the chapters are important, Part IV: Pain Care in Clinical Context speaks to specific care issues, such as pain emergencies, age-related challenges, addiction, and common chronic pain conditions. Each chapter outlines objectives to guide the reader toward specific learning outcomes. The case scenarios describe related real-world contexts with interprofessional and multiprofessional relevance. Review questions at the end of each chapter underline key takeaway points for the reader to remember. This organization of each chapter supports the learning experience and reflects best practices in health professions education. With this volume, Hogans and Barreveld successfully bridge the gaps between content and curriculum requirements, providing students and trainees with a foundation that supports empathic awareness, clinical skills development, compassion, and entry-to-practice competencies.

The Co-Editors are internationally and nationally known experts in the field of both pain care and pain education. Both Editors have had a remarkable influence on the field of pain at large.

Dr. Hogans is an Associate Professor of Neurology and Director of Pain Education at Johns Hopkins School of Medicine. She also serves as interim Associate Director for Evaluation and Education at the Geriatric Research Education and Clinical Center at the Veterans Administration Maryland Health Care System in Baltimore. She holds board certifications in Neurology, Clinical Electrophysiology, and Pain Medicine and is an experienced neurologist with a strong focus on providing patient-centered care. Known for comprehensive nonopioid management of painful neuropathies, headaches, and spine pain, Dr. Hogans has authored a book for those with low back pain entitled: *Take Back Your Back*. Dr. Hogans has been vigorous in interprofessional education collaborations and has served on the executive committees of the Interprofessional Pain Competencies (Fishman-Mayday) Project and contributed to the US Medical Licensing Examination Pain Competencies assessment project. She currently heads an interprofessional team working on the National Institutes of Health Pain Consortium Center of Excellence in Pain Education (CoEPE) at Johns Hopkins. Together with Dr. Debra Gordon, Dr. Hogans co-founded the Pain Education SIG for the US chapter of IASP and is the recently elected Chair of the IASP Pain Education Special Interest Group.

Dr. Antje M. Barreveld is Assistant Professor of Anesthesiology at Tufts University School of Medicine. She is Medical Director of the Pain Management Services, Director of the Substance Use Services (SUS), and Anesthesiologist with Commonwealth Anesthesia Associates at Newton-Wellesley Hospital in Newton, MA. Dr. Barreveld is also a Clinical Researcher at Harvard Medical School in the Department of

Anesthesiology, Perioperative and Pain Medicine at Brigham and Women's Hospital in Boston, MA.

Her clinical and research interests are in pain management education, chronic pelvic pain in men and women, acute and chronic postoperative pain, and safe practices in co-managing pain and addiction. She is Co-Principal Investigator of the Harvard School of Dental Medicine and Brigham and Women's Hospital Center of Excellence in Pain Education (CoEPE), designated by the National Institutes of Health Pain Consortium.

In summary, *Pain Care Essentials* is an excellent resource providing a comprehensive overview of the major components of pain care. The content is written by clinicians from across various professional designations and is relevant to any recently graduated health professional, or trainee, but also for those wanting further foundational understanding of pain. The Co-Editors are internationally respected for their clinical expertise and involvement in moving the pain education agenda forward. This is a major contribution to the field of pain education, including interprofessional pain education, and I highly recommend this book.

Judy Watt-Watson, RN, MSc, PhD
Professor Emeritus Lawrence S. Bloomberg Faculty of
Nursing Senior Fellow, Massey College University of Toronto
Associate Scientist, Sinai Health System
Canadian Pain Society, Past President

Preface

It may come as something of a surprise that pain, the most prevalent symptom in clinical practice, is not always addressed specifically in health professions training. Approximately one in six Americans lives with chronic pain, in addition to the millions who experience acute pain each day. Half of older adults live with chronic pain–associated conditions, and about half of all healthcare visits are initiated because of pain. Despite this, reports indicate that the vast majority of health professions schools in the United States do not teach required courses on pain, and the total amount of content pertaining to pain is a fraction of a percent of the total. Almost certainly, the lack of education in coordinated, comprehensive, compassionate care for pain-associated conditions contributed to pervasive opioid overprescribing and the ensuing wave of addiction and deaths that swept the country in the first part of this century. This book is our response to the pain care crisis—it is designed to prepare young clinicians to assess and treat a wide variety of pain conditions in a manner that balances competence and compassion, incorporating coordinated elements of pharmacologic and nonpharmacologic therapies.

The need for all clinicians to have a foundation knowledge of pain has become more critically important than ever, as the understanding of pain has undergone extraordinary development over the past 25 years. For example, it is increasingly evident that acute pain, if properly treated, is less likely to progress to chronic pain. This means that the leading cause of lost productivity in the home and workplace may be preventable if we take the time to teach and learn about treating pain. It seems that pain, an incredibly prevalent experience, suffers from being so much a part of all medical practice that none of the major traditional specialties, except anesthesiology, has claimed pain for its own. Because of a confluence of health system factors, many practitioners are unaware of scientific advances in the understanding of pain and the new approaches to pain management; as a consequence, many patients with pain remain inadequately treated and suffer needlessly.

Intended as a comprehensive introduction to pain for all entry-level healthcare practitioners, this book is written at a depth that highlights the principal features of pain management without being overwhelming in detail. It is clear that excessive detail leads to a loss of interest on the part of students and an actual decrease in the ability to retain fundamental information. This book focuses on the basics of pain care. Based on the structured approach to learning, each chapter begins with specific learning objectives and a clinical scenario. The content of the chapters parallels the learning objectives, and special points are highlighted through the use of text boxes and illustrations. At the end of each chapter, there is a summary paragraph and review questions that enable readers to test their knowledge. This organization reinforces learning by explicitly identifying, teaching, and testing the major learning objectives.

The topics for this introductory text were initially selected by a multidisciplinary team of Johns Hopkins pain specialists, including clinicians as well as researchers. Over the course of a year, this multidisciplinary team met and discussed the aims and objectives for educating our medical students about pain and pain care. The goal was to identify the essential knowledge that every medical graduate should possess at the completion of 4 years of medical training. Over the ensuing decade, the book changed in focus to include a broader expanse of learners. As more nurse practitioners, pharmacists, physician assistants, psychologists, and others are engaged in pain care, we have endeavored to include the content most useful to the entry-to-practice health professions student. Designed to be read during or after prelicensure training (e.g., medical, nursing, or pharmacy school) and to inspire students to learn more about painful conditions, this book is unique in its clinical focus and the level of detail that is included. The later chapters presuppose that the reader is familiar with the content of the earlier chapters but are self-contained. We believe that this book will be effective in improving pain care, most especially if used alongside a formal pain care course as part of prelicensure training, whether spread over four years or condensed into a shorter period. Through engagement in the interprofessional curriculum planning process, the content of the book has been shaped to align with the IASP interprofessional pain curriculum vision and to focus on the primary questions of: What is pain? How is pain assessed? How is pain managed? How does clinical context influence pain?

There are many people besides the authors and editors who have contributed to this book. We would like to acknowledge the contributions of some of those here. First and foremost, tremendous thanks go to Andrea Knobloch, whose consistent good will, vision, and encouragement made this book possible. Without Andrea's encouragement, this book would not be here. The editorial staff at Oxford University Press have provided consistent support and guidance. Our mentors in pain care and specifically in support of this project and our work together include Drs. Judy Watt-Watson, Rollin "Mac" Gallagher, Daniel Carr, and Dave Thomas. Dr. Hogans thanks professors James "Jim" Campbell, Richard "Dick" Meyer, Justin McArthur, Patricia Thomas, David Nichols, Jennifer Haythornthwaite, Gayle Page, Albert Wu, Sharon Kozachik, Marlis Gonzalez-Fernandez, Suzanne Nesbit, Luis Buenaver, Ahmet Hoke, Andrea Corse, Vinay Chaudhry, David Cornblath, and Glenn Triesman at Hopkins, and Professors David Yarnitsky, Stephen McMahon, Eloise Carr, Margaret Lloyd, Paul Wilkinson, Larry Driver, Sean Mackey, Scott Fishman, and Beth Darnall, as well as Dr. Christine Spellman for insights, feedback, and collaborations. Expert technical support from Dr. Lina Mezei and from Elizabeth Nenortas, Joseph Nugent, Merav Shor, and Kolade Fapohunda contributed to making this curriculum stronger and more vibrant. Dr. Barreveld would like to thank the following individuals: her mother Dorothee for inspiring her to pursue a career in pain medicine—and to always look for new ways to reduce suffering; her father Meenhard for being the most important role model in her life; Dr. Howard Fields for his stimulating lecture on the placebo effect and a launch into the field of pain medicine; Dr. Jake Joffe for his constant support of professional and clinical excellence and growth—and reminders that if you get confused, listen to the music play; her colleagues at Newton-Wellesley Hospital and the Pain Management Center for their collaborations and for being a simply awesome team; the NIH Pain Consortium for believing in (and funding!) pain education initiatives; Sebastian, Annika, and Julian for always being there in every way, every day; and to her patients for motivating her to inspire hope and never give up in the pursuit of defeating pain.

Beth B. Hogans
Baltimore
Antje M. Barreveld
Newton

Contributors

Bernard Abrams, MD
Department of Physical Medicine and Rehabilitation
Johns Hopkins School of Medicine
Baltimore, MD

Christopher R. Abrecht, MD
Department of Anesthesia & Perioperative Care
Division of Pain Medicine
University of California San Francisco
San Francisco, California

Paul Arnstein, RN, PhD, FAAN
Massachusetts General Hospital
Boston, MA

Antje M. Barreveld, MD
Medical Director, Pain Management Service
Department of Anesthesiology
Newton-Wellesley Hospital, Tufts University School of Medicine
Newton, MA

Staja Q. Booker, PhD, RN
Postdoctoral Fellow
University of Florida
Gainesville, FL

Matthew Digiusto, MD
Department of Anesthesiology and Critical Care Medicine
Department of Pediatrics
Johns Hopkins Hospital
Baltimore, MD

Susan G. Dorsey, PhD, RN, FAAN
Professor and Department Chair
Department of Pain and Translational Symptom Science
University of Maryland, School of Nursing
Baltimore, MD

Marlis Gonzalez-Fernandez, MD, PhD
Department of Physical Medicine and Rehabilitation
Johns Hopkins School of Medicine
Baltimore, MD

Keela A. Herr, PhD, RN, AGSF, FAAN
Kelting Professor in Nursing and Associate Dean for Faculty
University of Iowa, College of Nursing
Iowa City, IA

Beth B. Hogans, MS, MD, PhD
Associate Professor and Director of Pain Education
Department of Neurology
Johns Hopkins School of Medicine
Associated Director for Education and Evaluation
Geriatric Research, Education, and Clinical Center
VA Maryland Health Care System
Baltimore, MD

Valerie Jackson, PhD, MPH
Department of Anesthesia and
Perioperative Care
University of California, San Francisco,
Pain Management Center
San Francisco, CA

Robert N. Jamison, PhD
Departments of Anesthesia and
Psychiatry
Harvard Medical School,
Brigham and Women's Hospital
Boston, MA

Megan Keating, RN-BC, BSN
Massachusetts General Hospital
Boston, MA

Benjamin S. Kematick, PharmD
Clinical Pharmacy Specialist,
Palliative Care
Dana-Farber Cancer Institute
Boston, MA

Marc O. Martel, PhD
Faculties of Dentistry and Medicine
McGill University
Montreal, Quebec, Canada

Michele L. Matthews, PharmD, CPE, BCACP, FASHP
Associate Professor of Pharmacy
Practice
Massachusetts College of Pharmacy and
Health Science
Advanced Practice Pharmacist, Pain
Management
Brigham and Women's Hospital
Boston, MA

Amira Noles, MD
Johns Hopkins School of Medicine
Department of Physical Medicine and
Rehabilitation
Baltimore, MD

Tommy Rappold, MD
Department of Anesthesiology and
Critical Care Medicine
Department of Pediatrics
Johns Hopkins Hospital
Baltimore, MD

Cynthia L. Renn, PhD, RN
Associate Professor
Department of Pain and Translational
Symptom Science
University of Maryland, School of
Nursing
Baltimore, MD

Andrew Rubens, MD
Department of Anesthesiology
Newton-Wellesley Hospital
Newton, MA

Kristin Schreiber, MD, PhD
Professor of Anesthesia
Chief, Division of Pain Medicine
Department of Anesthesia and
Perioperative Care
University of California,
San Francisco
San Francisco, CA

Mark Schumacher, PhD, MD
Professor of Anesthesia
Chief, Division of Pain Medicine
Department of Anesthesia and
Perioperative Care
University of California,
San Francisco
San Francisco, CA

M-Irfan Suleman, MBBS, MD
Department of Anesthesiology and
Critical Care Medicine
Kennedy Krieger Rehabilitation
Institute
Baltimore, MD

Yi Cai Isaac Tong, MD
Pain Medicine Physician
Tricity Pain Associates
San Antonio, Texas

Katherine S. Wright, PhD
Department of Physical Medicine
and Rehabilitation
Johns Hopkins School of Medicine
Baltimore, MD

Ada L. Yao, MD
Department of Physical Medicine
and Rehabilitation
Johns Hopkins School of Medicine
Baltimore, MD

R. Jason Yong, MD, MBA
Medical Director, Brigham and Women's
Pain Management Center
Brigham and Women's Hospital/
Harvard Medical School
Boston, MA

Mark Young, MD
Department of Anesthesiology
Newton-Wellesley Hospital
Newton, MA

Nantthasorn Zinboonyahgooon, MD
Chief, Division of Pain Medicine
Siriraj Hospital
Mahidol University, Thailand

About the Cover

Demeter and Persephone, a mother–daughter pair in the Classical pantheon, are depicted in this 1st century Roman marble adaptation of an earlier Greek work, from the Metropolitan Museum of Art collection. Celebrated as patrons of rebirth, renewal, and growth, the placement of a firepot between the two subjects alludes to contemporaneous religious practices but hints at potential peril; the rightmost figure appears to caution the younger figure on the left, an allusion to the value of the mentoring relationships that inspired us to write "Pain Care Essentials."

—Beth B. Hogans and Antje M. Barreveld

Introduction

Antje M. Barreveld and Beth B. Hogans

Pain seems, at times, an inescapable feature of human existence; nonetheless, modern healthcare offers many modalities to mitigate and control pain. Enhancing human experience through the reduction of pain represents one of the great opportunities for good in the 21st century. Because of the traditional nature of educational systems, much of what has been discovered through basic and preclinical studies has not been delivered to the primary care setting. And the scientific understanding of pain has advanced dramatically faster than clinical trainees have been made ready. For diverse reasons, patients living with pain are still subject to extensive stigmatization, and pain is still relegated to being termed *subjective* and a *symptom*. What distinguishes pain from other experiences is the profound effect: reducing the sufferer's capacity to participate fully in productive activity and enjoy any single moment of life. Instead, existence becomes an unbearable torment, and some are willing to consider ending it all rather than endure another day in pain. Unfortunately, for many generations, the torment of pain itself was compounded by social ostracization; there was a linkage between virtuous conduct and freedom from pain; Dante's *Inferno* and Hugo's *Les Miserables*, among many works in the Western canon, promulgated the idea that pain was an inevitable punishment for moral transgressions.

Beginning 45 years ago, clinicians and researchers have made a concerted international effort to understand and communicate scientifically about pain. Although previous incremental insights hinted at the major features of ensuing studies, the research that followed 1973 has resulted in a dramatic reshaping of how we can conceptualize and reason clinically about pain. Pain is the manifestation of multifarious and exquisitely choreographed series of events in the nervous system. Pain is the primary reason that people seek out healthcare. Pain is a complex, intersubjective experience that can only be understood when both patient and clinician endeavor to communicate and understand it. Pain has profound impacts on quality of life and is the leading cause of years lost to disability globally. Pain is an important sign of disease but can also make disease recovery worse; pain can be a disease in and of itself as there are primary pain conditions as well as pain-associated conditions. The pain system in the body is far more pervasive and elaborate than was conceptualized 50 years ago, and so this book is our effort to bring pain out of the ivory tower and into the everyday clinical setting.

One of us, 10 years ago, undertook a study of North American medical schools and found that fewer than one in ten medical schools offered physicians-in-training a comprehensive view of pain. Dr. Watt-Watson and colleagues made similar observations across the spectrum of health professions schools in Canada, and although a similarly expansive study has not been carried out in the United States, there are indications that a paucity of pain education is a nearly global phenomenon [Shipton]. So despite the omnipresence of pain in clinical practice, healthcare providers have not been prepared to recognize and meet the challenges of pain. We began to assemble the ideas that became the outline for this book.

With this book, it was our vision to bring together experts in pain from a broad range of health professions, including those with primary training in medicine, nursing, pharmacy, and clinical psychology. Our goal is to give the prelicensure and early-stage healthcare professional a solid foundation in understanding the pain system and applying the foundational principles of interprofessional pain care in a primary care setting. Most of the available textbooks on "pain medicine" are prepared to address the needs of the advanced pain interventionalist, that is, the pain medicine fellow. The needs of these fellows are, at the present, primarily focused on the severest of chronic pain conditions and typically utilize a maximally invasive approach, such as pumps, nerve ablations, and epidural catheters. Undoubtedly appropriate in selected situations, there is strong evidence that pain is abundant in primary care settings and that appropriate, early proactive management of pain-associated conditions is effective and may prevent the establishment of more intractable, chronic pain.

The chapters of the book are organized into four parts that parallel the International Association for the Study of Pain (IASP) interprofessional curriculum organization to address the following "big questions" about pain: (I) What is pain? (II) How is pain assessed? (III) How is pain treated? (IV) How does context influence pain? Within each section, the chapters are organized with learning objectives, a clinical scenario to spur discussion, and content enhanced with figures, tables, and flowcharts, and each chapter closes with a few multiple-choice questions to check for understanding and selected references. To the extent possible, repetition is avoided wherever possible; however, we do reiterate the utility of assessing pain according to a standardize process of gathering information through active listening to the patient's pain narrative followed by extraction and generalized representation of cardinal pain characteristics. The characteristics are mapped onto a pain differential diagnosis, which guides treatment and diagnostic planning. We illustrate and encourage the coordinated use of pharmacologic and nonpharmacologic therapies, and we value above all pain self-management to the greatest extent possible while remaining safe. The chapters are part of a whole but may be read independently. Clinical conditions are organized using a somewhat novel approach of classifying pain-associated conditions according to acuity of needs: Emergent, urgent, acute, and chronic conditions are considered separately in chapters, along with a chapter entitled "Extremes of Pain," which is not comprehensive but endeavors to include many different forms of pain that illustrate the diversity and meaning of specific pain mechanistic processes. Although originally conceptualized from a curriculum designed for medical students, the text recognizes that other health professions are increasingly involved in delivering care to patients with pain. We have sought out a diverse authorship group, and wherever possible we have sought to include those actively involved in interprofessional educational innovation. The future for pain care is bright, and we hope you will enjoy traveling with us on this journey ahead.

PART I
THE MULTI-DIMENSIONALITY OF PAIN
NEUROBIOLOGY, SCOPE, AND IMPACT

1 Pain Pathways
Anatomic Organization and Development

Mark Schumacher and Beth B. Hogans

I believe all suffering is caused by ignorance.
—Dalai Lama

LEARNING OBJECTIVES

At the completion of this chapter, the learner should be able to discuss:

- The overall functional organization of pain pathways: transduction, transmission, perception, and modulation
- The basic properties of multiple classes of primary afferent neurons, especially nociceptive ones
- The organization of the spinal cord into Rexed laminae and the role of the specific laminae in pain signaling
- The multiple pathways of ascending pain transmission, the components of these pathways, and the ongoing revision of these pathways
- The occurrence of higher level pain processing in both the limbic and somatosensory regions of the brain and how the connections to basal ganglia may influence behavior
- The role of major specific nuclei in the brain and brainstem in controlling descending inhibition and facilitation of pain signals
- The major epochs in the establishment of the nociceptive processing system during development

CASE SCENARIO

A 49-year-old woman is admitted to same-day surgery for open reduction and internal fixation of a closed, displaced elbow fracture. The elbow was fractured 3 days earlier, and surgery was scheduled for the first available day, pending the arrival of specialty screws for the fixation. While waiting for the surgery, the patient was advised to rest, ice, compress, and elevate (RICE) the elbow, and opioid medication was offered. The patient requested an alternative to opioids, and tramadol was prescribed for preoperative control of pain associated with the fracture. Acetaminophen was held due to allergy to this medication. The morning of surgery, the patient was consented for a brachial plexus block for pain control, and the surgical procedure was performed under sedation. Upon awakening in the recovery room, the patient was aware of dense anesthesia of the arm—in fact, the arm was immobile and she was unable to move it for several hours. She was advised that this was not an uncommon experience. Acetaminophen and a nonsteroidal antiinflammatory medication was administered and scheduled. During overnight observation, the patient gradually became aware of deep aching in the arm as well as some stinging pain, both of which responded immediately to a modest dose of opioids, initially administered intravenously, as well as an ice pack. The patient was discharged with a several-day supply of oral oxycodone, which she took for 3 days but then discontinued because of resolving pain levels and constipation. The patient transitioned to time-contingent ice, with occasional use of a non-steroidal anti-inflammatory, e.g. ibuprofen, and completed a course of physical therapy without further substantive pain. The patient and surgeon were very pleased with the effectiveness of nerve block for acute pain control. Overall opioid utilization was modest. The addition of the conservative RICE protocol before and after surgery provided an extra measure of success to the fracture repair outcomes.

1. What is your experience with multimodal analgesia?
2. How many different pain prevention and treatment mechanisms can you identify in this uncomplicated surgical case?
3. How many healthcare providers do you think contributed to this good outcome, can you name some of the professions involved and their roles?

INTRODUCTION

Where Does "Pain" Normally Start?

Buried within most structures of the body are the tiny nerve endings of specialized sensory neurons, known as primary afferent nociceptors (PANs). These diverse cells are a subset of the larger class of sensory neurons known as primary afferent neurons. Developmentally, nociceptors arise from the edge of the neural plate during embryogenesis as one lineage of pluripotent neural crest cells that form an array of diverse cell types. These include neuronal and non-neuronal cells that form complex structures such as the dorsal root ganglion (DRG) and trigeminal ganglion (TG) that consist of sensory neurons and glia. Primary afferent neurons perform essential functions throughout the body by providing a real-time assessment of health and disease in various tissues and organs. Primed to detect potentially harmful stimuli, PANs are the initial portion of the pain pathway within the peripheral nervous system (PNS). PANs are phenotypically and functional variable; PANs may be specialized for the detection of noxious thermal, mechanical, and chemical stimuli, detected and encoded as action potentials though a process termed *transduction*.

The subsequent relay of nociceptive signals to the central nervous system (CNS) through action potentials and nerve synapses is termed *transmission*. The final interpretation of pain as a harmful and unpleasant experience in the brain is termed the *perception* of pain. A fourth component of the pain pathways involves controlling the pain signal, making the system more or less sensitive to external stimuli and internal activation event; this is termed *modulation*. This chapter will review clinically relevant aspects of the structures in the pain pathway and attempt to provide a conceptual framework on which clinical observations and pain management care are rationally developed. Finally, this chapter will cover the development of pain pathways in order to support enhanced understanding for the importance of pain control in the neonatal period and childhood.

TRANSDUCTION OF PAIN STIMULI

Somatic Nociceptors

Detection of noxious stimuli of the skin and underlying deep tissues (somatic) has been divided into three principle modalities—noxious thermal, mechanical, and chemical—based on exposure to various forms of noxious stimulants resulting in energy transfer at the molecular level. The behavioral and physiologic responses following exposure to noxious stimulation have traditionally served as the cornerstone for a classification scheme of nociceptors. Within this framework, the threshold for evoking the sensation of pain has been determined in human volunteers with certain external forces applied to the skin, such as noxious thermal stimuli (temperatures >43°–45° C) or intense mechanical stimuli. Criteria for noxious chemical stimuli have also been applied and rely on the sensation of pain in response to certain compounds, such as capsaicin, the pungent principle ingredient in hot chili peppers, or exposure to acidic solutions. Using these noxious stimuli in preclinical experiments, nociceptive responses, including electrophysiologic currents, neurotransmitter signaling, and axonal reflexes, have demonstrated how human pain thresholds are a response to the activation of various subpopulations of PANs.[1] The detailed molecular events relating to pain pathways will be presented in Chapter 2; here, the focus is on the structural aspects of nociceptive signaling.

PANs are typically neurons with small axon diameter, slow conduction velocity (CV), no or limited myelination, and small cell bodies. More recently, PANs have been further classified using immunochemical identification of specific proteins, receptors, and/or ion channels. PANs are a part of the broader class of neurons responsible for sensation, the Primary Afferent Neurons and fall into three distinct groups (Figure 1.1A): Aβ are large-diameter, 6- to 22-μm, heavily myelinated neurons with fast CVs of 33 to 75 m/s; Aδ fibers are thinly myelinated neurons with CVs of 5 to 30 m/s; and C fibers are 0.3- to 3-μm diameter, unmyelinated neurons with slow CVs of 0.5 to 2 m/s.[2] Most PANos are C fibers or thinly myelinated Aδ fibers (Figure 1.1B). In the periphery, nociceptive nerve endings are very minute, about 1 μm or less in diameter, and advanced microscopic techniques such as confocal or electron microscopy are required to visualize them. The miniscule dimensions of pain-sensing nerve

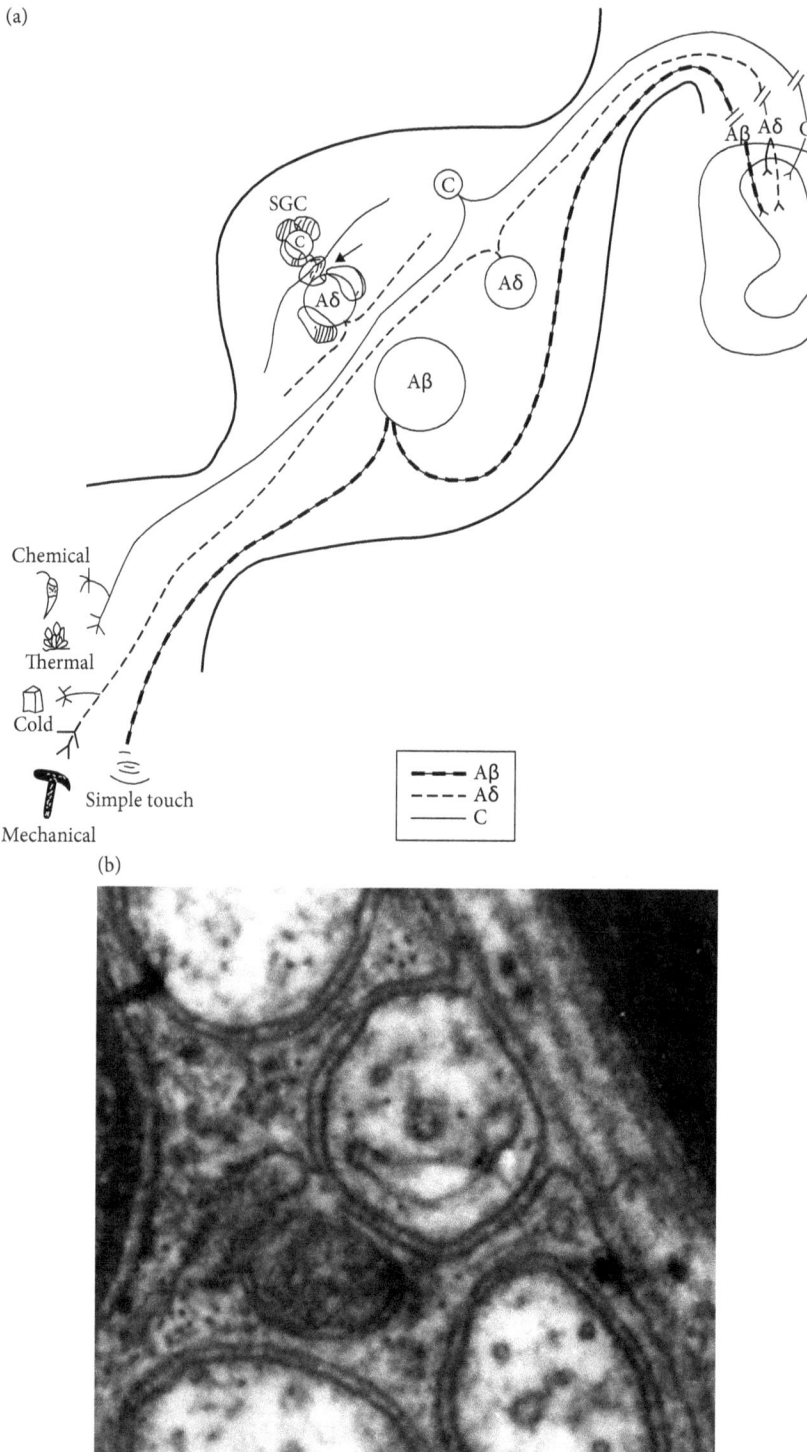

FIGURE 1.1 **Nociceptors and sensory ganglion. A,** Specialized primary afferent neurons dedicated to the transduction of noxious chemical, thermal, and mechanical stimuli (nociceptors) are identified by structural and functional features, including degree of myelination (C fibers—unmyelinated; Aδ—thinly myelinated), conduction velocity, neuronal diameter, and expression of receptor proteins. Together with large-diameter afferent neurons

endings have meant that scientific advances were needed before we could begin to appreciate the pervasive nature of pain nerve endings and truly appreciate how extensive the pain-sensing system is in the body. CV and DRG neuron diameter are loosely correlated so that smaller sensory neurons give rise to C and Aδ fibers. Correlation of nociceptor fiber type with modality of activation has resulted in additional subclassification. There are some PANs that are activated by multiple noxious stimuli, and these are referred to as *polymodal nociceptors*.

PANs are dynamically regulated across the life span, depending on internal and external factors.[3] PANs will respond by growing into an area if neurotrophic factors are released. Specifically, nerve growth factor (NGF) is released in response to injury and inflammation; it is trophic for a subset of PANs and may lead to increased pain in clinical settings. Examples include increased pain/touch sensitivity near a healing surgical site or burn, increased pain in chronically stressed or recurrently strained structures such as joints and vertebral disks, and compellingly, a treatment trial of NGF for peripheral neuropathy in the 1990s that led to increased pain and myalgias for those in the active treatment group. On the other end of the spectrum, patients with decreased PANs are at risk for repeated unintended injury, and this can occur as a congenital syndrome (Chapter 17) or more commonly in the setting of diabetic peripheral neuropathy with distal sensory loss (Chapter 15). Patients with decreased pain sensation, whether congenital or acquired, are at markedly increased risk for injury, infection, and even death.

Visceral Nociceptors

The notion that visceral nociceptors exist as an independent class of Primary Afferent Neurons compared with their somatic counterparts remains a point of intensive investigation.[4] Not all aspects of physiology are easily translated from somatic to visceral nociceptors. A case in point is the gastrointestinal system. As one examines nociceptive detection along the esophagus to the stomach, there is a proportionate decrease in the ability to detect noxious thermal stimuli. Remarkably, the entire length of the small intestine is insensitive to touch, thermal stimuli, cutting, or burning under normal conditions. However, under pathophysiologic conditions of inflammation, these same tissues sites are found to be sensitive to multiple noxious stimuli. In recent years, scientists have found evidence of nociceptive-type innervation in many viscera, including lung, pancreas, liver, heart, and the gastrointestinal tract. There is active research to better understand the role of the nerve endings in responding to injury, ischemia, and inflammation. The extent to which activation of these nerve endings is perceived as painful is very different from that of somatic nociceptors. Visceral nociception is characterized by far less precise localization. Nonetheless, there are common patterns that are clinically recognizable (Table 1.1).

FIGURE 1.1 Continued

(Aβ), nociceptor cell bodies reside in peripheral ganglion and are enveloped by satellite glia cells (SGCs) that provide a means to interconnect nociceptors within sensory ganglion. SGCs are believed to play important roles, especially under pathophysiologic conditions, to influence nociceptive input to the superficial dorsal horn of the spinal cord. **B,** Electron photomicrograph of peripheral nerve demonstrating multiple unmyelinated C fibers supported by a single Schwann cell. A small myelinated fiber and large myelinated fiber are located outside the frame of the picture on the left and right respectively. The *bar*, at the lower left, is 1 μm. (© Beth B. Hogans.)

Table 1.1 Classical Referred Pain Patterns of Selected Viscera

Viscera	Location of Referred Pain
Heart	Left upper chest, medial left arm, jaw line
Pancreas	Central epigastric, mid-back
Gallbladder, liver	Right shoulder and neck
Appendix	Periumbilical
Renal	Low back and flanks into lateral thigh
Uterus	Pelvis, thighs, back

TRANSMISSION OF PAIN
Sensory Ganglia

Activation of PAN nerve endings in the somatic structures leads to one or more action potentials that travel toward the center of the body, through the DRG, and into the protected spinal space by way of dorsal spinal roots. Distinct from the traditional view of neurons in the brain where action potentials activate dendrites, invade the cell body, and lead to an "outgoing" action potential when threshold is reached at the axonal hillock, the Primary Afferent Neuron is a pseudo-bipolar neuron in which the central process, connecting to the spinal dorsal horn, may be activated directly by the incoming action potential from the periphery without activation of the neuronal cell body.[5] This may offer the advantage of rapid signaling but also means that the role of the sensory ganglion in pain processing is distinct from CNS neurons, which are often viewed as "mini-computers." Potentially, the influence of the ganglion on pain signaling is more diffuse than computational per se. Consistent with this, the somatotopic organization of cells in the DRGs is modest.[6]

In the DRG, Primary Afferent Neurons are surrounded by satellite glial cells (SGCs). Although historically overlooked, the past decade has shown a resurgence of interest in the role of SGCs in nociception. Since PANs in the DRG and TG do not form synaptic connection between themselves, investigators have turned their attention to SGCs, which provide the structural elements for intraganglionic signaling. As shown in Figure 1.1A, SGCs envelop nociceptors and are interconnected through gap junctions. Therefore, SGCs are now accepted to be playing critical roles in nociceptive signaling, especially under pathophysiologic conditions such as neuroinflammation.[7] Although the basis of signaling between ganglionic SGCs and nociceptors remains under study, it is believed that purinergic signaling (adenosine triphosphate) serves a predominant role.

Nociceptive Transmission Into the Central Nervous System

Despite many decades of anatomic and physiologic investigation of the spinal dorsal horn, new insights into the structure and function of its cellular features continue to evolve. As shown in Figures 1.1 and 1.2, the majority of the body's nociceptive input into the CNS arrives into the spinal dorsal horn through the dorsal nerve roots. A confluence of nociceptive and non-nociceptive primary afferent nerve

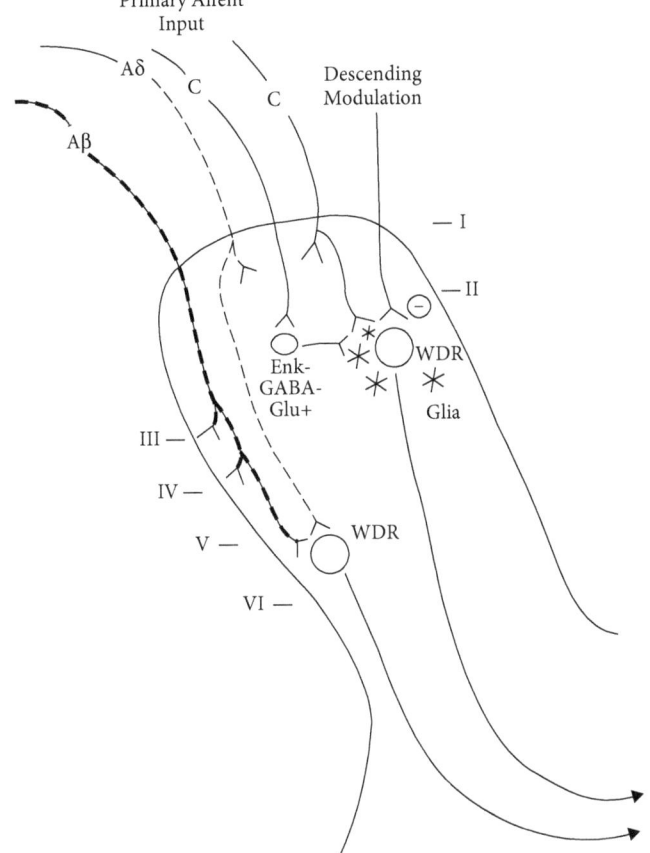

FIGURE 1.2 **Spinal dorsal horn.** The majority of peripheral sensory input to the central nervous system arrives within the superficial layers of the dorsal horn of the spinal cord. Nociceptor input primarily terminates in laminae I and II as well as in the deeper laminae V. Overlapping connections of both Aδ and Aβ fibers to second-order neurons deep in laminae V provide opportunities for integration of innocuous (simple touch) and nociceptive signaling. Synaptic connections with second-order spinal neurons represent important sites of nociceptive integration. Key components include (1) spinal, wide dynamic range (WDR) neurons that help integrate noxious stimuli into phenomena of temporal and spatial pain summation that exhibit plasticity changes such as central sensitization and "wind up"; (2) interneurons that provide excitatory (glutamate) or inhibitory (enkephalin, GABA) nociceptive modulation; (3) spinal glia (*insert icon*) that mediate important pathophysiologic states such as neuroinflammation and neuropathic pain; and (4) descending inhibitory modulation that can be influenced by both endogenous and exogenous opioids.

fibers from the adjacent DRG subsequently synapse with second-order neurons and are roughly divided into those signaling primarily nociceptive input (synapse in Rexed laminae I and II) (substantia gelatinosa) and inputs that also contain non-nociceptive afferents such as warmth and simple mechanical touch (Rexed lamina V) (Figure 1.2). Importantly, great attention has been afforded to the second-order neurons in laminae I, II, and V that subserve broad nociceptive integrative function. Anatomic and physiologic studies of wide dynamic range (WDR) neurons correlated to human pain biophysical tests have identified WDR neurons as critically important for the phenomenon of temporal and spatial pain summation. Clinically, they represent perhaps one of the first steps of the CNS to amplify the sensation of pain. Following extensive tissue injury, the spinal dorsal horn is bombarded with nociceptive afferent activity of increasing frequency and intensity. In response to persistent nociceptive input, the WDR neurons exhibit plasticity that results in facilitation and prolongation of nociceptive signaling.[8] In addition to the plasticity of second-order sensory neurons that amplifies nociceptive signaling, at least two other structural components can play critical roles in fine-tuning nociceptive signaling: (1) inhibitory interneurons (GABA) linking PANs with second-order spinal neurons (such as WDRs) and (2) spinal glia (Figure 1.2). The role of spinal glia has emerged as a dominant force in the regulation of nociceptive signaling in the development of chronic pathophysiologic pain states such as neuropathic pain.[9] As shown in Figure 1.2, glia residing in key spinal laminae, consisting of two predominant glial subtypes (astrocytes and microglia), are proposed to modulate nociceptive input through their interposition in synaptic transmission—between PANs and second-order dorsal horn neurons. There are multiple processes occurring in the spinal dorsal horn that contribute to amplification of pain signals, collectively referred to as *central sensitization*.

Signaling Nociception to Higher Centers Through Spinothalamic Tracts

Just as there is functional diversity among the PANs and their connections to second-order (projection) neurons in the dorsal horn, there also is hierarchical organization of ascending nociceptive input to the brain. The spinothalamic tract (STT) has long been recognized to transmit the discriminative and localization features of pain. However, ascending nociceptive signaling utilizes multiple tracts. The familiar STT is split into two tracts. The first is the neospinothalamic tract, drawing the majority of fibers from nociceptive specific neurons in the superficial dorsal horn laminae (I and II). Following its contralateral projection, the neospinothalamic tract ascends through the anterolateral column, terminating in the ventral posterior lateral (VPL) region of the thalamus, and is subsequently relayed to the somatosensory cortex. The second is the paleospinothalamic tract (PSTT), also referred to as the *reticulospinothalamic tract*. The PSTT draws on superficial and deeper dorsal horn laminae (V) WDR neurons transmitting a mixture of noxious and non-noxious stimuli. Following a complex course and projection to several key structures, such as the rostroventral medulla, pons, and midbrain, the PSTT ultimately connects to the midline thalamus and then relays fibers to the limbic cortex. Compared with the neospinothalamic tract, the complex signals derived from the PSTT involve behavioral experiences of pain, including arousal, emotion, motivation, and motor integration.[10] The primary importance of this portion of the pain pathway is that thalamic projections to the somatosensory, prefrontal, and motor cortex allow simultaneous integration and response to painful stimuli. This is possible through the processing of both somatic and visceral afferent signaling, allowing temporal and spatial summation of nociceptive input and amplifying the stimulus initially detected by peripheral nociceptors.[11]

PERCEPTION OF PAIN
Cortical and Subcortical Nociceptive Processing

Where does the sensation and emotional experience of pain reside? Our experience of pain is inherently complex, utilizing wide-ranging neural networks that attempt to help us integrate both internal and external nociceptive signaling and place this information into a meaningful social context. In short, the sensation of pain resides in multiple brain regions. Among these, the conscious awareness of pain is typically associated with cortical function. As shown in Figure 1.3, our ability to localize and discriminate pain from nociceptive input travels from the neospinothalamic tract and projects through the VPL of the thalamus to both the primary and secondary somatosensory cortex (SI and SII). Subsequent interconnections between SI, SII, insula,

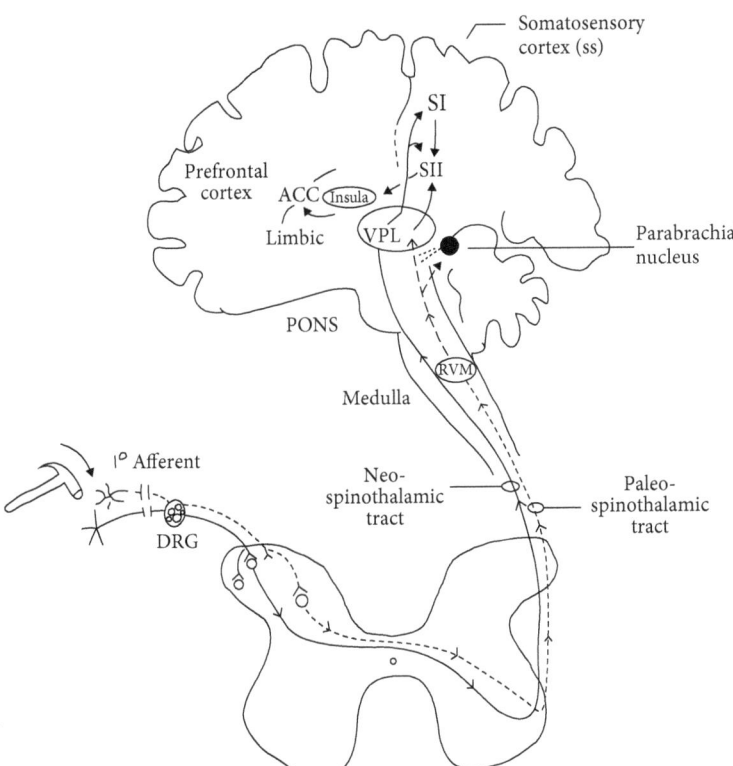

FIGURE 1.3 **Ascending pain pathways.** The perception of nociceptive pain can be elicited by activation of peripheral nociceptors with central input to superficial and deeper laminae of the spinal dorsal horn. Following crossover, nociceptive signaling is transmitted to higher centers by two components of the spinothalamic tract: The neospinothalamic tract conveys afferent input from superficial spinal laminae to the ventral posterior lateral (VPL) thalamus, whereas afferent input from deeper spinal layers (e.g., laminae V) ascend through the paleospinothalamic tract, with connections to the rostral ventromedial medulla (RVM) and parabrachial nucleus, terminating within the thalamus. Subsequently, thalamic-cortical, limbic (anterior cingulate cortex [ACC], insula, amygdala), and prefrontal signaling are further relayed and integrated, and together help form the perception of pain. Central pain pathway integration allows for pain modulation, where distraction can decrease activation of the thalamus, somatosensory cortex (SI), and insula. Conversely, anxiety or states of hypervigilance can produce exaggerated perceptions of pain.

and cingulate cortex/gyrus contribute to the increasing complexity of an unpleasant perception.

The attention to pain may be another way to understand how various brain regions work together to either reduce or enhance the perception of pain. For example, distraction reduces pain-related activation of the somatosensory cortex (SI), thalamus, and insula.[12] Concomitantly, other brain regions are recruited and activated in the attempt to decrease the experience of pain, including the prefrontal cortex, anterior cingulate cortex, and periaqueductal gray (PAG).[13] Conversely, states of hypervigilance, as observed with anxiety disorders and/or cognitive distortions such as catastrophizing, produce the opposite effect—promoting exaggerated or persistent perceptions of pain.[14]

MODULATION OF PAIN

The enhancement or amplification of painful sensations can be considered a process that recruits one or more of the components of the pain pathway, including peripheral, central (spinal), and supraspinal modulation. The modulation of pain is dependent on repeated biochemical and/or molecular themes involving inflammation, post-translational modification, and/or changes in gene expression conspiring on peripheral, spinal, and supraspinal elements of the pain pathway.

Positive Modulatory Pathways

Peripheral sensitization has been defined as the "[d]evelopment of a persistent dysfunction of the PNS including the dorsal root ganglion often typified by lowering nociceptor activation thresholds or spontaneous activation."[15] It is a process that encompasses the biology of PANs. For example, in PAN-mediated hyperalgesia following a sunburn, warm temperatures are perceived as hot and painful because of a "resetting" of the peripheral nociceptor threshold.[16] As discussed elsewhere, peripheral sensitization is invoked through local changes in target tissues, with the concurrent release of multiple molecular factors transiently activating specific ion channels and proteins responsible for the transduction of peripheral painful sensations. In addition, peripheral sensitization also lead to semipersistent phenotypic change through protein signaling and gene expression, resulting in sustained sensitization of selected Primary Afferent Neurons to both noxious and non-noxious stimuli.

Central (spinal) sensitization has been defined as "abnormalities of nociceptive signaling and plasticity in the spinal cord dorsal horn."[8] Such enhancements of nociceptive processing have been found to rely on modulation of second-order (projection) neurons, especially those that receive broad afferent input such as WDR neurons. The process of central (spinal) sensitization can be blocked in part by N-methyl-D-aspartate (NMDA) antagonists such as ketamine as well as by peripheral nerve blocks, which can prevent pain signals from entering the CNS.

Supraspinal modulation describes a third process involving signaling alterations in cortical projections to the midbrain and medulla, subsequently dedicated to descending inhibition of second-order dorsal horn neurons.[17] Undesirable supraspinal modulation is linked to syndromes of cognitive distortions such as catastrophizing, which can uncouple the descending inhibitory pain pathway (see later) to the dorsal horn. Clinically, this is seen as states of hypervigilance to pain or painful stimuli such that catastrophizing reduces the descending inhibitory tone, allowing nociceptive input relayed through the dorsal horn to become more pronounced. Conversely, cognitive behavioral therapy and acceptance commitment therapy target supraspinal modulation processes to enhance beneficial pain modulation.

Negative Modulatory Pathways

Overlapping negative regulatory pathways that serve to decrease the intensity of nociceptive signaling and the perception of pain have been described. At spinal segmental levels, inhibitory interneurons, predominant in laminae I and V, synapse on PANs and second-order (projection) neurons. As a result of nociceptor activation, these inhibitory interneurons are themselves activated and release GABA and enkephalin that function to dampen or inhibit primary afferent signaling (Figure 1.2). This segmental inhibitory circuit is superimposed on a more complex descending system. As illustrated in Figure 1.4, whether as a result of pain or the expectation of painful

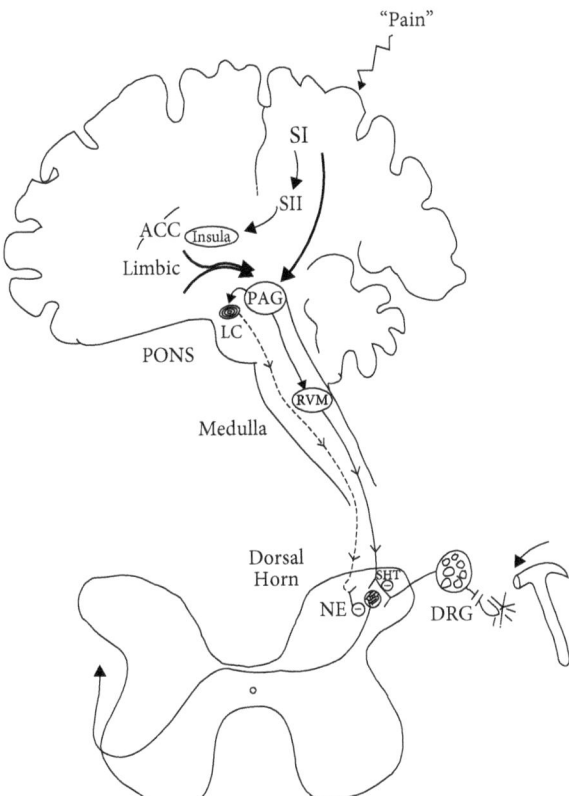

FIGURE 1.4 **Descending pain pathways.** Whether as the result of a painful event or its expectation, a complex descending inhibitory pathway can be recruited to reduce nociceptive input. Cortical and corticolimbic activation of the midbrain periaqueductal gray (PAG) evokes release of endogenous opioid peptides that serve to enhance descending inhibitory signaling through the rostral ventromedial medulla (RVM) (nucleus raphe magnus neurons: serotonin—5HT) and locus coeruleus (LC) (norepinephrine—NE) at the level of the dorsal horn. ACC = anterior cingulate cortex; DRG = dorsal root ganglion.

stimuli, corticolimbic brain regions activate neurons in the midbrain PAG, evoking a release of endogenous opioid peptides that in turn enhance descending inhibition through projections to the locus coeruleus (norepinephrine [NE]) and the rostral ventral medulla (nucleus raphe magnus—5HT). As a result of PAG activation and release of endogenous opioid peptides, NE and 5HT participate in the inhibition of nociceptive transmission at the level of the dorsal horn[18] (Figure 1.4). Curiously, another inhibitory network has emerged, termed *diffuse noxious inhibitory control* (DNIC), representing a pathway that does not require higher level brain input but rather is constitutively active within the spinal–medulla–spinal axis. More recently, studies have shown that the nucleus raphe magnus tonically inhibits trigeminal nociceptive inputs and is involved in the neuronal network underlying DNIC.[19] Importantly, dysfunction of the DNIC is being examined as a mechanism underlying certain widely dispersed pain states such as fibromyalgia or gender differences in pain processing. Suprapsinal, pharmacologic interventions such as the use of selective norepinephrine and serotonin reuptake inhibitors can blunt or reverse abnormalities in function of the descending inhibitory pain pathways. They may also be helpful in patients with centrally sensitized chronic pain syndromes and associated history of depression and/or anxiety.

EMERGING TRENDS AND THERAPEUTIC DEVELOPMENT

Despite recent advances in some areas of medicine, there remains a shortfall of effective analgesics. As shown in Figure 1.5 and described later, overlap between analgesic actions can, in part, be explained by the broad distribution of analgesic targets (receptors—ion channels) throughout the nervous system. In response, the trend of repurposing established analgesic agents, sometimes at lower concentrations (ketamine), and the combination of different classes of nonopioid analgesic compounds (e.g., acetaminophen, gabapentinoids, nonsteroidal anti-inflammatory drugs) show promise to improve patient satisfaction and analgesic outcomes. Appropriate use of regional techniques with local anesthetics can reduce opioid use and enhance mobility in the perioperative setting. While we wait for a new generation of antinociceptive agents targeting specific pain processing centers, transducing receptors, and channels, technologic advances are allowing more discrete application of agents (transdermal systems). Therapies for persistent painful conditions may also shift to neuromodulation of both central and peripheral neuronal targets, avoiding complex and unwanted systemic pharmacology.[20] Finally, as we gain additional insight into plasticity changes occurring hours, days, or weeks following tissue injury, it may be possible one day to interrupt or reverse the progression of acute to chronic pain at the level of gene expression.

THE DEVELOPING PAIN SYSTEM

At the point of birth, a sophisticated pain-sensing system is already taking shape in the newborn; however, the nascent pain-processing system is far from fully functional at this stage. The myelination of peripheral axons, so essential to rapid and accurate transmission of electrical signals, is only partially complete. The myelination of the brain is barely begun at birth, accounting for the ability of parts of the neonatal brain to function independently and asynchronously. Synaptogenesis and synaptic

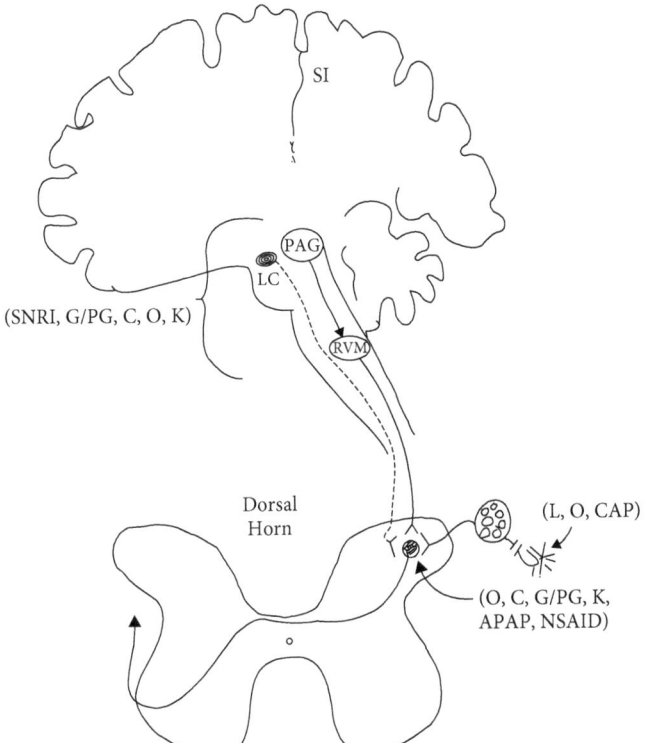

FIGURE 1.5 **Neuroanatomy of analgesic action.** Although pain may arise from a distinct anatomic location, treatment options often rely on the collective action of an analgesic agent (opioids) at all of its major nervous system binding sites (supraspinal, spinal, and peripheral). This property includes not only opioids but also other agents, such as gabapentin/pregabalin [G/PG], serotonin-norepinephrine reuptake inhibitors (SNRIs), ketamine (K), and α_2-agonists like clonidine (C) that can enhance midbrain descending inhibitory pathways. Analgesic agents with anti-inflammatory properties (acetaminophen/paracetamol [APAP], nonsteroidal anti-inflammatory drugs [NSAIDs]) represent yet another therapeutic choice to direct an even broader range of action, including inhibition of cyclooxygenase pathways in the central and peripheral nervous system as well as in peripheral tissues. At the spinal dorsal horn, presynaptic inhibition has been demonstrated for opioids (O), α_2-agonists, and gabapentin/pregabalin, whereas ketamine blocks postsynaptic NMDA receptor signaling. Agents that may have undesired effects if administered systemically, such as local anesthetics (sodium channel blockade—lidocaine [L]), opioids (O), or capsaicin (CAP), have also been used effectively when administered adjacent to peripheral nerves or applied to the skin topically for the local relief of painful symptoms.

pruning are just starting what will be a period of intense plastic development lasting throughout childhood. In many ways, the newborn, with limited peripheral myelination, low brain myelination, and rudimentary synaptic connections, is not able to perceive pain in the same way an adult would, and it is probably inaccurate to say that newborns "feel" pain in a way that is analogous to the adult experience.[21] It is more precise to state that newborns and infants "respond to" pain. Given the limitations of neurotransmission at birth, conscious awareness of painful stimuli is likely to be limited, and the pain behavior is probably mediated by spinal reflexes and subcortical (nonconscious) responses.

The distinctive way in which neonates process and respond to pain does not diminish the importance of aggressive pain control but rather changes the way we understand the reasons for controlling early pain. The fundamental reasons for early pain control are to promote survival and to ensure normal pain processing later in life. Not providing analgesia during major procedures in infants was the standard of care before the late 1980s because infants were held to be incapable of "experiencing" pain. However, research showed that not controlling noxious stimulation resulted in increased mortality for neonates. In animal models, researchers continue to show that aggressive early pain control prevents neuroplastic changes that promote overactive pain signaling later in life.[22] Similarly, neonates receiving no pain control for early procedures demonstrated prolonged crying and signs of pain with subsequent procedures. There is overwhelming evidence that strong pain experiences imprint the developing nervous system, leading to enhanced pain perception later in life. Clearly, it is very important to protect newborns, infants, and children from preventable pain.

Neuronogenesis and Migration

The neuronal elements of the nociceptive system are derived from ectoderm through a series of steps beginning early in gestation (Figure 1.6). On day 18, the notochord induces the ectoderm to organize the neural fold. The neural fold evolves into the neural groove and then into the neural tube, which closes caudally on day 27. The rostral end of the neural tube, the rostral neuropore, forms the floor of the fourth ventricle (medulla) and other cranial structures. The DRG neurons are derived from neural crest cells. The neural crest cells are located at the dorsal edge of the neural groove, just at the point where the neural tube closes. With tube closure, the neural crest cells migrate laterally and ventrally from the dorsal midline. Recent studies indicate that some neural crest cells cross the midline and migrate to the contralateral DRG. The

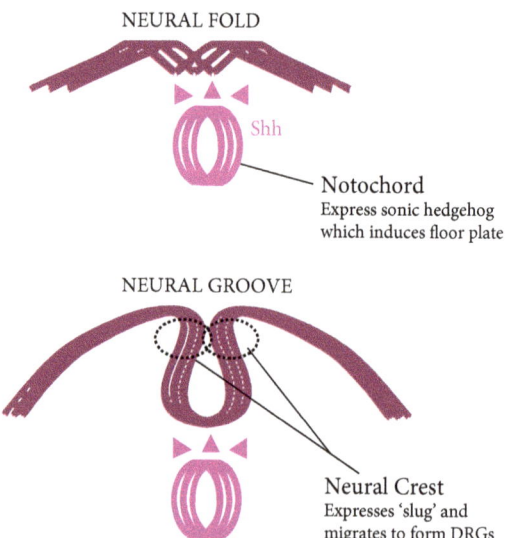

FIGURE 1.6 Schematic diagram of neural fold and neural crest formation, demonstrating early development of dorsal root ganglion (DRG), including primary afferent nociceptors and satellite Schwann cells.

cells in the DRG consist of nascent neurons, neuronal progenitors, and glia elements (Schwann cells). The DRG neurons and precursors undergo mitosis and development under the control of neurotrophins such as NT-3 and NGF through receptor molecules such as TrkC, TrkB, and TrkA as well as other cell signaling molecules. The enteric neurons (innervating and controlling the gut) arise from vagal and sacral neural crest progenitors. The process of enteric neuronal migration is lengthy, requiring up to 3 weeks during gestation.

The neural tube is organized into a ventrally located basal plate, which gives rise to motor neurons under the direction of Shh (sonic hedgehog) and a dorsally situated alar plate. Shh is initially expressed by the notochord inducing the neural fold but is eventually expressed by the basal plate itself and contributes to the differentiation of motor neurons from the basal plate. Sensory structures, including the dorsal horn (and sensory cortex more rostrally), arise from the alar plate and are under the control of bone morphogenic protein 4 (BMP4) and BMP7. These migration events occur simultaneously with ongoing cell division and neuronogenesis. The neural crest cells express "slug." Non-neuronal cells also derive from the neural crest; specifically, glia develop from neural crest progenitor cells following activation of Notch. The sympathetic ganglia also arise from neural crest cells at about this time, under separate control. With the beginning of limb formation (limb bud stage), the first neurons begin to extend peripheral neurites that elongate further as the limbs lengthen and grow. The complex events that occur during morphogenesis lead to sophisticated structural inter-relationships of nerves, bones, muscles, tendons, and other tissues. This underlies the major challenges to repair after injury and accounts in part for the difficulties in restoring effective innervation and function after trauma.

Peripheral Myelination During Development

Initially, sensory axons are all unmyelinated and clumped together (Figure 1.7). These axons can only send signals very slowly (<1 m/s) and have little capacity for localizing

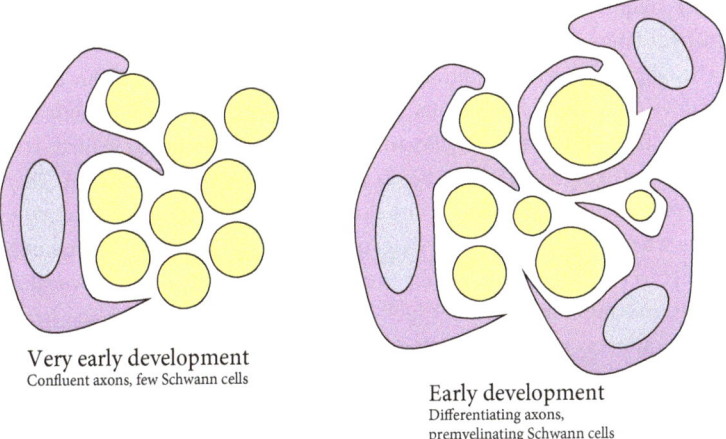

Very early development
Confluent axons, few Schwann cells

Early development
Differentiating axons,
premyelinating Schwann cells

FIGURE 1.7 Schematic diagram of early events in peripheral nerve development relevant to pain pathways. Axons are confluent in early development and are later separated by Schwann cells; selected axons undergo myelination depending on phenotype.

the sensory information they transmit. Gradually, dividing Schwann cells migrate into and along the nerve, insinuating cytoplasmic processes between the confluent young axons. As development continues, many axons increase in diameter, others will remain small in diameter, and still others will undergo atrophy and degeneration. Although the largest diameter axons will be dedicated to transducing and transmitting proprioceptive information, the smaller diameter axons will transduce and transmit sensations such as warmth, heat, cold, and pressure, many of these smaller diameter axons are the processes of "nociceptive" primary afferents. The myelination of axons increases the rate at which action potentials can pass over the axon; this rate is the CV. Axonal diameter is also correlated with increased CV. In addition to increasing the CV, myelination increases the reliability of action potential propagation, the so-called safety factor. The process of Schwann cells dividing and wrapping around axons is termed *peripheral myelination*. Neuregulin 1, an epidermal growth factor–like signaling molecule, binds to ErbB class receptors (transmembrane tyrosine kinases) to modulate the proliferation, development, and myelination of Schwann cells. Peripheral myelination is actively occurring at the time of birth but is a process that continues throughout childhood, and children do not attain adult speeds of peripheral neurotransmission until the age of 10 years.

Central Myelination

A process similar to peripheral myelination occurs in the CNS but at an even later stage of development. The myelinating cells of the CNS are called oligodendrocytes. Myelination in the CNS is very limited at birth, occurring mostly in the auditory pathways and some other brainstem structures; myelination occurs earliest in the PNS. This accounts for the fact that it is possible to test the hearing of newborns using "evoked potentials," that is, synchronous action potentials occurring in brainstem nuclei and measurable on the surface of the skull. By contrast, it is not possible to assess vision in the same way at this stage of development because myelination of visual pathways occurs quite late. Important pain-processing structures are unmyelinated at birth: The thalamic radiations, responsible for carrying pain signals to the cortex (required for conscious perception of pain) are unmyelinated, as are the intracortical fibers that make conscious awareness and integration of stimuli possible. The cingulated gyrus is almost fully myelinated by 1 year, probably accounting for the developing ability of infants to detect and respond appropriately to emotional cues. The advanced myelination of peripheral pain pathways at birth accounts for the vigorous responses of newborns and infants to noxious stimuli. There are multiple reflex arcs in the spinal cord that allow for potentially protective motor responses when painful stimuli are detected. In addition, the myelination of brainstem structures makes it possible for the reflex responses to include vocalization, grimacing, and autonomic changes such as increased blood pressure and heart rate. These reflex systems are highly plastic and subject to "learning" in the form of long-term potentiation (LTP), wind-up (enhancement of C-fiber responses with repeated stimulation), and long-lasting facilitation. Vigorous prophylaxis of pain in neonates and infants is currently the standard of care among pediatric pain specialists. Pain assessment is discussed in Chapter 4, and pediatric pain treatment is covered in Chapter 15.

Aging and Pain Pathways

The prevalence of pain increases with age, but this is due to a variety of factors, including the accumulation of changes such as deteriorating musculoskeletal function associated with osteoarthritis and sarcopenia as well as inflammatory processes associated with decreased lean body mass. With normal aging, following mid-life, there are some general patterns that influence pain signaling: The innervation of distal structures declines slowly, peripheral nerves conduct signals less well in late life, and brain processing is less crisp both temporally and spatially with advanced age. There is considerable effort directed toward separating the changes associated with healthy aging from those resulting from common medical conditions associated with age, such as hypertension, hyperlipidemia, and even diabetes. Hypertension has clear deleterious effects on the CNS, and diabetes can sensitize nerves in a manner so that pain signaling is increased and patients experience more pain even as the feet are more numb. Studies of aging adults indicate that while young adults have more effective central pain modulation systems that are capable of suppressing pain from conscious awareness, these pain suppression systems are less effective with aging. There are several reasons that pain is a prominent feature of aging, and further research and more determined efforts at comprehensive treatment are needed to improve quality of life across the life span.

SUMMARY

The pain-processing system is extensive, being present in most structures of the body, and complex, being under constant bidirectional control so that pain awareness and sensitivity can be increased or decreased according to circumstances. Transduction, transmission, perception, and modulation are all essential to the experience of pain, and these functional components of pain processing represent potential therapeutic opportunities. Although neonates do not experience pain in the same manner as older children and adults, it is clearly important to optimize pain control in the vulnerable youngest patients because long-term increased pain sensitivity may otherwise arise. Older adults are at increased risk for pain because of factors both intrinsic and extrinsic to the pain pathways. Understanding of the neuroanatomic basis of the pain experience can aid clinicians in detecting pain and in developing effective pain treatment plans with their patients.

REVIEW QUESTIONS

1. A 48-year-old woman with peripheral neuropathy was referred for nerve biopsy, a procedure typically done using lidocaine for local anesthesia. The patient had told her local neurologist that she was insensitive to lidocaine and that another anesthetic should be used. On closer questioning by the surgeon, it appeared that the patient had recently undergone local injections of lidocaine in the foot in an effort to alleviate her neuropathic foot pain. The injections had been completely ineffective, and the patient concluded that she must be insensitive to lidocaine. The surgeon drew a different conclusion and found during surgery that the patient responded normally to lidocaine. Using the idea of "identify the pain generator,"

can you explain why injections of lidocaine into the foot did not work to relieve pain for this patient?
   a. The patient is insensitive to lidocaine.
   b. The patient's nerves no longer reach the foot, so lidocaine injected there is not effective.
   c. The lidocaine used for the previous injections must have been expired or diluted.
   d. The patient requires competency evaluation because lidocaine unresponsiveness does not occur.

2. Which of the following is not a recognized functional part of the pain pathways?
   a. Transmission
   b. Reduction
   c. Transduction
   d. Perception

Match the following:

3. PANs a. thalamus

4. Secondary afferent neuron b. dorsal root ganglion

5. Tertiary afferent neuron c. spinal dorsal horn

REFERENCES

1. Schumacher MA. Transient receptor potential channels in pain and inflammation: therapeutic opportunities. Pain Pract. 2010;10(3):185–200.
2. Fields HL, ed. Pain Syndromes in Neurology. London, Boston: Butterworths-Heinemann Ltd; 1990.
3. Levine JD, Fields HL, Basbaum AI. Peptides and the primary afferent nociceptor. J Neurosci. 1993;13(6):2273–2286.
4. McMahon SB. Are there fundamental differences in the peripheral mechanisms of visceral and somatic pain? Behav Brain Sci. 1997;20(3):381–391; discussion 435–513.
5. Amir R, Devor M. Electrical excitability of the soma of sensory neurons is required for spike invasion of the soma, but not for through-conduction. Biophys J. 2003;84(4):2181–2191.
6. Prats-Galino A, Puigdellívol-Sánchez A, Ruano-Gil D, Molander C. Representations of hindlimb digits in rat dorsal root ganglia. J Comp Neurol. 1999;408(1):137–145.
7. Watkins LR, Hutchinson MR, Milligan ED, Maier SF. "Listening" and "talking" to neurons: implications of immune activation for pain control and increasing the efficacy of opioids. Brain Res Rev. 2007;56(1):148–169.
8. Woolf CJ. Central sensitization: implications for the diagnosis and treatment of pain. Pain. 2011;152(3 Suppl):S2–15.
9. Milligan ED, Watkins LR. Pathological and protective roles of glia in chronic pain. Nat Rev Neurosci. 2009;10(1):23–36.
10. Peschanski M, Besson JM. A spino-reticulo-thalamic pathway in the rat: an anatomical study with reference to pain transmission. Neuroscience. 1984;12(1):165–178.

11. Peyron R, Laurent B, García-Larrea L. Functional imaging of brain responses to pain: a review and meta-analysis (2000). Neurophysiol Clin. 2000;30(5):263–288.
12. Tracey I, Mantyh PW. The cerebral signature for pain perception and its modulation. Neuron. 2007;55(3):377–391.
13. Wiech K, Ploner M, Tracey I. Neurocognitive aspects of pain perception. Trends Cogn Sci. 2008;12(8):306–313.
14. Koyama T, McHaffie JG, Laurienti PJ, Coghill RC. The subjective experience of pain: where expectations become reality. Proc Natl Acad Sci U S A. 2005;102(36):12950–12955.
15. McGreevy K, Bottros MM, Raja SN. Preventing chronic pain following acute pain: risk factors, preventive strategies, and their efficacy. Eur J Pain Suppl. 2011;5(2):365–372.
16. Caterina MJ, Leffler A, Malmberg AB, et al. Impaired nociception and pain sensation in mice lacking the capsaicin receptor. Science. 2000;288(5464):306–313.
17. De Felice M, Sanoja R, Wang R, et al. Engagement of descending inhibition from the rostral ventromedial medulla protects against chronic neuropathic pain. Pain. 2011;152(12):2701–2709.
18. Budai D, Fields HL. Endogenous opioid peptides acting at mu-opioid receptors in the dorsal horn contribute to midbrain modulation of spinal nociceptive neurons. J Neurophysiol. 1998;79(2):677–687.
19. Chebbi R, Boyer N, Monconduit L, et al. The nucleus raphe magnus OFF-cells are involved in diffuse noxious inhibitory controls. Exp Neurol. 2014;256:39–45.
20. Borsook D, Veggeberg R, Erpelding N, et al. The insula: a "hub of activity" in migraine. Neuroscientist. 2016;22(6):632–652.
21. Verriotis M, Chang P, Fitzgerald M, Fabrizi L. The development of the nociceptive brain. Neuroscience. 2016;338:207–219.
22. Schwaller F1, Fitzgerald M. The consequences of pain in early life: injury-induced plasticity in developing pain pathways. Eur J Neurosci. 2014;39(3):344–352.

2 Nociceptive Processing
Neurochemistry and Neurophysiology

Cynthia L. Renn and Susan G. Dorsey

Pain is a symphony—a complex response that includes not just a distinct sensation but also motor activity, a change in emotion, a focusing of attention, a brand-new memory.
—Atul Gawande, *Complications*

LEARNING OBJECTIVES

At the completion of this chapter, the learner should be able to discuss:

- The major molecules and receptors involved in peripheral transduction of pain
- The principle neurotransmitters and receptors/molecular pathways responsible for nociceptive signaling in the dorsal horn and at higher centers
- The role of opioid, cannabinoid, and other relevant receptors at multiple levels
- The mediation of descending inhibition by specific neurotransmitters released in response to excitation of neurons in specific supraspinal nuclei
- The occurrence of descending facilitation of pain processing through distinct neurotransmitters
- The impact of nociceptive stimuli on the systemic physiology

CASE SCENARIO

A 68-year-old woman is undergoing chemotherapy for multiple myeloma. Until her diagnosis, she was healthy and active, and although her fasting glucose was slightly elevated, she did not have diabetes. Since starting chemotherapy, she developed mild numbness of the toes, and more recently she has developed burning pain in both feet, most noticeable at bedtime. Her primary care provider started her on gabapentin 300 mg at bedtime for neuropathic pain. She is referred to the neurology clinic where you are rotating for 3 months as a resident. You interview her and learn that she is doing well but still has some bothersome burning in both feet. Unfortunately, she is also quite dizzy in the morning and has almost fallen a couple of times when getting up. This is problematic because she needs to rush to the bathroom to urinate first thing in the morning, so she gets moving even though she is aware of being lightheaded.

1. What neurotransmitter system is being modulated by gabapentin?
2. What other neurotransmitter systems are active in reducing pain at the spinal dorsal horn level?
3. Can you recommend an alternative to her current medication?

INTRODUCTION

While pain is an unpleasant experience and source of suffering, it is also a vital physiologic element that alerts us when tissue injury occurs. Often, pain is acute and resolves with recovery from an illness or injury. Unfortunately for many, pain is a chronic pain condition. A key contributor to the development of chronic pain is poorly managed acute pain. There are several contributing factors to poorly managed acute pain, including inconsistent pain assessment, inadequate preemptive analgesia before procedures, as needed (PRN) analgesic administration in lieu of time-contingent medication dosing, and a lack of awareness regarding clinical implications of pain physiology. In addition, there are both heritable and acquired pain-associated conditions and forms of chronic pain that arise as a result of molecular events and changes in nociceptive processing. This chapter will address the pain physiology knowledge gap by discussing the key molecular mediators, neurotransmitters, and ligand receptors that are involved in nociceptive transmission along the ascending and descending pain processing pathways.

ASCENDING NOCICEPTIVE TRANSMISSION

Pain is a complex sensory process. It involves activation of neurons within the peripheral nervous system (PNS) that transmit nociceptive information to the central nervous system (CNS). Within the CNS, the nociceptive input is transmitted along ascending pathways to regions within the brainstem and cerebral cortex for processing of the information, recognizing that the stimulus stems from actual or potential tissue damage in the periphery and leading to a cognitive and affective experience of pain. At each phase of the ascending nociceptive system, neurotransmitters and their receptors play a vital role in the pain transmission process.

Molecular Machinery of Nociception

Mechanical nociceptors are the specialized sensory neurons in the PNS that typically have a high threshold of activation, and the mechanisms underlying mechanically induced nociception remain somewhat unclear. However, the transduction of mechanical stimuli is generally thought to result from deformation of the cell membrane, which mechanically alters the quaternary structure of ion channels, opens the pore to allow the movement of ions (e.g., sodium and potassium) across the cell membrane, and results in depolarizing the neuron to generate an action potential.[1] There is evidence suggesting that members of the acid-sensing ion channel (ASIC), potassium channel, and transient receptor potential (TRP) families play a role in mechanical nociception.[2] Recently, studies have found that other structures, such as the cytoskeleton and extracellular matrix proteins, also contribute to mechanical transduction.

By comparison, the mechanisms underlying thermal (hot and cold) nociception are more clearly understood. Members of the TRP channel family are the key components for the transduction of innocuous and noxious thermal stimuli.[1] TRP channels are nonselective ion channels that are ubiquitously expressed in a broad range of cell types and tissues and allow the movement of cations such as sodium and calcium across the cell membrane.[3] There nearly 30 members of the TRP channel family[4]; however, only a small subset of the TRP channels (vanilloid 1 and 2 [TRPV1, TRPV2], melastatin 8 [TRPM8], and ankyrin 1 [TRPA1]) play a role in thermal nociception.[3-5] The thermosensitive TRP channels are expressed in primary somatosensory neurons and sense a range of temperatures from noxious cold to noxious hot (Table 2.1).[5,6] Within this broad range of temperatures, noxious cold (<17° C) elicits a pain response by activating TRPA1 and TRPM8, while noxious hot (>43° C) elicits a pain response by activating TRPV1 and TRPV2.[1,7-9] Warm temperatures that are not in the noxious range are sensed by TRPV3, TRPV4, TRPM4, and TRPM5.[6]

Chemically induced nociception can occur as a result of exogenous chemicals causing tissue damage and/or directly activating nociceptors by binding to their respective cell surface receptors (e.g., acid-activating ASICs; Table 2.2). In addition to their role in transducing thermal stimuli, the TRP channels also play a role in chemical activation of nociceptors by responding to contact with plant-derived ligands such as mustard and garlic (TRPA1), capsaicin (TRPV1), and menthol (TRPM8).[10-14] However, the primary source of noxious chemical stimuli is the release of endogenous substances when tissue is injured by any of a variety of mechanisms (e.g., mechanical trauma, ischemia, infection). Endogenous chemical mediators are released from the damaged cells, sympathetic efferent discharge, and inflammatory cells (e.g., macrophages, lymphocytes, mast cells) that are recruited to the site of injury.[14] The release of these substances forms what is thought of as the inflammatory "soup" that initiates a cascade of events involved

Table 2.1 Temperature and Chemical Mediators of TRP Channel Activation

Activation Temperature	TRP Channel	Chemical Agonists
≥ 52°C	TRPV2	2-Aminoethoxydiphenyl Borate, Mechanical Stimuli
≥ 42°C	TRPV1	Chili Pepper (Capsaicin), Garlic, Camphor, Ethanol, Acidic pH (H$^+$)
> 33°C	TRPV3	Oregano, Thyme, Clove, Camphor
< 35°C	TRPM4 TRPM5	Soy Sauce, Sugar
~ 27–35°C	TRPV4	Hypotonic Material, Mechanical Stimuli
≤ 25°C	TRPM8	Mint, Menthol, Eucalyptol
≤ 17°C	TRPA1	Icillin, Cinnamon, Garlic, Wasabi, Mustard Oil, Mechanical Stimuli

Table 2.2 Chemical Mediators of Nociception: Their Sources and Their Receptors

Source	Mediator	Receptor
Tissue Damage	Bradykinin	BK_2
	Hydrogen Ions (H^+)	Acid Sensing Ion Channel (ASIC)
	Prostaglandin-E_2 (PGE_2)	Prostanoid Receptor E2 (EP_2)
	Adenosine Triphosphate (ATP)	Purinoceptor 3 (P2X3)
Macrophages	Interleukin-1β (IL-1β)	IL-1R Type I and Type II
	Nerve Growth Factor (NGF)	Tropomyosin Receptor kinase A (TrkA)
	Interleukin-6 (IL-6)	IL6R
	Tumor Necrosis Factor-α (TNF-α)	Tumor Necrosis Factor Receptor 1 (TNFR1)
	Bradykinin	BK_2
Mast Cells	Nerve Growth Factor (NGF)	Tropomyosin Receptor kinase A (TrkA)
	Bradykinin	BK_2
	Prostaglandin-E_2 (PGE_2)	Prostanoid Receptor E_2 (EP_2)
Platelets	Adenosine Triphosphate (ATP)	Purinoceptor 3 (P2X3)

in the inflammatory process, including nociceptor activation.[2,15] The mediators composing the inflammatory soup change the chemical milieu at the site of tissue injury, bind to their respective cell surface receptors, and sensitize nociceptors by lowering their threshold of activation and increasing their responsiveness.[13–15]

Key constituents of the inflammatory soup include bradykinin, hydrogen ions (protons, H^+), adenosine triphosphate (ATP), interleukin-1β (IL-1β) and IL-6, nerve growth factor (NGF), tumor necrosis factor-α (TNF-α), and prostaglandin E_2 (PGE_2).[2,13,15] Bradykinin is released by disrupted cells, macrophages, and mast cells, binds to the BK2 cell surface receptors, and sensitizes nociceptors. BK2 is a G protein–coupled receptor that exerts its effect through activation of intracellular signaling pathways to trigger the release of additional inflammatory mediators from the nociceptor, including PGE_2, NGF, and cytokines, to further sensitize the neuron.[14] Protons are released when the cytosol and its constituents leak from damaged cells, leading to acidification of the extracellular milieu, which can enhance the activity of TRPV1 channels as well as bind to ASICs on the surface of the nociceptor to contribute to the transduction of noxious mechanical stimuli.[14] ATP is also released from damaged cells as well as from macrophages and platelets, and it binds to the P2X3 receptor on nociceptors. The P2X3 receptor is an ion channel that is gated by the binding of ATP to allow the influx of cations, resulting in depolarization of the neuron and modulation of TRPV1 to increase its activity. Macrophages recruited to the site of injury release the cytokines IL-1β, IL-6, and TNF-α.[8] While cytokines exert a direct action on nociceptors, their chief contribution to hyperalgesia is to stimulate increased production and release of other inflammatory mediators such as bradykinin, NGF, and prostaglandins that further enhance peripheral sensitization.[14,15] IL-1β is a potent proinflammatory agent that binds the IL-1 receptor (IL-1R) and induces both mechanical and thermal hyperalgesia. Neurons lack membrane-bound IL-6R, the receptor for

IL-6; however, when IL-6 is bound to the soluble form of IL-6R, it can interact with glycoprotein 130 (gp130) on the surface of nociceptors to exert a pronociceptive effect. TNF-α is a proinflammatory cytokine that exerts its effect by binding to the TNFR1 and TNFR2 receptors, which triggers a cascade of intracellular signaling events that sensitize other cell surface receptors and ion channels. TNF-α binding to both receptor subtypes contributes to the activation of nociceptors and the development of hyperalgesia and allodynia. PGE_2 is a product of damaged cells when arachidonic acid from the ruptured lipid bilayer is acted on by the enzyme cyclooxygenase.[16] It is also released from mast cells[14,15] and binds to the prostanoid receptor E2 (EP2), which is a G protein–coupled receptor that can directly activate nociceptors as well as potentiate the effects of other inflammatory mediators such as ATP and bradykinin. NGF, a member of the neurotrophin family, is released by macrophages and mast cells at the site of tissue injury and inflammation.[14,15] NGF binds to its receptor tropomyosin receptor kinase A (TrkA) and triggers an intracellular signaling cascade that sensitizes the nociceptor to both thermal and mechanical stimuli.[17]

The majority of the activity resulting from the action of inflammatory mediators on nociceptors is through the interaction of intracellular send messenger signaling pathways that serve to enhance the function of other cell surface receptors and ion channels or by increasing the production and release of additional quantities of the mediators.[13,15] An active area of ongoing research is directed at finding ways to inhibit the effects that these inflammatory mediators have on nociceptors, thus reducing the amount of nociceptive input from an area of injury.

Two fiber types carry nociceptive input in the primary afferent nerve. The first type are the Aδ fibers, which are thinly myelinated, are fast transmitting, and produce the sharp or pricking first pain that is felt immediately after injury.[2,15] Aδ fibers are stimulated by noxious thermal and mechanical stimuli.[15] The second type are the C fibers, which have a small-diameter, unmyelinated axon that conducts action potential more slowly than Aδ fibers produce the dull or burning second pain that develops after the first pain subsides.[2,15] C fibers are polymodal and respond to noxious mechanical, thermal, and chemical stimuli.[15] Nociceptive information is transmitted from the peripheral terminal to the central terminal of the nociceptor as an electrical signal in the form of action potentials. The generation and transmission of action potentials depend on the opening of voltage-gated sodium channels to allow sodium to enter the cell.[2,15] Repolarization of the cell membrane after an action potential is dependent on voltage-gated potassium channels.[13,15]

SPINAL DORSAL HORN IN ASCENDING TRANSMISSION

Within the spinal cord, the primary afferent C fibers enter the spinal cord and terminate in laminae I and II, and Aδ fibers terminate predominantly in laminae I and V of the dorsal horn (Figure 2.1A and B).

When nociceptors are in the resting polarized state, voltage-gated calcium channels (VGCCs) are closed and vesicles containing neurotransmitters are sequestered in the cytosol of the presynaptic nerve terminal (Figure 2.2A). As action potentials reach the central presynaptic nerve terminal of the nociceptor, the terminal membrane depolarizes and VGCCs open to allow the influx of calcium. The calcium influx triggers trafficking of the vesicles to the synaptic membrane, where they dock and release neurotransmitters into the synaptic cleft (Figure 2.2B). The neurotransmitters cross the synaptic cleft and bind with their receptors on the surface of the postsynaptic cell body, which activates intracellular signaling pathways, depolarization of the neuron, and propagation of action potentials to continue the transmission of the nociceptive information to the brainstem and cerebral cortex.[2] Nociceptors function as excitatory neurons and predominantly release the primary excitatory neurotransmitter glutamate. In addition to glutamate, nociceptors also release other excitatory neurotransmitters, including substance P, calcitonin gene–related peptide (CGRP), and brain-derived neurotrophic factor (BDNF).[2,18,19]

Glutamate is a major amino acid neurotransmitter expressed in widely in neurons, including nociceptors, that functions as a fast excitatory neurotransmitter.[18] Glutamate binds with high affinity to α-amino-3-hydroxy-5-methyl-4-isoxazole propionate

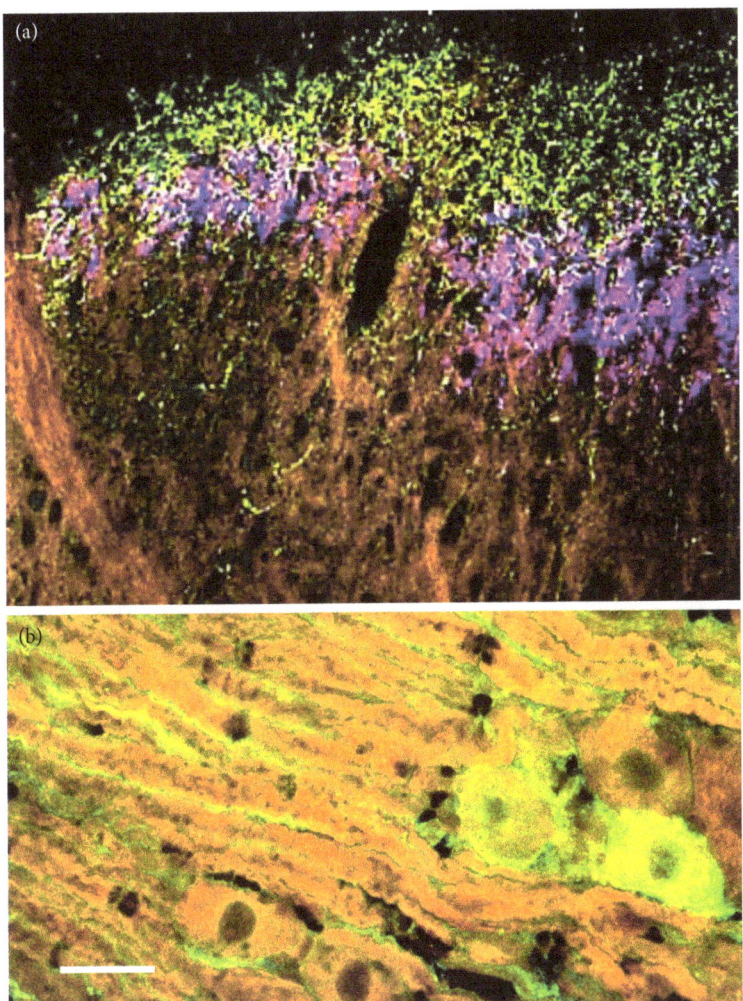

FIGURE 2.1 Immunostaining and fixation of spinal dorsal horn and dorsal root ganglion (DRG). **A,** Spinal dorsal horn viewed using combination immunofixation and glutaraldehyde autofluorescence. The superficial dorsal horn (laminae I and II outer portion) is stained for calcitonin gene–related peptide (CGRP) with green immunofluorescence. The inner portion of lamina II binds avidly to isolectin B4 (IB4), demonstrating phenotypic (functional) separation in the superficial dorsal horn. *Inset* demonstrates minimal overlap between CGRP and IB4 staining. Bar = 80 μm. **B,** The DRG is stained here for CGRP (green-yellow) together with glutaraldehyde-induced myelin autofluorescence, illustrating that diverse cells are not segregated in the DRG (strongly, moderately, and weakly CGRP-staining cells are seen together in this section). Bar = 40 μm. (© Beth B. Hogans.)

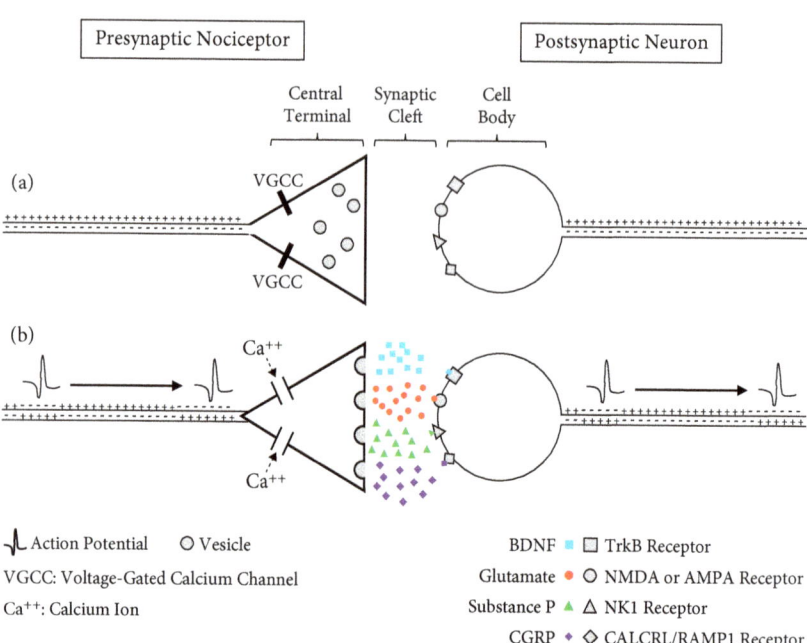

FIGURE 2.2 Transmission of nociceptive input from the presynaptic nociceptor to a postsynaptic neuron in the spinal dorsal horn. **A,** In the resting state, the cell membrane of the presynaptic nociceptor is negatively charged on the intracellular side and positively charged on the extracellular side. Voltage-gated calcium channels (VGCCs) in the cell membrane of the central terminal of the nociceptor are closed, and neurotransmitters are sequestered in vesicles in the cytosol. The cell membrane of the postsynaptic neuron is also negatively charged on the intracellular side and positively charged on the extracellular side. Cell surface receptors are not bound with their neurotransmitter ligands, and ion channels are closed. There are no action potentials being propagated along the axon of either the presynaptic or postsynaptic neuron. **B,** As action potentials are propagated along the axon of the presynaptic nociceptor, the cell membrane depolarizes and becomes positive on the intracellular side and negative on the extracellular side. After an action potential passes, the membrane repolarizes and returns to its resting state. When the action potentials reach the central terminal of the nociceptor and depolarize the cell membrane, VGCCs open to allow the influx of calcium ions (Ca^{++}), which triggers intracellular signaling mechanisms and trafficking of neurotransmitter vesicles to the synaptic membrane, where they fuse and release their contents into the synaptic cleft. The neurotransmitters diffuse across the synaptic cleft and bind with their receptors in the cell membrane of the postsynaptic neuron, which triggers intracellular signaling mechanisms, opening of ion channels, depolarization of the cell membrane, and propagation of action potentials along the axon to higher centers in the central nervous system.

(AMPA), kainite (KA), and *N*-methyl-D-aspartate (NMDA) ionotropic receptors on the cell body of the second-order neuron, causing the influx of calcium and the generation of postsynaptic action potentials. Glutamate also binds to several members of the metabotropic glutamate receptor (mGluR) G protein–coupled receptor family, activating intracellular signaling pathways such as phospholipase C (PLC), protein kinase C (PKC), and extracellular signal–related kinase (ERK) to mediate ongoing cellular activity associated with central sensitization.

Substance P is a member of the neurokinin family of peptides and binds to the neurokinin 1 (NK1) receptor, which is a G protein–coupled receptor that activates intracellular signaling pathways, produces a prolonged membrane depolarization, and sensitizes other receptors in the postsynaptic cell membrane.[18] CGRP is a peptide that binds to a complex of its G protein–coupled receptor, CGRP receptor–like receptor (CRLR), and receptor activity–modifying protein 1 (RAMP1), which activates protein kinase A (PKA) and PKC intracellular signaling pathways, potentiates the activity of substance P, increases BDNF release, and sensitizes the neuron. BDNF is a member of the neurotrophin family, is released from the central terminal of nociceptors, and binds to its cognate receptor tropomyosin receptor kinase B (TrkB), which activates ERK and PKC intracellular signaling pathways to enhance NMDA receptor activity and sensitize the neuron.

Nociceptive transmission is typically thought of as an anterograde process with information moving from the peripheral to the central terminal of the neuron.[13,15] However, nociceptors also exhibit retrograde transmission and release of neurotransmitters from the peripheral terminal that contribute to peripheral sensitization of the nociceptor and the development of neurogenic inflammation.[13,15] Nociceptors are also capable of regulating the release of neurotransmitters from their central terminal by autocrine signaling mechanisms through neurotransmitter receptors located on the cell membrane adjacent to but outside the synapse. While much progress has been made in recent decades, additional research is needed to further elucidate the mechanisms of action of neurotransmitters and their receptors, and perhaps others yet to be discovered, in the process of pain transmission. As these mechanisms become clearer, new therapeutic strategies can be designed to block the function of these neurotransmitters, reduce the flow of nociceptive transmission, and decrease pain.

Ascending Tracts

The second-order projection neurons receive the nociceptive signal from the primary afferent nociceptor and transmit the nociceptive information to higher regions in the CNS. When the second-order neurons reach their target structures, they synapse with third-order neurons that transmit the nociceptive signal to cortical and limbic structures. While many of the neurotransmitters discussed previously are involved in the ascending transfer of nociceptive input from second-order to third-order neurons, glutamate binding to ionotropic (AMPA, NMDA, KA) and metabotropic (mGluR) receptors plays a key role.

DESCENDING PAIN MODULATION

A large volume of knowledge regarding pain perception and modulation has been gained over the past century. The theory that nociception is affected by modulatory influences from higher centers within the CNS was first proposed by Head and Holmes.[20] Further evidence of endogenous inhibitory modulation of pain was put forth by Beecher, who found that nearly 75% of soldiers wounded on the battle field in World War II reported only minimal to moderate pain and often refused pain medication.[21] Head and Holmes' theory and Beecher's observations were later confirmed by studies demonstrating that several supraspinal sites exert tonic inhibitory control of neurons in the spinal dorsal horn, affecting the flow of ascending nociceptive input. In recent decades, many research studies have focused on understanding the mechanisms involved in descending modulatory processes. Descending projection neurons release neurotransmitters in the spinal dorsal horn onto the central terminal of the primary afferent and/or onto the cell body of intrinsic interneurons and second-order neurons (Figure 2.3). The descending modulatory effect can alter either the release of

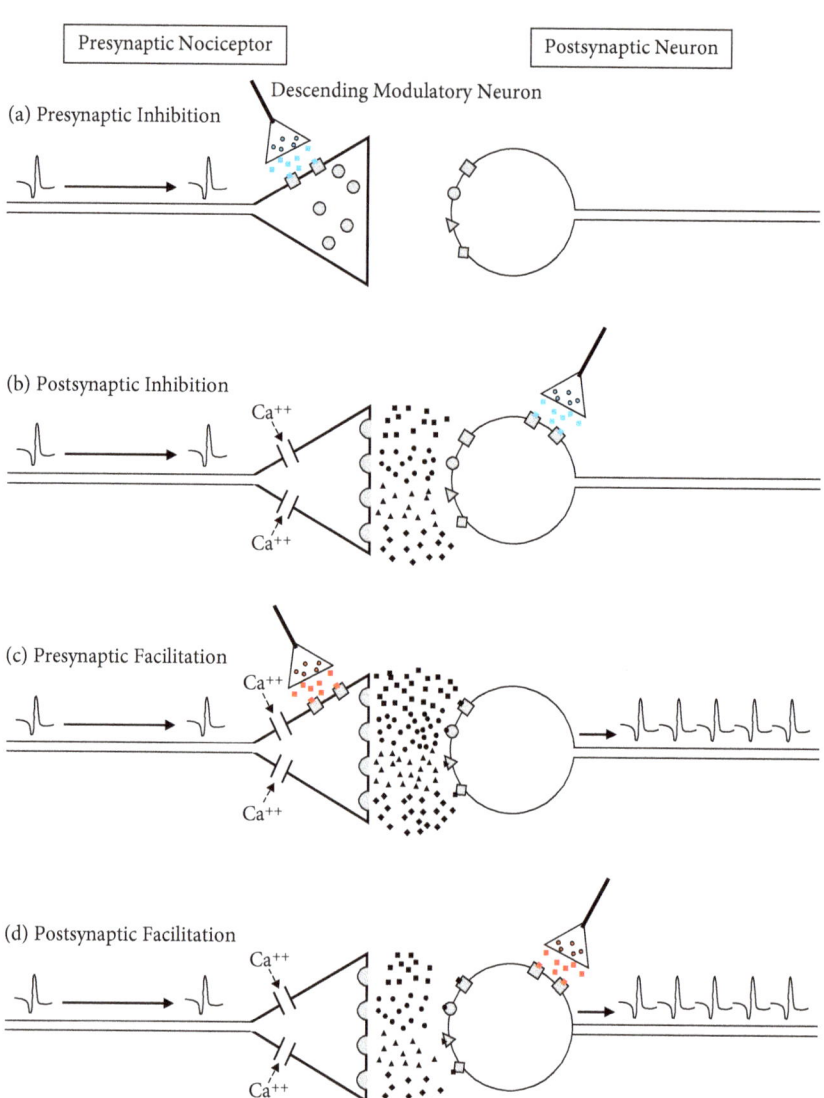

FIGURE 2.3 Presynaptic and postsynaptic modulation of nociceptive transmission in the spinal dorsal horn. **A,** Presynaptic descending inhibition. The descending modulatory neuron synapses with the central terminal of the nociceptor and releases inhibitory neurotransmitters that bind with cell surface receptors triggering intracellular signaling mechanisms that prevent vesicular trafficking and neurotransmitter release into the synaptic cleft. As a result, the postsynaptic neuron remains quiescent and in its polarized resting state. No action potentials will be propagated in the postsynaptic neuron, and nociceptive transmission will be attenuated. **B,** Postsynaptic descending inhibition. The descending modulatory neuron synapses with the postsynaptic neuron and releases inhibitory neurotransmitters that bind with cell surface receptors triggering intracellular signaling mechanisms that inhibit the function of neurotransmitter receptors and ion channels on the synaptic membrane and regions adjacent to the synapse. As a result, the postsynaptic neuron remains quiescent and in its polarized resting state. No action potentials will be propagated in the postsynaptic neuron, and nociceptive transmission will be attenuated. **C,** Presynaptic descending facilitation. The descending modulatory neuron synapses with the central terminal of the nociceptor and releases excitatory neurotransmitters that bind with cell surface receptors triggering intracellular signaling mechanisms that enhance vesicular trafficking and neurotransmitter release into the synaptic cleft. As a result, additional neurotransmitter receptors will be recruited to the synaptic membrane of the postsynaptic neuron to bind the increased

neurotransmitter from the primary afferent terminal (Figure 2.3A and C) or the function of neurotransmitter receptors on the postsynaptic neuron (Figure 2.3B and D).

Two brainstem sites play a critical role in descending modulation of nociception: the mesencephalic periaqueductal gray (PAG) and the rostral ventromedial medulla (RVM).

Periaqueductal Gray

The PAG surrounds the cerebral aqueduct throughout the mesencephalon (Figure 2.4A) and was the first region found to exert inhibitory control of pain.[22,23] Reynolds first reported the ability to perform abdominal surgery on a rat in the absence of anesthesia while stimulating the PAG with electrical current. These findings were replicated and expanded by others and established that the PAG is an essential element of pain modulatory circuitry.

The PAG is activated by input from higher regions of the CNS such as the thalamus, hypothalamus, and cerebral cortex as well as from collateral projections from ascending spinothalamic tract neurons. Few PAG neurons project directly to the spinal dorsal horn. Instead, the PAG acts indirectly through projections to other brainstem structures, such as the RVM, and other brainstem nuclei. The RVM is enriched in serotonergic neurons projecting to the spinal dorsal horn, whereas noradrenergic neurons from the brainstem are widespread and include locus coeruleus and the A5 and A7 cell groups.[22] The PAG has been shown to be a key source of opioid-mediated descending inhibition of nociception that is naloxone-reversible. Further, owing to its high concentration of opioid receptors,[15] morphine injections into the PAG exert a greater analgesic effect than injections into other CNS regions. In the absence of nociception, neurons within the PAG are under tonic inhibitory control by gamma-aminobutyric acid (GABA) released from inhibitory interneurons. Projection neurons from higher regions of the CNS such as the anterior cingulate cortex (ACC) and amygdala release endogenous opioids in the PAG that inhibit the action of the GABAergic interneurons, which releases the tonic inhibitory control of the PAG neurons and allows them to be activated by excitatory neurotransmitters (e.g., glutamate and substance P) that are also released by afferent projection neurons. When projection neurons in the PAG are excited, they in turn release neurotransmitters in other brainstem regions to excite neurons that project directly to the spinal dorsal horn, where they exert their modulatory effect.

FIGURE 2.3 Continued

volume of neurotransmitters in the synaptic cleft, and the generation of increased numbers of action potentials propagated in the postsynaptic neuron and nociceptive transmission will be accentuated. **D,** Postsynaptic facilitation. The descending modulatory neuron synapses with the postsynaptic neuron and releases excitatory neurotransmitters that bind with cell surface receptors triggering intracellular signaling mechanisms that enhance the binding of neurotransmitters and activation of receptors. As a result, additional neurotransmitter receptors will be recruited to the synaptic membrane of the postsynaptic neuron to bind the increased volume of neurotransmitters in the synaptic cleft, and the receptors will be sensitized such that they produce a larger response when the bind with their ligands. This will lead to the generation of increased numbers of action potentials propagated in the postsynaptic neuron, and nociceptive transmission will be accentuated.

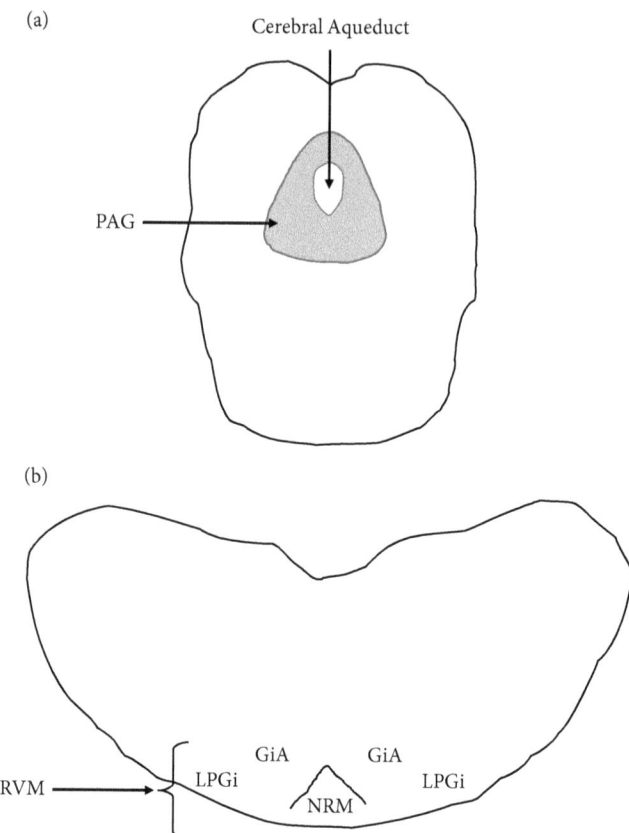

FIGURE 2.4 Diagrams of the structure of the periaqueductal gray (PAG) and rostral ventromedial medulla (RVM). **A,** Diagram of a cross section of the midbrain showing the location of the PAG matter surrounding the cerebral aqueduct. **B,** Diagram of a cross section of the rostral medulla showing the region of the RVM and its subdivisions (nucleus reticularis gigantocellularis pars alpha [GiA], nucleus paragigantocellularis lateralis [LPGi], and the midline nucleus raphe magnus [NRM]).

Rostral Ventromedial Medulla

The RVM is the second major region in the pain modulatory circuit and the primary source of projection neurons to the spinal dorsal horn. The RVM can exert its own modulatory effects as well as relay the modulatory signals from higher brainstem sites. It is a large region of the rostral ventral aspect of the medulla with two bilateral subregions (the nucleus reticularis gigantocellularis pars alpha [GiA] and the nucleus paragigantocellularis lateralis [LPGi]) and the midline nucleus raphe magnus (NRM; Figure 2.4B). Efferent projections from the RVM have been identified in all levels of the spinal cord.

While all of the constituents of the descending modulatory circuitry are important, the RVM is the final common relay point for descending pain modulatory signals. The RVM is a functionally complex region that exerts a bidirectional modulatory effect on nociception.[22] Descending modulatory signals can be both excitatory (pronociceptive) and inhibitory (antinociceptive).[15] The RVM contains a heterogeneous mix of two types of cells that have been identified as on-cells and off-cells. Just before a nocifensive withdrawal reflex, on-cells markedly increase their firing in response to noxious stimulation (Figure 2.5A), whereas off-cells pause their firing after a noxious stimulus (Figure 2.5B) but before a nocifensive withdrawal reflex. It is generally thought that on-cell activity results in facilitation and that off-cell activity results in inhibition of nociception. Further evidence of their respective roles in pain modulation is that the cells in the RVM express high levels of opioid receptors,[8] and opioids binding to the receptors inhibit on-cell activity and stimulate off-cell activity. GABA also plays an important role in the RVM pain modulation process. Off-cells are under tonic inhibition by GABAergic interneurons within the RVM and projections from the PAG. Opioids bind their receptors on the GABAergic neurons to inhibit their activity, which then disinhibits the activity of off-cells. On-cells are not under tonic control by interneurons and are directly excited by cholecystokinin to increase their activity after a noxious stimulus.

The bidirectional modulation of the spinal dorsal horn by the RVM is carefully balanced to titrate the amount of facilitatory and inhibitory effects that are exerted.[15] The pain modulatory effect from the RVM is dependent on the intensity and nature of the intra-RVM stimuli that trigger it. Although the circuitry underlying the generation of the facilitatory and inhibitory modulation may be distinct, an anatomic and neurochemical differentiation of the bimodal modulatory structures has not been determined. It is the balance between inhibition and facilitation that determines the net

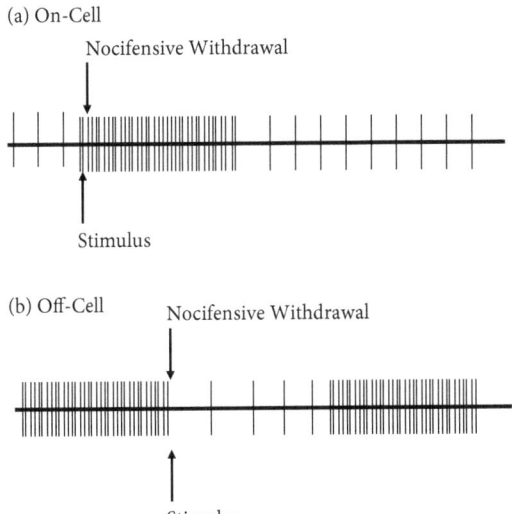

FIGURE 2.5 Diagram of the functional activity of on-cells and off-cells in the rostral ventromedial medulla (RVM). **A,** On-cell action potentials being fired in response to a noxious stimulus. In the resting state, on-cells are quiet and fire very few action potentials. When a noxious stimulus occurs, on-cells immediately fire a rapid burst of action potentials just before a nocifensive withdrawal reflex occurs (e.g., hind paw withdrawal from noxious heat). **B,** Off-cell activity pauses in response to a noxious stimulus. In the absence of nociceptive stimulation, off-cells are tonically active and firing action potentials. When a noxious stimulus occurs, off-cells immediately stop firing action potentials just before a nocifensive withdrawal reflex occurs (e.g., hind paw withdrawal from noxious heat).

effect of descending modulation on nociceptive transmission. The neurochemistry of descending modulation from RVM projection neurons remains unclear. However, it is known that the RVM is the major source of serotonergic projection neurons as well as populations of GABAergic and glycinergic projection neurons.

Spinal Dorsal Horn in Descending Modulation

There is strong evidence that serotonin is released and binds actively in the spinal dorsal horn, either directly from projection neurons or indirectly from intrinsic interneurons. Serotonin exerts both an excitatory and inhibitory effect, depending on which 5-hydroxytryptamine (5-HT) receptor subtype it binds. Serotonin activating the 5-HT1A, 5-HT1B, 5-HT1D, and 5-HT7 receptors has been shown to exert an antinociceptive effect, while activation of the 5-HT2A and 5-HT3 receptors facilitates nociception. However, there is no direct correlation between on-cells, off-cells, and whether the serotonin they release binds specifically to excitatory or inhibitory 5-HT receptors. While a majority of the projections to the spinal dorsal horn are serotonergic neurons from the RVM, there are also noradrenergic projection neurons that originate in the brainstem noradrenergic A5, A6 (locus coeruleus), and A7 (Kolliker-Fuse) cell groups.[22] When dopamine binds to $α_2$-adrenergic receptors, the effect is antinociceptive, while binding to $α_1$-adrenergic receptors is pronociceptive. Opioids, GABA, and glycine, the major inhibitory neurotransmitters, also play important roles in nociceptive modulation in the spinal dorsal horn.[15] When opioids, GABA, and glycine bind to their receptors, it results in hyperpolarization of the cell membrane of the central terminal of the nociceptor, second-order neurons, or postsynaptic interneurons. The hyperpolarization of the cell membrane prevents the propagation of action potentials, thus decreasing the transmission of nociceptive input.

In clinical practice, pharmacologic control of various neurotransmitters, active at the spinal dorsal horn and elsewhere, is often beneficial in relieving pain. Selective serotonin/norepinephrine reuptake inhibitors (SNRIs) are widely used for the management of chronic neuropathic pain. Opioids relieve pain by action at cortical, spinal, and peripheral levels but exhibit highly problematic coactivation of reward pathways contributing to addiction. Also, the gabapentinoids (e.g., gabapentin) have been found to be active in decreasing pain signal entry to the CNS by blocking calcium currents at the presynaptic nerve terminals of PANos in the spinal dorsal horn.

SUMMARY

Pain processing in the PNS and CNS is a complex phenomenon that is bidirectionally regulated by specific molecular events. Nociceptive signals are transmitted from peripheral nerve endings (nociceptors) to the brain for interpretation through complex ascending pathways (comprising second- and third-order neurons). As ascending nociceptive transmission passes through the brainstem and reaches the cerebral cortex, it triggers the activation of a multistage process of pain modulation. The modulatory circuitry projects to the spinal dorsal horn where the modulatory effect constrains or enhances the transfer of nociceptive information from the primary afferent to the second-order neuron. This entire process requires the interplay of inflammatory mediators, neurotransmitters, and their receptors.

REVIEW QUESTIONS

1. The following receptor and sensory mediation phenomena pairings are correct:
   a. Heat pain and TRPV1; chemical pain and TRPA1; chemical pain and Acid-sensing ion chanel (ASIC)
   b. Heat pain and TRPA1; chemical pain and TRPV1; chemical pain and Base-sensing ion chanel (BSIC)
   c. Heat pain and ASIC; chemical pain and Chemical-sensing ion chanel (CSIC); chemical pain and TRPV4

2. The following is not an inflammatory mediator contributing to enhanced pain signaling in the context of inflammatory or tissue destruction:
   a. Protons
   b. Bradykinin
   c. NGF
   d. TNF-α
   e. Isolectin-B4

3. The following is not a key neurotransmitter involved in descending modulation of pain signaling:
   a. Norepinephrine
   b. Acetylcholine
   c. Serotonin
   d. Endogenous opioid
   e. Cannabinoid

REFERENCES

1. Del Valle ME, Cobo T, Cobo JL, Vega JA. Mechanosensory neurons, cutaneous mechanoreceptors, and putative mechanoproteins. Microsc Res Tech. 2012;75(8):1033–1043. doi:10.1002/jemt.22028.
2. Dubin AE, Patapoutian A. Nociceptors: the sensors of the pain pathway. J Clin Invest. 2010;120(11):3760–3772. doi:10.1172/JCI42843.3760.
3. Venkatachalam K, Montell C. TRP channels. Annu Rev Biochem. 2007;76(1):387–417. doi:10.1146/annurev.biochem.75.103004.142819.
4. Ramsey IS, Delling M, Clapham DE. An introduction to TRP channels. Annu Rev Physiol. 2006;68(1):619–647. doi:10.1146/annurev.physiol.68.040204.100431.
5. Stucky CL, Dubin AE, Jeske NA, et al. Roles of transient receptor potential channels in pain. Brain Res Rev. 2009;60(1):2–23. doi:10.1016/j.brainresrev.2008.12.018.
6. Vay L, Gu C, McNaughton PA. The thermo-TRP ion channel family: properties and therapeutic implications. Br J Pharmacol. 2012;165(4):787–801. doi:10.1111/j.1476-5381.2011.01601.x.
7. Cortright DN, Krause JE, Broom DC. TRP channels and pain. Biochim Biophys Acta—Mol Basis Dis. 2007;1772(8):978–988. doi:10.1016/j.bbadis.2007.03.003.
8. Julius D. TRP channels and pain. Annu Rev Cell Dev Biol. 2013;29:355–384. doi:10.1146/annurev-cellbio-101011-155833.
9. Mickle AD, Shepherd AJ, Mohapatra DP. Nociceptive TRP channels: sensory detectors and transducers in multiple pain pathologies. Pharmaceuticals. 2016;9(4):1–27. doi:10.3390/ph9040072.

10. Bandell M, Story GM, Hwang SW, et al. Noxious cold ion channel TRPA1 is activated by pungent compounds and bradykinin. Neuron. 2004;41(6):849–857. doi:10.1016/S0896-6273(04)00150-3.
11. Caterina MJ, Schumacher MA, Tominaga M, et al. The capsaicin receptor: a heat-activated ion channel in the pain pathway. Nature. 1997;389(6653):816–824.
12. Jordt SE, Bautista DM, Chuang HH, et al. Mustard oils and cannabinoids excite sensory nerve fibres through the TRP channel ANKTM1. Nature. 2004;427(6971):260–265. doi:10.1038/nature02282.
13. Gold MS, Gebhart GF. Nociceptor sensitization in pain pathogenesis. Nat Med. 2010;16(11):1248–1257. doi:10.1038/nm.2235.
14. Basbaum AI, Bautista DM, Scherrer G, Julius D. Cellular and molecular mechanisms of pain. Cell. 2009;139(2):267–284. doi:10.1016/j.cell.2009.09.028.
15. Hudspith MJ. Anatomy, physiology and pharmacology of pain. Anaesth Intensive Care Med. 2016;17(9):425–430. doi:10.1016/j.mpaic.2016.06.003.
16. Emanuela Ricciotti P, Garret A, FitzGerald M. Prostaglandins and inflammation. Arterioscler Thromb Vasc Biol. 2011;31(5):986–1000. doi:10.1161/ATVBAHA.110.207449.
17. Mantyh PW, Koltzenburg M, Mendell LM, et al. Antagonism of nerve growth factor-TrkA signaling and the relief of pain. Anesthesiology. 2011;115(1):189–204. doi:10.1097/ALN.0b013e31821b1ac5.
18. Latremoliere A, Woolf CJ. Central sensitization: a generator of pain hypersensitivity by central neural plasticity. J Pain. 2009;10(9):895–926. doi:10.1016/j.jpain.2009.06.012.
19. Zhou XF, Rush RA. Endogenous brain-derived neurotrophic factor is anterogradely transported in primary sensory neurons. Neuroscience. 1996;74(4):945–951. doi:10.1016/S0306-4522(96)00237-0.
20. Head H, Holmes G. Into sensory disturbances from cerebral lesions. Brain. 1911;34(2-3):102–254. doi:10.1016/S0140-6736(00)51693-6.
21. Beecher HK. Pain in men wounded in battle. Pain. 1945;123(1):96–105. doi:10.1213/00000539-194701000-00005.
22. Mantyh PW, Peschanski M. Spinal projections from the periaqueductal grey and dorsal raphe in the rat, cat and monkey. Neuroscience. 1982;7(11):2769–2776. doi:10.1016/0306-4522(82)90099-9.
23. Yaksh TL, Rudy TA. Narcotic analgesics: CNS sites and mechanisms of action as revealed by intracerebral injection techniques. Pain. 1977;4(C):299–359. doi:10.1016/0304-3959(77)90145-2.

3 Impact of Pain on the Individual and Others
Implications for Healthcare Professionals

Paul Arnstein and Megan Keating

It is easier to find men who will volunteer to die, than to find those who are willing to endure pain with patience.
—Julius Caesar

LEARNING OBJECTIVES

At the completion of this chapter, the learner should be able to discuss:

- The multidimensional effects of pain on the individual
- The societal impact of chronic pain
- The global disease burden of chronic pain

CASE SCENARIO

A 74-year-old retired basic scientist with decades of chronic migraine headaches, abdominal pain attributed to irritable bowel syndrome, and a recent small hemorrhagic embolic stroke with minimal deficits is seen by her primary care physician in follow-up. Since the stroke she has been unable to eat because of severe gastritis symptoms shortly after eating as well as abdominal bloating. Her migraine headaches have increased in intensity and frequency. She has been unable to sleep because of pain. This insomnia and pain have led to rising anxiety. Her family notes her significant irritability, emotional lability, and drastic weight loss because she is unable to tolerate food. Her workup has been negative for any cancer or other concerning findings, and her neurologic status has been stable. Over the years she has tried numerous medications, naturopathic strategies, behavioral approaches including therapy and meditation, physical therapy, and other treatments without significant improvement in her chronic pain symptoms. She frequently experiences side effects from the medications and treatments recommended to her, causing her to doubt her providers. She often has to cancel appointments and social activities because of severe pain and other physiologic symptoms. She spends most of her day, when she is able to, coordinating her medical care and specialists and researching her symptoms, and she has very little time and energy to enjoy any activities. On physical exam she is in pain, cachectic, and exhausted, and she has a distended, mildly tender but nonsurgical abdomen.

1. What are some of the individual and societal impacts of chronic pain for Maria and other patients suffering from this disease?
2. How will you gauge the impact Maria's pain is having on her and her family? How will you address this with Maria?
3. How can you gain Maria's trust as a provider knowing that she feels she has been negatively affected by many recommendations made to her in her care?
4. How will you inspire Maria's hope and will to live as fulfilling a life as is possible?
5. What ethical challenges do you face as a provider in managing chronic pain and disability in general?

INTRODUCTION

Transient pain is a natural part of birth, life, and the dying process. Serving as a vital warning system, it motivates people to avert serious illness, injury, or impending death. Strategies to control it are available throughout the life span, but this biopsychosocial phenomenon is unique to the individual, accounting for variable responses to pain and its treatment. Damaged nerves or maladaptive responses can transform pain into a chronic disease, burdening the person and others who struggle to understand and relieve it.

Pain sends ripples through the nervous system that can hijack the person's attention, personality, activities, and valued roles or relationships (Figure 3.1). Pain signals can be amplified, spread, and persist to the point of chronification through a variety of biopsychosocial mechanisms. The person's genetic makeup, culture, past experiences, and current thoughts and feelings, and pain's anticipated future impact, all shape its perception and a wide variation in responses to the same treatment.

Pain is encountered in most healthcare settings. Patients, professionals, and the public overestimate the benefits and safety of pain treatments (e.g., medications, invasive procedures, or nondrug modalities) without acknowledging the high degree of variability in patient response to any pain treatment.[1] Lacking an evidence-based "precision medicine" approach to pain, a personalized treatment plan followed by vigilant monitoring and refinement to balance safe, effective pain reduction with improved functioning is considered the best practice. Unpredictable treatment responses raise ethical concerns that weigh the benefits of compassionate alleviation of suffering against the potential for immediate or long-term harm. This chapter introduces the reader to the impact pain has on the individual, family, and society, while exploring the ethical and practice-based challenges that many professionals face when trying to help the person seeking pain relief.

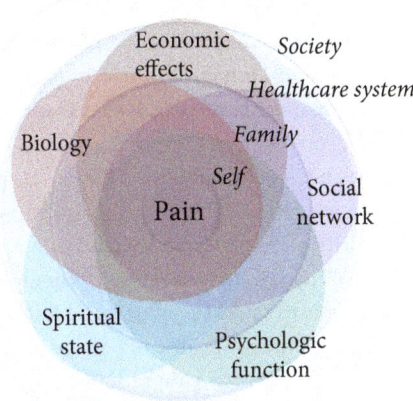

FIGURE 3.1 The rippling effect of pain. Pain effects individuals in many dimensions including biological, psychological, spiritual, social, and economic. In addition, pain impacts those around the individual, including family or close ones, the healthcare system, and society.

IMPACT OF PAIN ON THE INDIVIDUAL

Intense ongoing pain creates degenerative changes throughout the nervous system. This can progress to high-impact chronic pain that harms the person's mind, body, spirit, and social interactions.[1] This disabling pain produces financial hardships, despair, and medical frailty and shortens life. In newborns, repeated exposure to untreated pain affects brain mass, learning abilities, and pain sensitivity years later.[2] In adults, gray matter changes linked to persistent pain greatly outpace those seen with normal aging and can explain the learning, memory, and emotional difficulties experienced by many living with pain.[3]

Severe or prolonged pain permeates the very essence of the person, where it may erode core beliefs and values. This spiritual aspect of pain affects a person's innermost concerns, including the perceived purpose, meaning, and driving force of life. Pain may have a religious meaning for some, such as a deity-dispensed form of punishment, or an opportunity to demonstrate strength that will be rewarded after death. Spirituality is not limited to the confines of religious traditions and may involve tapping into sources of energy that bond the person with other people, animals, a community, nature, or the universe. To the extent that pain affects the essence of the person, it can be a source of spiritual distress and suffering, or a source of strength and motivation. Exploring patients' innermost concerns and values and the endorsed ways of honoring their spiritual needs can help diminish their pain and related suffering.[4]

Anticipation of or exposure to severe pain often triggers undesirable psychological states such as anxiety, fear-avoidance behaviors, learned helplessness, or depressed mood. Anxiety can worsen pain and interferes with healing. When the pain is unexplained, poorly responds to treatment, or signals an inability to continue valued roles and relationships, the anxiety worsens.[4] Unproductive rumination, ritualistic behaviors, or difficulties with problem-solving often accompany this highly anxious state. Uncontrolled, pain predisposes the patient to a spectrum of anxiety disorders, such as obsessive-compulsive or post-traumatic stress disorders.[5] Depression can also worsen pain. The risk for depression increases 10-fold if pain persists beyond 6 months.[4] These sources of distress in persons disabled by pain, combined with feeling defeated or a burden to others, drive many to consider or attempt suicide.[6]

How pain and planned treatments are perceived is shaped by culture and ethnicity. Many cultures stigmatize people with pain, especially when it is chronic. Demographic, socioeconomic, physical and mental capacity, lifestyle, geographic, environmental, and a host of other characteristics are historically linked to discrimination, exclusion, and pain care disparities.[1] To better understand pain and its treatment options, these vulnerable individuals need to have access to culturally and linguistically appropriate services. Opportunities to improve cultural and linguistic competence in pain care are evident by studies showing that 20% of patients with chronic pain sever ties with professionals who didn't take their pain seriously and that 80% of primary care practices have discharged patients with chronic pain.[7]

IMPACT OF PAIN ON CLOSE SOCIAL NETWORK

The physical and social environments surrounding the person with pain have a profound effect on their perception and observable pain behaviors. Behaviors may be reflexive, emphatically expressed, or stoically suppressed.[8] People with pain often withdraw from social interactions and work, becoming isolated and unable to join in meaningful activities or to fulfill valued social roles.[4] Pain can motivate the person to seek and accept help from others, which can strengthen bonds or create conflicts given the stigma attached to expressing pain and seeking relief.

People closest to the person with pain who initially help often become frustrated or burdened when pain interferes with role functioning, finances, companionship, and intimacy. Statements that are punishing or critical or that blame the individuals for their pain often increase pain sensitivity. Similarly, solicitous responses by overly protective loved ones also increase sensitivity to pain.[9] Most studies have focused on the negative impact that maladaptive beliefs (e.g., catastrophizing) have on interpersonal outcomes rather than how to optimize the positive effects of informational, emotional, and social support.

Validating concerns and using humor, distraction, and prompts to cope have been shown to reduce pain and promote adaptive responses.[9] This form of social support is highly valued by chronic pain patients and has a protective role in the individual's health, serving as a buffer to the negative impact of a stress. Additionally, support that validates emotions, aids in problem-solving, and persuades patients to take action enhances self-efficacy beliefs that foster task persistence and autonomy.[9] Thus, professionals can help by counseling loved ones to minimize punishing or solicitous responses and use helpful forms of psychosocial support to lessen pain and emotional distress, while enhancing social engagement, autonomy, and quality of life.[10]

Those closest to the person experiencing pain can also be profoundly affected. Alleviating pain and suffering, especially at the beginning or end of life, can strengthen the person's bonds. In contrast, unsuccessful attempts to console a loved one with intolerable pain can leave emotional scars. Caregivers are also burdened with assessing pain, deciding which drug to give and in what dose, and interpreting the side effects. These are decisions that even professionals struggle with.[11]

As upsetting as this journey can be, loved ones are best positioned to help the team provide needed relief. Some caregivers hold the fatalistic belief that people are destined to suffer and that caregivers should not interfere with the experience of pain. When faced with that outlook, professionals need to address the treatment of pain in a culturally sensitive way to prevent well-intentioned pain-relief acts from becoming a source of existential suffering.[11] Some cultures have assigned healthcare proxies based on family role. Barring those cultural factors, discussions are needed to resolve any conflicts regarding the goals of therapy and the best method to achieve them. Programs are in development to help educate family caregivers to engage them in care, enhance their knowledge and skills about pain and its treatment, and augment communication with health professionals.

Outside the supportive social network, chronic pain patients face stigma, shaming, and shunning that make it difficult to access care and live a productive life with dignity. This stigma has worsened in recent years as mass media increasingly presupposes that all pain is about opioids and all opioids are about substance misuse or addiction. Thus, many seeking help for their pain are labeled as "drug seekers," and their reports of pain are discredited. Very young or old; those with HIV, sickle cell, or substance use disorder; the poor or homeless; and ethnic minorities and others marginalized by society encounter disparities in pain treatment.[1,12] A balanced approach to managing pain, reducing harm, overcoming stigma, and using evidence-based practices will stand up in the era of scrutiny.

IMPACT OF PAIN ON SOCIETY

Pain is a leading reason that patients seek healthcare. An estimated 50 million Americans experience acute pain from major trauma or surgical procedures annually.[1] Globally, more than 230 million people undergo surgery each year, with 75% reporting moderate, severe, or extreme postoperative pain.[13] Poorly controlled severe pain increases the risk for complications, delayed recovery, and the development of persistent postoperative pain. The severity of acute pain 3 days after surgery is the factor most strongly associated with the transition from acute to chronic postsurgical pain, with up to 50% of orthopedic surgery patients continuing to have pain 2 years later.[14]

Impact of Pain on Society

- 100 million American adults are living with chronic pain.
- Low back pain has ranked as the most burdensome cause of disability globally by the World Health Organization (WHO).
- Back and neck pain account for more years lived with disability than cancer, heart attacks, and diabetes combined.

In America, at least 50 million adults are living with chronic pain[15] Of those, 20 million Americans endure high-impact chronic pain that substantially restricts their ability to participate in work, social interactions, and self-care activities.[1,15] Most prevalent is chronic back pain, which afflicts approximately 20% of people across age groups in developed nations. The prevalence of musculoskeletal pain increases with age, including one-fourth of older adults who have persistent upper extremity pain. Chronic widespread pain and neuropathic pain each afflicts close to 10% of the population, with as many as 30% of people with cancer reporting pain with neuropathic characteristics. Chronic pain is increasingly prevalent given recent trends, including a longer life expectancy, more obesity and sedentary lifestyles, and medical advances that improve survival but result in chronic pain. Those at highest risk for developing chronic pain are traumatized children, older adults, persons whose acute pain is not adequately controlled, and those with specific psychosocial risks.

Cancer is the leading cause of death worldwide, with 14 million people diagnosed with the disease and 8 million dying from cancer in 2012. Prevalence studies show that half of patients actively being treated for cancer, one-third of cancer "survivors," and 80% at the end of life endure strong cancer pain, with 33% reporting moderate or severe intensity. Sadly, evidence-based approaches are underutilized even with the distressing, intolerable suffering of advanced disease. Despite considerable advances in other areas of cancer treatment, there has not been a corresponding development of better pain therapies. In fact, new cancer treatments have produced new forms of iatrogenic cancer pain.[16] Unfortunately, strong analgesics are now frequently withheld from the estimated 10 million Americans with cancer pain until the final weeks of life.

The WHO monitors large international databases of more than 350 diseases to calculate a "global burden of illness" representing the number of person-years lived with a disability.[17] For the past three decades, low back pain has ranked as the most burdensome cause of disability globally, accounting for more than 57 million years lived with disability (YLD), closely followed by migraine headaches in the most recent estimations.[17] Neck pain, other musculoskeletal conditions, and anxiety and depression are also in the top 10 sources of disability. Back and neck pain accounts for more YLD than cancer, heart attacks, and diabetes combined. Arthritis pain has risen from number 23 to 15 to 11 in recent decades and is expected to become the fourth pain type on this top-10 list of most disabling afflictions.[17]

The cumulative economic burden of chronic pain is considerable. Estimates in the United States and Australia are similarly calculated at more than $10,000 per person with chronic pain. In Europe, an estimated 1.5% to 3% of the gross domestic product is spent on back pain.[17] Given 2010 cost estimates in the United States ranging from $560 to $635 billion, this economic burden exceeds that of heart disease, cancer, and diabetes combined.[1,17] The downstream effects of opioids prescribed for pain are not included in those calculations. Combining the impact of prescribed and diverted pharmaceutical opioids plus illicit opioids, the opioid crisis in America in 2015 was a similarly costly problem.

IMPACT OF PAIN ON HEALTHCARE PROFESSIONALS

The control of pain is considered a basic human right by the WHO, United Nations, National Academy of Sciences, and 64 nations and is recognized by law in 20 American states.[1] All professionals have a clinical responsibility to take the patient's report of pain seriously and either treat it or refer the patient to an appropriate professional for help. Unfortunately, clinicians often fall short of what is considered the core interprofessional competencies related to pain: understanding the multidimensional nature of pain; using valid, reliable pain assessment methods; preventing opioid-related harm;

and taking a collaborative approach to pain management across the life span and the continuum of care.[18]

Although opioids have been a cornerstone of treating severe pain, there are known to be significant risks associated with their use even when taken exactly as prescribed. Over time, many patients developed new physical and psychosocial problems, including a paradoxical increase in pain. Public health problems of substance use disorders and overdose deaths involving opioids have grown at an alarming rate, ultimately being labeled an epidemic and public health emergency. Information about this crisis is based on available public health data that do not distinguish use that adheres to the prescribed regimen from nonmedical use or from use of illicit opioids for purposes other than pain. Toxicology results indicate that 25% of overdose deaths involve more than one opioid and that 66% of overdoses are likely linked to illicit opioids.[19] This problem worsened the most during a time of an unprecedented drop in the amount of opioids prescribed.[19] Even hospice patients with cancer pain have become collateral damage too afraid to take analgesics, while clinicians often delay prescribing opioids to dying patients until the final weeks of life.[20]

Assuming irresponsible prescribing of opioids is to blame for the opioid epidemic, policy changes that restrict patient access are increasingly enacted and often supersede clinical judgment. A small minority of patients with chronic pain are prescribed chronic opioids, and the vast majority of that therapy is in keeping with federal and state policies. Opioids do help a subset of pain patients, with 2% of patients prescribed long-term therapy developing an opioid use disorder (OUD).[21] Opioids aside, there are a plethora of other ways to manage pain, including an interprofessional team approach. Avoiding the problem by undertreating pain or discharging patients with chronic pain[7] results in many patients self-managing their pain with alcohol or illicit opioids.[21]

Health system initiatives designed to save costs and promote efficiency with short visits and simple medical algorithms have favored prescribing opioids over an integrated multidisciplinary approach for strong or persistent pain. This application of a simple biomedical solution to a complex biopsychosocial phenomenon, along with other medical, social, and economic trends, contributed to more liberal prescribing patterns. Aggressive marketing by the opioid pharmaceutical industry and their lobbying activities and influence on professional education promoted an overestimation of benefits and underestimation of related iatrogenic addiction that blurred the line between medically necessary and nonmedical opioid use.[20] Guidelines suggest avoiding opioids in favor of nonopioid and adjuvant drugs,[13] which has resulted in a push to prescribe only opioid alternatives. This fails to acknowledge the lack of efficacy, high cost, and potentially deadly effects of these opioid alternatives.[22,23] Thus, a more balanced multimodal, multidisciplinary approach tailored to the individual is advised.[13]

Although the moral imperative to ensure that pain is addressed has been established,[18] training programs, regulators, and practice policies do not facilitate the fulfillment of this duty. Instead, health professionals are held accountable for productivity and efficiency standards that incentivize seeing more patients and doing more billable interventions. This limits time and access to noninvasive, nondrug interventions while increasing exposure to potentially dangerous treatments. Denying appropriate care to people with chronic pain, whether or not opioids are prescribed, is unethical because it can lead to physical, mental, and socioeconomic harm and premature death.[24] This is especially true in certain vulnerable populations, including people with limited access to healthcare services, racial and ethnic minorities, people with low income or education, children, older adults, and those at increased risk because of where they live or work or because of limited communication skills. Respecting the patient's communication style, decision-making, treatment choices, and emotional expressions will improve access to multimodal treatment of pain and comorbid behavioral health conditions.[1]

ETHICAL ASPECTS OF PAIN TREATMENT

Pain-related ethical conflicts can arise at the individual, organizational, and societal levels. These conflicts involve choosing between equally defensible actions, such as providing compassionate care without harming the patient (beneficence vs. nonmaleficence); choosing treatments aligned with professional but not patient preferences (paternalism vs. autonomy); being truthful and trusting the truthfulness (veracity) of the patient; and prudent and consistent use of resources to reduce disparities (justice). The primary ethical principle, nonmaleficence, refrains from harming others, including third parties not prescribed opioids through accidents or unauthorized exposure. Before dismissing any pain therapy as too harmful, consider potential harm from pain itself or desperate acts people take to relieve it. Relative risks need to be determined on an individual basis because any single therapy (e.g., chronic opioid therapy, chronic nonsteroidal anti-inflammatory drugs, epidural steroids) can create significant harm or can be less harmful than alternatives.[22,23]

"Effective pain management is a moral imperative, a professional responsibility, and the duty of the people in the healing professions."[1]

A common dilemma faced when treating pain is balancing concerns regarding the overuse of opioids, the fear of addiction, and the misuse of the medication. "Effective pain management is a moral imperative, a professional responsibility, and the duty of the people in the healing professions."[1 (p.17)] Many health professionals and patients lack knowledge about adequate pain control beyond medication management. When patients request a specific drug and dose they believe is needed for pain, they should neither be labeled "drug-seekers" nor be allowed to dictate therapy. Patients displaying this type of behavior should neither be shamed nor shunned, which adds to the stigma they face gaining access to care. Professional judgment and patient experience should be balanced when these "paternalism versus autonomy" conflicts arise. The current knowledge gap can be bridged through education and facilitating access to appropriate multimodal resources.

Professional treatments may be influenced by concerns over litigation related to overtreatment or undertreatment or may be driven out of a business model focusing on the most lucrative practices. Profits, not efficacy or humanity of care, sometimes drive decisions that undermine the trust between patients, providers, and society. The moral obligation to alleviate pain and suffering is often overlooked through a biomedical or business lens. Treating pain is difficult because it evades the biomedical notion that disease is a broken part that could be fixed with the appropriate medication, surgery, or technology. Effective treatment can be costly when multiple, multidisciplinary treatments, extensive education, and counseling are required. These needs are often unmet given a lack of reimbursement for multidisciplinary pain programs, which is a deterrent for organizations faced with financial pressures.

SUMMARY

Given genetic, psychosocial, economic, and other reasons that first-line pain therapy may provide inadequate relief, patient input during the treatment planning process is essential. This promotes autonomy and engagement rather than the shame and isolation that result when patients are labeled pejoratively if standard therapy fails. A patient-centered team approach tailored to their responses, balanced with professional judgment, resolves the classic paternalism-autonomy conflict. Current payer policies, administrative priorities, and overregulation, however, have eroded the therapeutic relationships, and teamwork is needed to overcome these challenges. Instead, when standard therapy fails, patients face stigma or are discharged to suffer in silence and cope with whatever means are available.[7,12] Some benefit from sequential specialty consultations, but if problematic behaviors or comorbidities persist, a program using an interprofessional team approach is best. These best practice models are becoming more accessible to facilitate collaboration among professionals who share different understandings, assessments, and critical thinking about pain to best serve patients.[1]

As a nation, we are investing our resources in extending life over the alleviation of pain and the burden it poses for individuals and society. Deaths from cancer, HIV, and heart disease have declined over the past 10 years, but those related to pain and its treatment have increased. Research dollars spent by the National Institutes of Health have remained low relative to the prevalence and disabling nature of pain especially when compared to other diseases with a lower burden to society. This significant need for increased research funding for pain management is being addressed in the Federal Pain Research Strategy.[1,17] To eliminate the threat of the problems posed by uncontrolled pain to a just, compassionate, and productive society will require political will as well as an investment of resources and collaborative efforts between federal agencies, industry, clinicians, scientists, and the public.

A public health approach across the continuum of pain care can be accomplished without worsening the opioid crisis. This strategy begins with preventing and effectively treating acute pain while avoiding unnecessary exposure to opioids (primary prevention), followed by early identification and effective treatment (secondary prevention) of chronic pain or OUD and then with preventing morbidity and mortality from high-impact chronic pain or OUD (tertiary prevention).[1] A good start is to fully implement and fund the 2016 National Pain Strategy, and support team-based, patient-centered care for those with pain refractory to standard approaches of providing relief. Acknowledging the magnitude and complexity of pain, we cannot do everything at once; but we must do something at once to help the multitude who are suffering from this burden of disease.

REVIEW QUESTIONS

1. All of the following statements are true *except*:
   a. Chronic back pain is the number-one global burden of disease as designated by the WHO.
   b. US government funding for pain research exceeds funding for cancer research.
   c. Back and neck pain accounts for more years lived with disability than cancer, heart attacks, and diabetes combined.
   d. Less than 5% of patients prescribed long-term opioid therapy develop an OUD.
   e. In adults, gray matter changes linked to persistent pain greatly outpace those seen with normal aging.

2. The personal dimension most significantly affected by pain is:
   a. Physiologic
   b. Psychological
   c. Economic
   d. Social
   e. All of the above

REFERENCES

1. US Department of Health and Human Services (USDHHS). National Pain Strategy: A Comprehensive Population Health-Level Strategy for Pain. Washington DC: National Institutes of Health; March 2016. Accessed August 29, 2017 at: http://iprcc.nih.gov/docs/HHSNational_Pain_Strategy.pdf.
2. Duerden EG, Grunau RE, Guo T, et al. Early procedural pain is associated with regionally-specific alterations in thalamic development in preterm neonates. J Neurosci. 2018;38(4):878–886.
3. Coppieters I, Meeus M, Kregel J, et al. Relations between brain alterations and clinical pain measures in chronic musculoskeletal pain: a systematic review. J Pain. 2016;17(9):949–962.
4. Okifuji A, Turk DC. The influence of psychosocial environment in pain comorbidities. In Giamberardino MA, Jensen TS, eds. Pain Comorbidities: Understanding and Treating the Complex Patient (pp. 157–174). Seattle: IASP Press; 2012.
5. Ziadni MS, Sturgeon JA, Darnall BD. The relationship between negative metacognitive thoughts, pain catastrophizing and adjustment to chronic pain. Eur J Pain. 2018;22(4):756–762.
6. Racine M. Chronic pain and suicide risk: A comprehensive review. Prog Neuropsychopharmacol Biol Psychiatry. 2018;87(Pt B):269–280.
7. O'Malley AS, Swankoski K, Peikes D, et al. Patient dismissal by primary care practices. JAMA Intern Med. 2017;177(7):1048–1050. doi:10.1001/jamainternmed.2017.1309.
8. Craig KD. Social communication model of pain. Pain. 2015;156(7):1198–1199.
9. Bernardes SF, Forgeron P, Fournier K, et al. Beyond solicitousness: a comprehensive review on informal pain-related social support. Pain. 2017;158(11):2066–2076.
10. Jongen PJ, Ruimschotel RP, Museler-Kreijns YM, et al. Improved health-related quality of life, participation, and autonomy in patients with treatment-resistant chronic pain after an intensive social cognitive intervention with the participation of support partners. J Pain Res. 2017;10:2725–2738.

11. Oliver DP, Wittenberg-Lyles E, Washington K, et al. Hospice caregivers' experiences with pain management: "I'm not a doctor, and I don't know if I helped her go faster or slower." J Pain Symptom Manage. 2013;46(6):846–858.
12. Cagle J, Bunting M. Patient reluctance to discuss pain: understanding stoicism, stigma, and other contributing factors. J Soc Work End Life Palliat Care. 2017;13(1):27–43.
13. Chou R, Gordon DB, de Leon-Casasola OA, et al. Management of postoperative pain: a clinical practice guideline. J Pain. 2016;17(2):131–157.
14. Simanski CJ, Althaus A, Hoederath S, et al. Incidence of chronic postsurgical pain (CPSP) after general surgery. Pain Med. 2014;15(7):1222–1229.
15. Dahlhamer J, Lucas J, Zelaya C, et al. Prevalence of chronic pain and high-impact chronic pain among adults—United States, 2016. MMWR Morb Mortal Wkly Rep. 2018;67(36):1001–1006.
16. National Cancer Institute (NCI). 2017 Cancer Pain PDQ –Health Professional Version. Accessed May 19, 2017 at: https://www.cancer.gov/about-cancer/treatment/side-effects/pain/pain-hp-pdq.
17. GBD 2017 Disease and Injury Incidence and Prevalence Collaborators. Global, regional, and national incidence, prevalence, and years lived with disability for 354 diseases and injuries for 195 countries and territories, 1990-2017: a systematic analysis for the Global Burden of Disease Study 2017. Lancet. 2018;392(10159):1789–1858.
18. Fishman SM, Young HM, Lucas Arwood E, et al. Core competencies for pain management: results of an interprofessional consensus summit. Pain Med. 2013;14(7):971–981. doi:10.1111/pme.12107.
19. Saloner B, McGinty EE, Beletsky L, et al. A public health strategy for the opioid crisis. Public Health Rep. 2018;133(1 Suppl):24S–34S.
20. Bohnert ASB, Guy GP Jr, Losby JL. Opioid prescribing in the United States before and after the Centers for Disease Control and Prevention's 2016 Opioid Guideline. Ann Intern Med. 2018;169(6):367–375.
21. Han B, Compton WM, Blanco C, et al. Prescription opioid use, misuse, and use disorders in U.S. adults: 2015 National Survey on Drug Use and Health. Ann Intern Med. 2017;167(5):293–301.
22. US Food and Drug Administration. Drug Safety Communication: FDA Requires Label Changes to Warn of Rare but Serious Neurologic Problems After Epidural Corticosteroid Injections for Pain. April 23, 2014. Accessed December 24, 2017 at: https://www.fda.gov/downloads/Drugs/Drug-Safety/UCM394286.pdf.
23. Solomon DH, Husni ME, Libby PA, et al. The risk of major NSAID toxicity with celecoxib, ibuprofen, or naproxen: a secondary analysis of the PRECISION Trial. Am J Med. 2017;130(12):1415–1422.
24. Arnstein P, Herr K, Butcher HK. Evidence-based practice guideline: persistent pain management in older adults. J Gerontol Nurs. 2017;43(7):20–31.

4 Pain Appraisal
Classification, Measurement, and Nomenclature

Chris R. Abrecht, Beth B. Hogans, and Antje M. Barreveld

... [L]et a sufferer try to describe a pain in his head to a doctor, and language at once runs dry.
—Virginia Woolf

LEARNING OBJECTIVES

At the completion of this chapter, the learner should be able to discuss:

- The International Association for the Study of Pain (IASP) definition of pain
- The formal definitions of the mechanism-based classification of pain, including nociceptive, inflammatory, and neuropathic
- The major historical landmarks in the evolution of pain terminology and assessment
- A variety of pain assessment tools used commonly today
- Basic principles of pain measurement, recognizing that accurately recording the patient's pain level is essential for care
- Factors influencing how pain assessment tools are used as outcome measures in clinical studies of pain
- Different strategies for communicating about pain with special populations

CASE SCENARIO

You are taking care of a patient in the perioperative acute care unit. The patient is just awakening from nasal fracture repair surgery, and discharge home is planned after the patient is awake and able to ambulate safely. The patient is still exhibiting reduced alertness from anesthesia but is moaning intermittently, suggesting pain. You want to ask the patient about the pain so that you can determine whether additional pain medication is needed because, based on your behavioral assessment that includes wincing with movement and moaning, the patient is currently experiencing pain that requires treatment.

1. What is the most efficient way to communicate about pain intensity?
2. If your options are a numeric scale ranging from 0 to 10, or a verbal descriptor scale ranging from no pain to severe pain, which do you prefer? Which do you think your patient would prefer? Can you see an advantage to using pain scales consistently across different healthcare settings?
3. Do you think it is practical in this setting to base the assessment on pain interference, that is, whether the pain in question is interfering with activities such as normal work and sleep?

INTRODUCTION

Pain assessment is perhaps uniquely challenging compared with other spheres of clinical practice because pain has real effects on health outcomes and yet aspects of pain (i.e., the internal experience) are subjective. This subjectivity places special demands on patients and clinicians as they strive to communicate with each other, as noted by Virginia Wolfe in the chapter opener quotation. Clinicians also perceive this difficulty: As the pediatric pain psychologist L. Kuttner observed, "attempting to assess and measure another person's pain is like trying to speak a foreign language that you don't understand."[1] The patient, who may or may not have external signs of disease, and who typically does not have any special training, must convey to the clinical practitioner as precisely as possible what is happening. The clinician, in turn, is forced to rely on the patient for key information that will guide diagnosis. At times, the clinician and patient may struggle to understand each other, and the negative emotions naturally associated with pain can interfere with rapport-building in the pain-focused encounter. Successful pain appraisal thus requires clinical proficiencies in both the cognitive and emotional domains, ensuring the relevant details of the pain are adequately understood while also ensuring that the patients' emotional experience of pain is empathetically interpreted.[2] With so many demands placed on clinicians and so many variables in place, simple tools to assist diagnosis are needed and welcome. Here, we briefly consider some basic terms and ideas applied to the study and care of pain as well as some valuable pain assessment tools used at all levels of pain assessment from clinical trials and the most experienced pain-expert clinicians to the first-year health professions student.

INTERNATIONAL ASSOCIATION FOR THE STUDY OF PAIN DEFINITION OF PAIN

The IASP definition of pain was developed by a consensus panel of pain specialists from multiple areas of interest, including surgeons, anesthesiologists, psychologists, psychiatrists, and basic scientists (see the following box). The real value of having an agreed-on definition is that clinicians, scientists, and patient alike can have a basis for communicating about pain.

IASP Definition of Pain

"An unpleasant sensory and emotional experience associated with actual or potential tissue damage, or described in terms of such damage."[3]

There are multiple critically important features of the IASP definition of pain. First, pain is unpleasant. Second, there are two principal aspects to the experience of pain: It is both sensory and emotional. Third, there are three possible associations: with actual tissue damage, with potential tissue damage, or with being described in terms of such damage. As of 2019, the IASP is considering a revision of the definition of pain, the current version proposes that pain is an "aversive sensory and emotional experience typically caused by, or resembling that caused by, actual or potential tissue injury."

CLASSIFICATION OF PAIN

Pain can be divided into many different categories; however, at the most basic level, pain is usefully categorized into three major classes: nociceptive, inflammatory, and neuropathic.[4] Categorizing pain in this way helps to focus clinical reasoning on class of mechanism, in which, despite some overlap, particular pathways and molecules lead to common features of a pain class. For example, neuropathic pain is often characterized by burning or shock-like pain and does not respond well to nonsteroidal anti-inflammatory drugs (NSAIDs); inflammatory pain involves increased sensitivity to normally nonpainful pressure and responds, at least temporarily, quite well to NSAIDs; and mild nociceptive pain may respond to ice temporarily, but more severe nociceptive pain requires local anesthetics or even opioids. This is a mechanism-based approach to classifying pain. Determining that a specific pain condition falls into one of these classes also has important implications for both diagnosis and treatment, as we will discuss later. As illustrated in Figure 4.1, nociceptive, inflammatory, and neuropathic pain can occur separately or together, depending on the condition.

Nociceptive Pain

Nociceptive pain is pain in response to an injury. It is typically acute in nature. Nociceptive pain, although varying from person to person, results from the activation of pain-sensing afferent neurons, or nociceptors, to painful stimuli. The intensity of nociceptive pain is typically proportional to the intensity of the painful stimulus, and this proportional relationship defines the so-called stimulus–response curve. The stimulus–response curve is a graphic plot of the amount of pain stimulation presented to a person on the x-axis and the intensity of pain experienced plotted on the y-axis. For each type of pain stimulus presented, an individual person will have a fairly stable set of responses; in other words, the individual's stimulus–response curve is relatively reproducible. Factors can make people more or less sensitive to pain, and these factors will shift the curve left or right, respectively. There are many published studies showing that nociceptive stimulus–response curves are a reliable and reproducible way to assess pain experience. This is part of the robust evidence base that support the use of pain scales, which will be described in more detail later in this chapter. Nociceptive responses principally occur in response to painful heat or mechanical force, but certain

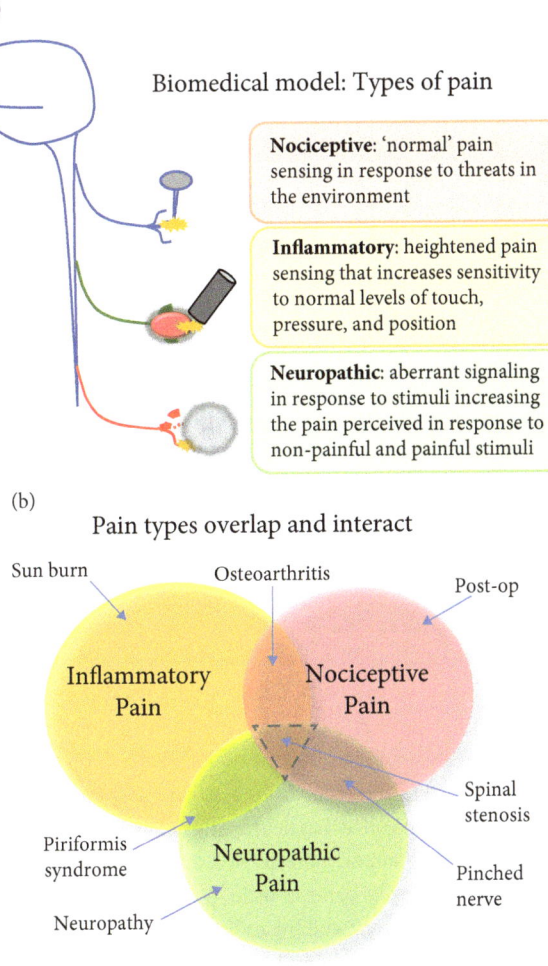

FIGURE 4.1 Relationship of nociceptive, inflammatory, and neuropathic pain mechanism classes. Conditions may have pain mechanisms that arise from multiple. Some conditions represent primarily one class or another. For example, osteoarthritis may be primarily inflammatory, but if there is new or ongoing injury to the joint involved, a component of nociceptive pain may be present as well.

other stimuli (e.g., chemical, biochemical) can also directly activate nociceptors and thus be referred to as nociceptive.

Inflammatory Pain

Inflammatory pain is pain associated with changes in nociception in response to inflammatory mediators under conditions of infection, late-phase injury response, or inflammation. It is initiated by the upregulation of inflammatory mediators and an influx of inflammatory cells, both of which can directly activate and sensitize nociceptive peripheral afferent terminations. Inflammatory pain can be acute, as when it is associated with infection or response to an injury (e.g., burn response), or chronic, as when it is associated with a chronic inflammatory process such as arthritis. It is often associated symptomatically with allodynia or the experience of pain in response to a normally nonpainful stimulus. Normally nonpainful stimuli such as light touch or mild pressure can produce pain when inflammatory mediators have acted on the relevant nervous system elements. Think of the painful pressure a favorite pair of shoes can cause if your toe has a blister: This feels painful in a way that it did not before the blister forming. Inflammatory pain is typically characterized by the upregulation of inflammatory mediators such as prostaglandins, cytokines, and nerve growth factor, as described in Chapter 2, and may respond to treatment strategies that interrupt the sensitization of peripheral nociceptors.

Neuropathic Pain

Neuropathic pain was formally defined by the IASP as pain that is "initiated or caused by a primary lesion or dysfunction in the nervous system."[3] As such, neuropathic pain can result from an injury to the nervous system or may result from some other process that has caused the nervous system to function abnormally in a way that is interpreted by the body as painful. Neuropathic pain can occur acutely or may develop more slowly over hours, days, or months. Neuropathic pain is typically characterized by distinct sensations, such as burning, deep cold, or shock-like jolts; it is resistant to treatment with anti-inflammatory agents such as NSAIDs; and it may be treatment resistant generally. A research-oriented revised definition of neuropathic pain specifies the need to identify a specific lesion to the nervous system in association with the pain condition. This excludes conditions that are neuropathic at the molecular level, a controversial assertion and one that necessitates the introduction of yet another class of pain conditions. It is important for the clinician to recognize that neuropathic pain can arise from macroscopic, microscopic, and molecular changes in the nervous system; in many cases, the key characteristics of pain quality, temporal patterns including persistence, and responsiveness to treatment will be similar, consistent with the utility of this classification system.

The three pain classes can overlap and interact with each other. In patients who have pain from multiple classes, e.g., inflammatory and neuropathic (Figure 4.1B), it is typically necessary to prescribe medications and recommend nonpharmacologic therapies that can address either and both forms, Table 4.1. Approaching a pain-associated problem with the pain classification method allows the provider to begin treatment based on utilizing therapies that are likely to be effective based on pain class, even while the diagnostic process is underway and the diagnosis is being refined.

Other systems of classifying pain focus on specific aspects of the pain experience. These can serve a complementary purpose. For example, pain can be classified as central versus peripheral in origin, malignant versus nonmalignant, acute versus chronic, or somatic versus visceral.

HISTORICAL PERSPECTIVES ON PAIN, PAIN TERMINOLOGY, AND PAIN ASSESSMENT

Pain has long been recognized as a central feature of the human condition. As early as 500 B.C.E., the **Buddhists** acknowledged the relief of pain and suffering as a primary goal. Early Greek philosophers had substantial interest in pain, and the meaning of pain played a central role in defining major schools of philosophic thought.[5] The

Table 4.1 Application of Mechanisms-of-Pain Classification System to Etiology, Diagnosis, and Treatment

Pain Type	Specifics of Mechanism	Examples	Nonpharmacologic Treatments	Pharmacologic Treatments
Nociceptive	Activation of nociceptive afferents using ordinary mechanisms of sensing	Cuts, pricks, burns, blows, breaks, crushes, chemical exposures	Cold or cooling Rubbing (counterirritant) Distraction	NSAIDs Local anesthetics Opioids (severe + acute)
Inflammatory	Activation of afferents following modification in response to inflammatory mediators	Arthritis, inflammation, blister, infection (e.g., abscess)	Warmth (heating pad, Epsom salts) or cooling Gentle exercise PT: strengthening stretching, bracing	NSAIDs Acetaminophen (not anti-inflammatory) Disease modifiers Minimize opioid use
Neuropathic	Activation of nociceptive processing pathways due to disease or dysfunction of nervous system	Neuropathy, MS, transverse myelitis, spinal cord injury, nerve damage	Distraction Self-management CBT/ACT PT, empathetic support	Pain-active antidepressants Pain-active anticonvulsants Local anesthetics Minimize opioid use

ACT = acceptance commitment therapy; CBT = cognitive behavioral therapy; NSAID = nonsteroidal anti-inflammatory drug; PT = physical therapy.

well-known dictum of **Hippocrates,** "primum non nocere," instructs the physician to do no harm but does not explicitly address pain. The **Epicureans** held that the avoidance of pain was a noble goal in itself, while the **Stoics** cultivated the tolerance of pain in the pursuit of virtue. The Stoics had a profound influence on the subsequent development of Roman culture and later civilization. The fundamental paradigm of valuing the pursuit of virtue over the avoidance of pain dominated society through much of the Middle Ages. Not until the late 12th century does a concern for pain re-emerge, when it is expressed in the work of **Maimonides,** a physician-philosopher residing in North Africa. **Descartes,** known most famously for his statement, "I think therefore I am," was a keen student of nerves as well as brain and proposed that pain sensations are transmitted by activation of fluid traveling in little tubes (Figure 4.2).

Unfortunately, even into the 19th century, pain alleviation methods were rudimentary to nonexistent, and surgical and dental procedures were dreaded, almost barbaric ordeals. More recently, the complicity of some physicians in the tragic events of the mid-20th century compelled an intense re-examination of medical ethics and yielded ethical platforms such as the **Nuremberg code** and **Helsinki declaration,** compelling the avoidance of unnecessary physical suffering in the conduct of medical research. Nevertheless, to this day, none of the principal codes of medical ethics bind physicians in practice to pursue the relief of pain.

The evolution of pain terminology took an interesting turn about 100 years ago. In 1904, **Sherrington** coined the term *nociceptive,* derived from *nocere,* taken to mean

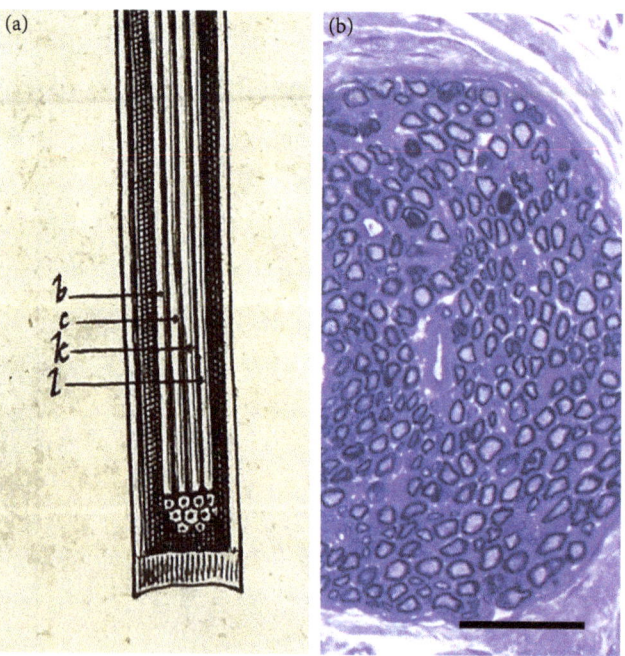

FIGURE 4.2 Views of the nerves, a conduit for pain signaling in antiquity and today. **A,** Descartes described the microscopic structure of peripheral nerves as consisting of densely packed double-walled tubes containing liquid involved in signaling. (This rendering was photographed by the author [BBH] from the collection of Dr. Thomas Brushart.) **B,** Modern photomicrograph of peripheral nerve prepared by plastic resin embedding and toluidine blue staining. Bar = 0.5 mm. (© Beth B. Hogans.)

"pain perceiving."[6] This linguistic innovation has remained popular and lead to the terms *nociceptor* (pain receptor), *nociception* (pain perception), and *nocifensive* (pain producing). Other word roots in use pertaining to pain include *algo* used in the words *algogen*, or pain-producing substance, and *analgesia*, or pain relief; however, attempts to adopt the name *algology* for the field of pain medicine did not succeed.

The adoption of pain assessment in clinical settings has been glacially slow by some accounts. It was long recognized by astute clinicians that pain should be assessed for quality, region, and intensity as well as temporal course and exacerbating and relieving factors, but approaches were not standardized. A prescient clinician, Dr. Kenneth **Keele**, reported the utility of close attention to pain ratings in 1948 as "the first steps in rendering pain intelligible to the observer."[7] Unfortunately for many, it was not until the late 1970s that systematic pain assessment was undertaken by clinicians and researchers in a more quantitative and qualitative fashion. In 1975, Ron Melzack published a description of the **McGill Pain Questionnaire**, an intensively developed, highly structured tool to evaluate the sensory-discriminative and emotional aspects of pain as well as pain intensity and other features.[8] Subsequently, as part of studies to evaluate the effects of analgesia and placebo treatments, it became very important to have reliable methods of "measuring" what is in part a subjective experience—pain.[9] This led to the widespread use and comparison of various scales for measuring pain intensity and the development of more complex instruments to measure various aspects of pain.

PAIN ASSESSMENT TOOLS

Pain assessment tools can be divided into those that are unidimensional and those that are multidimensional; the unidimensional pain assessment tools measure single aspects of pain, the most common of which is pain intensity. Multidimensional pain assessment tools attempt to measure multiple aspects of pain, including pain intensity, pain quality, the amount of distress associated with pain, the degree to which pain interferes with normal function, and the impact of pain on overall functioning.

Unidimensional Pain Assessment Tools

Pain intensity is generally measured by one of three approaches: an analog scale, a numeric scale, or a verbal descriptor scale; these are described in detail later.[10] Pain intensity (severity) assessment tools have been extensively validated in experimental, preclinical studies. The numeric pain rating scale, for example, is strongly correlated with heat-evoked brain activation in controlled pain experiments.[11] The scales described here demonstrate exceptional reliability, reproducibility, and validity. When trained in the use of scales, people use pain scales very consistently to report pain severity. The scales can be used in all different settings, including home, hospital, clinic, and triage. The scales are easily understood and do not require literacy for use.[12] The principle limitation is that the scales do not function with complete linearity at the upper ranges because people seem to have difficulty distinguishing the relative intensity of the most severe pain experiences, not unlike the difficulties with distinguishing extremes of color, sound, or taste. The numeric rating scale (NRS) is the most widely used in clinical practice.

Among the first tools used to assess patient self-report of pain intensity is the visual analog scale (VAS) (Figure 4.3). With the VAS, patients are presented a 10-cm line labeled "no pain" on one end, and "worst pain ever"—or something similar—on the other. Between these end labels, there are no markings. Patients are asked to identify with a mark where on this line their pain falls. The distance from the zero point to the mark in centimeters is the pain score; because there are no reticulations (scaling marks), it is necessary for the clinician using this scale to measure the distance from zero to the patient's mark in order to convert the VAS mark to a reportable number.

In contrast to the VAS is the NRS (Figure 4.3), in which patients are presented with a graduated scale labeled from 0 to 10 and asked to mark the point describing their pain. A response of "0" in this scale signifies "no pain," and one of "10" represents "worst pain imaginable." In the NRS, equally spaced markings identify each value from 0 to 10 along the scale. The numeric markings facilitate the process of assigning a numeric score to the patient's pain. The ease of scoring the NRS relative to the VAS makes it appealing in clinical practice, and generally the VAS and NRS are equally sensitive for measuring changes in pain. The NRS is much easier to use in practical terms. Despite good reproducibility and reliability, the scales are not infinitely sensitive to changes. A two-point improvement in the NRS scale is termed the minimally clinically significant improvement. Importantly, the NRS is robust for use in many populations and in one study was more reliable for illiterate patients than was the VAS.[12]

The patient's report of pain intensity is sometimes measured through the use of a verbal descriptor rating scale (VRS), in which, instead of numeric scales, patients are presented with a series of adjective descriptors and asked to indicate which best describes their pain (Figure 4.3). A common example of such a scale includes the words "mild," "moderate," and "severe" and instructs patients to select only one. Although the

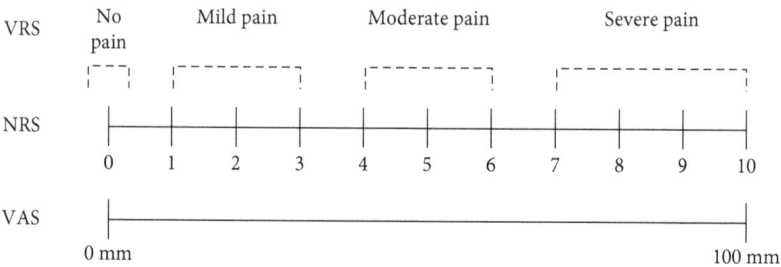

Note: In comparing the VRS to the NRS, "no pain" usually corresponds to 0, "mild pain" to 1–3, "moderate pain" to 4–6, and "severe pain" to 7–10.

FIGURE 4.3 Common pain intensity scales. **A,** Using the visual analogue scale (VAS), a horizontal line without any scaling marks, the provider must measure the distance from zero to the patient's pain mark to be able to record a numeric values. Psychometric properties are similar to the numeric rating scale (NRS). **B,** With the NRS, vertical marks make interpretation and recording of a numeric pain score easier in clinical practice. The NRS is highly reproducible, reliable, and robust across diverse populations. The minimum clinically meaningful change is about 2 points for each scale.

VRS is favored by some patients, it is recognized as being less sensitive to changes in pain intensity.

Multidimensional Pain Assessment Tools

Multidimensional pain scales measure multiple aspects of a pain complaint, such as the quality of pain and the impact of the pain on mood or function. The principle multidimensional pain scales include the McGill Pain Questionnaire (MPQ), the Brief Pain Inventory (BPI), and the Memorial Pain Assessment Card (MPAC); these are described briefly here.

The MPQ represents a survey tool that is significantly more extensive—and time-consuming—than three described previously. The MPQ is a multidimensional measure that divides pain into three dimensions—sensory, affective, and evaluative.[8] Patients are presented with 20 sets of words, containing anywhere from two to six descriptors, and are asked to mark any that are relevant to their situation or describe their experience. Each of these descriptor sets is aimed to specifically address a specific dimension of pain, with the first 10 dedicated to sensory-discriminative aspects (e.g., stabbing, crushing, scalding); the next five dedicated to affective aspects (e.g., exhausting, terrifying, grueling); the next one to evaluative aspects (e.g., annoying, intense); and the remaining four to all three areas.

The BPI is another useful and well-validated pain tool often utilized to obtain a multidimensional understanding of the impact of pain on the patient.[13] The motivation behind its use is to assess pain intensity and pain-associated disability. The BPI is characterized by a series of NRS scales—again ranging from 0 to 10—that prompt patients to provide ratings of pain intensity (worst pain, least pain, average pain, current pain) and the impact of pain on daily function and activity. This measure often additionally contains a diagram of the body on which patients are asked to identify all areas in which pain are felt. The BPI requires slightly more time to complete than the VAS, NRS, or VRS, but it also approaches pain as a multidimensional issue.

The MPAC is designed to explore the multidimensionality of pain through the use of a series of unidimensional measures and qualitative pain descriptors.[14] As such, the MPAC features a sequence of VASs aimed to quantify three key variables—pain, pain relief, and mood—on the standard 0 to 10 continuum. The MPAC additionally includes a list of descriptors related to pain intensity from which patient are asked to select. Thus, this assessment tool allows for a quick and relatively straightforward multidimensional measure of pain.

Communicating About Pain With Special Populations

Alternative strategies for communicating about pain vary with the needs of the population to be evaluated. Pediatric patients should be evaluated with tools that are appropriate to the developmental stage of the patient.[10] Young and very young children can be asked about pain using the depictions of pain such as the Faces Pain Scale.[15] In depiction-based scales, patients are shown a series of faces ranging in emotional intensity and asked to select that which best describes their pain. Another scale often used, though most

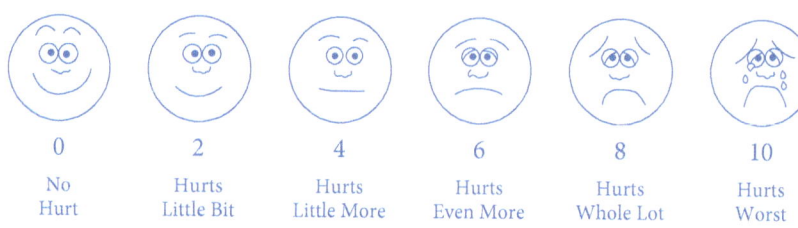

FIGURE 4.4 Wong-Baker FACES Pain Rating Scale. (Reproduced with permission.)

often with children, is the color scale, in which patients are instructed to select the color that best represents their pain. By about 8 years of age, most children can utilize a numerical rating scale (NRS). Infants must be evaluated using behavioral assessment tools.[16-18]

To measure pain in the pediatric population, a number of scales are available. Arguably the most well-known and most frequently used is the Faces Pain Scale-Revised (FPS-R), which consists of six faces ranging in emotional intensity corresponding to different levels of pain. Patients are asked to select that which best describes their pain.[16] Multiple studies comparing the FPS-R to the VAS found that the FPS-R is validated for measuring acute pain in children 4 years and older. This scale is "revised" from a previous Faces Pain Scale that contained seven faces; the use of six faces allows easier comparison to the NRS and VAS. Another pediatric pain measurement tool frequently used is the Wong-Baker FACES Pain Rating Scale. Figure 4.4 displays this scale and its instructions for use. Another scale often used, though most often with children, is the color scale, in which patients are instructed to select the color that best represents their pain. Younger children, those with developmental delay, and infants must be evaluated using behavioral assessment tools. Behavioral pediatric pain measurement tools include the FLACC (face, legs, activity, cry, consolability) tool validated for pediatric patients 2 months to 7 years of age with acute pain.[16] The CRIES Pain Scale (crying, oxygen saturation, blood pressure, heart rate, facial expressions, amount of sleep) is a validated measure of pain in pediatric patients from 32 gestational weeks to 6 months.[17] See Table 4.2 for more information on scoring pain with the FLACC and CRIES scales. Measurement scales also exist for nonverbal populations. The COMFORT pain scale, for instance, measures pain in ventilated infants, children, and adolescents using a scoring system that includes alertness, respiratory distress, crying, muscle tone, blood pressure, and more.[8]

In addition to these, a number of tools have been developed to allow the self-reporting of pain by elderly people, foreign language speakers, those with cognitive impairments, and others who may struggle with more complicated measures. These tools include the PAIN-AD and the MOBID-2 pain scales, which assess patients with dementia or geriatric patients in nursing homes.[19] It is essential to ensure that patients are able to use the scale presented to them, so a guide to selecting scales based on patient characteristics should be available in your practice environment. An example of this process is illustrated in Figure 4.5.

Basic Principles of Pain Appraisal

The basic principles of pain measurement can be divided into those factors that are the responsibility of the physician, those factors that are intrinsic to the pain assessment tool in use, and those factors under control of the patient. These factors are summarized in the following box.

Table 4.2 Pain Measurement in the Pediatric Population: FLACC and CRIES

FLACC	Face	Legs	Activity	Cry	Consolability
0	No particular expression or smile	Normal position or relaxed	Lying quietly, normal position, moves easily	No cry	Content, relaxed
1	Occasional grimace or frown; withdrawn, disinterested	Uneasy, restless, tense	Squirming, shifting back and forth, tense	Moans or whimpers, occasional complaint	Reassured by occasional touching, hugging, or being talked to; distractible
2	Frequent to constant frown, clenched jaw, quivering chin	Kicking or legs drawn up	Arched, rigid, or jerking	Crying steadily, screams or sobs; frequent complaints	Difficult to console or comfort

CRIES	Crying	Requires Oxygen for Saturation >95%	Increased Vital Signs	Expression	Sleepless
0	No	No	Heart rate and blood pressure equal to or less than preop. levels	None	No
1	High pitched	<30%	Heart rate and blood pressure increased by less than 20% of preop. levels	Grimace	Wakes at frequent intervals
2	Inconsolable	>30%	Heart rate and blood pressure increased by greater than 20% of preop. levels	Grimace, grunt	Constantly awake

In both the FLACC and CRIES scales, the patient's score ranges from 0 to 10, meant to mirror the commonly used numeric rating scale. The FLACC scale was created by Merkel, Voepel-Lewis, Shayevitz, and Malviya and published in *Pediatric Nursing* in 1997; the CRIES scale was created by Krechel and Bildner and published in *Pediatric Anesthesia* in 1995.

Patient population	Clinical scenario	Appropriate pain scales
Thirty-two-year-old man without cognitive deficit or any other significant past medical history. 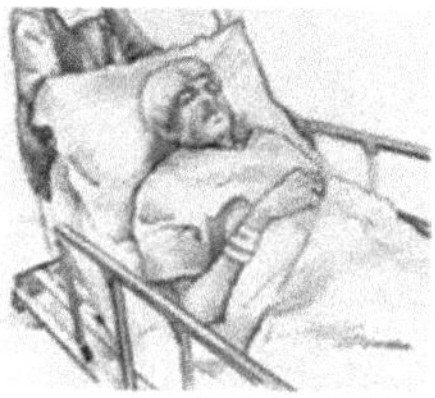	Admitted with vomiting and severe pain in his right lower abdomen, found to have appendictis.	NRS, VRS, VAS
Four-week-old boy with severe bacterial gastroenteritis. 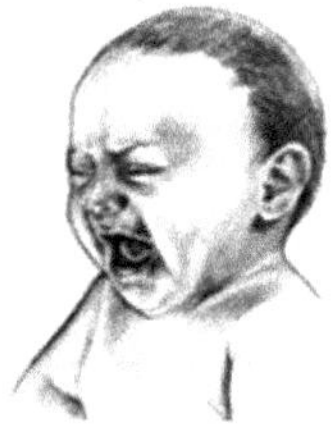	In-patient admission after prolonged vomiting and diarrhea, for volume resuscitation and antibiotics.	CRIES
Seven-year-old boy with sickle cell disease. 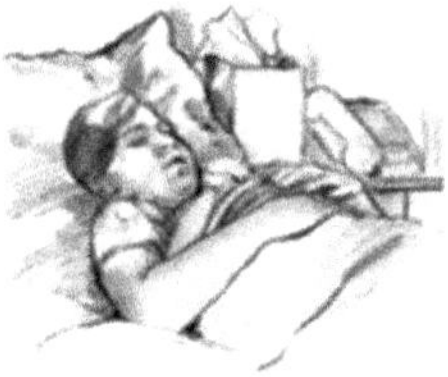	In-patient admission for sickle cell crisis, with severe pain in fingers, toes, and back, treated with intravenous opioids.	FPS-R, FLACC, NRS, VAS
Forty-year-old woman with chronic pelvic pain. 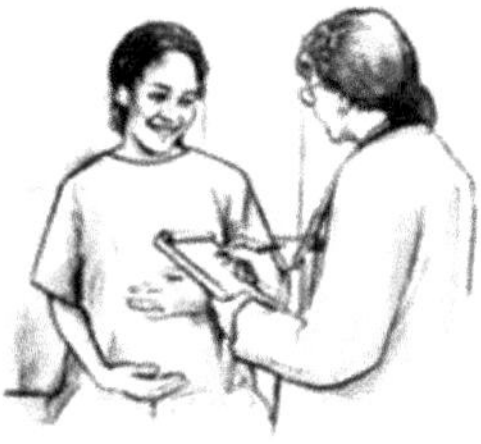	Clinical trial to determine the efficacy of a new medication to treat chronic pelvic pain.	MPQ, SF-MPQ, BPI, NRS, VRS, VAS

FIGURE 4.5 Choosing an appropriate pain scale based on patient characteristics.

Principles of Pain Measurement Summary

The clinicians' responsibilities include:
1. Accept the patient's report of pain
2. Respond to reports of pain effectively
3. Reassess frequently if pain is present

The pain assessment tool must be:
4. Easily understandable
5. Sensitive to changes in pain level
6. Reliable and reproducible

The patient (when able) is responsible to:
7. Learn to use a basic pain assessment tool
8. Respond accurately about the pain
9. Keep contemporaneous records when asked

The first principle of pain assessment is: Accept the patients' report of their pain. People are remarkably diverse in terms of pain experienced in response to the same stimulation (Figure 4.6), but it is a clinical truth that severe pain produces suffering and is very real to the person experiencing it. Several decades of research support the patient's self-report of pain as the most accurate readily available measure of pain.[7,8,10–12] The acceptance of pain self-reporting has been somewhat controversial in media sources and therefore is discussed here in detail. One important reason for using the patients' self-report of pain is that there are no other robust methods for accurately measuring pain in clinical settings; behavioral signs of pain vary widely between cultures, the amount of pain experienced in response to a particular stimulus varies widely between individuals, and physiologic responses to pain can vary systematically with gender, age, and other factors. Even with the advent of functional magnetic resonance imaging and electrical measures of brain activity associated with pain stimuli,

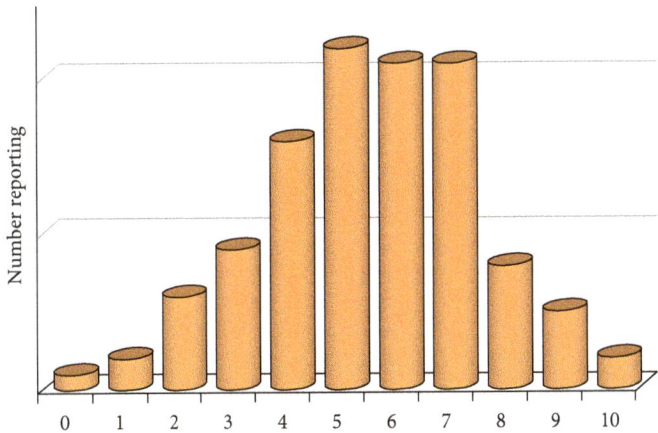

FIGURE 4.6 Pain varies widely from one individual to the next. In this figure, young adults were exposed to cold pressor (ice water) stimulus for 2 minutes, and pain ratings were collected. Pain ratings ranged from mild to severe with a mode of moderate to severe intensity.

there is currently no more quick, reproducible, reliable, and readily available measure of pain intensity than the patient's communicated perception.

With time and experience, accepting the patient's report of pain has achieved wider validation. Within the past 20 years, pain assessment and education have been identified by **The Joint Commission (TJC)**, the agency that certifies hospitals, as a key performance measure.[20] This means that pain needs to be screened routinely, recorded accurately, assessed and reassessed, and responded to promptly in both inpatient and ambulatory care settings. This also implies that underreporting someone's pain is akin to distorting the medical record. As part of recommended care, all providers should educate patients about pain assessment methods and actively enquire about current and recent pain levels. Additionally, TJC requires that healthcare providers learn about pain and pain management, including nonpharmacologic approaches, the risks of opioids, and the need to exercise additional caution in those patients with respiratory compromise.

Frequently, medical students and others express the concern that patients will try to manipulate pain scores in an attempt to obtain powerful pain medications. In fact, research studies show that both doctors and nurses have routinely underestimated pain in their patients, recording, on average, a pain score two to three points lower (on a 10-point scale) than that reported by the patient.[21] The reasons for pervasive **pain underestimation** are not known but may reflect worries about overtreatment of drug-seeking patients or a simple failure to recognize someone else's suffering. Although the percentage of patients who exaggerate pain to obtain medications is unknown, underestimating pain scores does not solve the problem. The fallacy that pain underestimation will correct for pain-exaggerating patients is illustrated in Figure 4.7. The most serious negative consequence of underestimating pain is that those patients who are genuinely seeking care will have their pain undertreated, and in most settings, these patients are the vast majority. The further consequence of underestimating pain is that the patient who is exaggerating or manufacturing a pain complaint to obtain narcotics will still require expenditure of healthcare resources and will still receive treatment—albeit at a lower level of intensity. Thus, relying on pain underestimation as a strategy to avoid prescribing medications to exaggerating patients is unlikely to be effective.

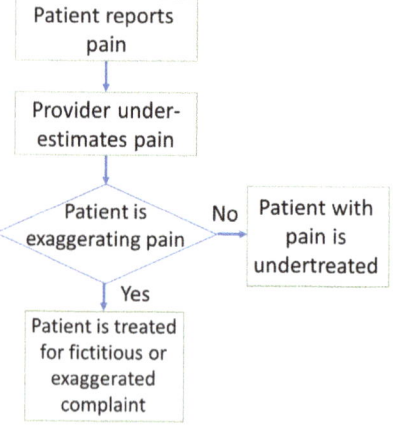

FIGURE 4.7 Flow chart illustrating the consequences of pain underestimation, a commonly adopted approach that leads to undertreatment of most patients; see details in text.

The preferred method to address concerns about pain-exaggerating patients is to accept the pain score as reported by the patient but to make treatment contingent on other clinical criteria. We recommend affirmation of three important questions: (1) Are the history and exam consistent with a known pain process? (2) Does the patient have an adequate social support network and no evidence of past or present substance abuse? (3) Does the patient demonstrate conscientious behavior in keeping follow-up appointments and complying with treatment recommendations? This contingency-based approach to assessment and treatment is illustrated in Figure 4.8. Failure to satisfy any of the three contingency questions raises serious concerns and should lead the physician to modify the treatment plan as follows: If the history and exam are not consistent with a known pain process, this may be because the pain condition is rare, represents a rare presentation of a common condition, or is "functional" in nature. In any of these cases, referral to a pain medicine specialist will be of benefit. If the patient has a readily recognizable pain condition but lacks a strong social support network or demonstrates evidence of substance abuse (e.g., self-report, positive urine drug screen, aberrant medication use, physical stigmata suggestive of drug use), involvement of an addiction specialist will be beneficial. Last, if the patient fails to demonstrate accountability in follow-up and management of interim pain relief prescriptions, then it is likely that extra caution should be exercised in providing additional prescriptions; strategies could include scheduling very frequent follow-up appointments, limiting or avoiding opioid use, contracting for responsible prescription use, and maintaining contact with the pharmacist. The advantage of the contingency management approach is that the

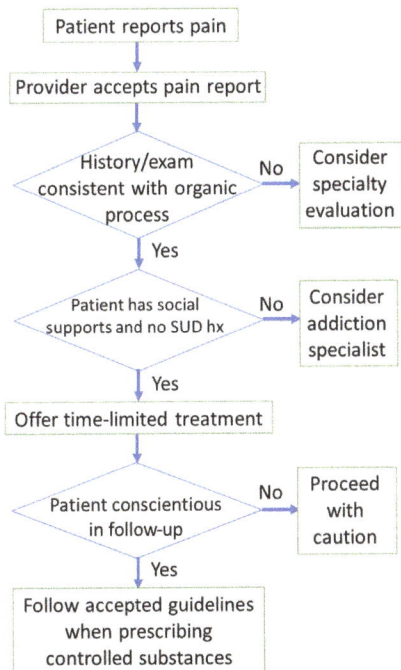

FIGURE 4.8 Flow chart for responding to pain ratings. The pain rating is one piece of information that is gathered about a patient reporting pain. The clinical assessment is further detailed in Chapters 6 and 7 in terms of information gathering and diagnostic reasoning that lead ultimately to the provider's response to a pain rating. SUD hx = substance use disorder history.

majority of patients who are genuinely suffering from pain-associated conditions are likely to receive appropriate treatment. Those who, for various reasons, are exaggerating pain will be identified and will also receive appropriate referral.

The second principle of pain assessment is to provide a supportive environment.[22] Pain perception is a complex, integrative process that relies on a variety of factors, including environment. Some patients will underreport pain in an effort to please healthcare providers.

The third principle of pain measurement is to reassess pain frequently, if present. This is important for several reasons. First, pain reassessment is critical to ensure that effective treatment measures are being taken. Second, knowing the temporal characteristics of a pain complaint will aid in formulating the differential diagnosis. Third, contemporaneous reports of pain are more accurate.

The fourth, fifth, and sixth principles of pain assessment pertain to the tools used for pain assessment. These are that the tool must be easily understood, must be sensitive to changes in pain levels, and must consistently produce reliable and reproducible results. The tools typically used to measure pain were discussed in the preceding section. The commonly used pain assessment tools, such as the NRS, meet the criteria established by these principles of pain assessment.

The seventh, eighth, and ninth principles of pain assessment describe the responsibilities of the patient. The first is that the patient must make an effort to learn how to use a basic pain tool to communicate about their pain. The second is that the patient has a responsibility to report the pain accurately. The third patient-oriented principle is that when requested, patients should record their pain at reasonable intervals.

Pain Assessment Tools as Outcome Measures for Clinical Trials

Pain assessment tools have become vitally important as outcome measures for clinical trials of pain treatments. Pain treatments represent a multibillion-dollar market in the United States alone; thus, there is tremendous pressure to develop new, effective forms of treatment and to demonstrate in clear terms the effectiveness of new and established treatments. Tools such as the NRS are easily understood, have been extensively validated, and show sensitivity to changes in pain levels. However, the design of pain treatment trials involves added levels of complexity. For one, all pain treatments are subject to large and variable placebo effects, a topic discussed in detail in Chapter 7. Therefore, most pain treatment trials must include a placebo treatment group. In general, because of the prevalence and magnitude of placebo effects, the criteria for treatment trial success are more stringent than the absolute level of detectable change. Thus, although the NRS can detect changes in pain as small as 20%, it has generally been observed that a 30% reduction in pain intensity is necessary for a change to be significant within the context of a treatment trial. A second consideration in the design of pain treatment trials is that current standards of evidence-based medicine require rigorous trial design. For treatment trials, this means that treatment effects must be demonstrated in randomized, controlled, double-blinded studies. Last, modern standards of statistical analysis require that outcome measures be determined in advance (a priori) of beginning the trial. The considerations for pain treatment trials are summarized in Table 4.3.

Table 4.3 Factors Affecting Pain Clinical Trials

Properties of pain assessment scale	Reliability, reproducibility, speed of administration, and sensitivity
Placebo effect	Consistency (presence in all members of the study population) and magnitude
Randomized control design	Safety, unmasking, existing alternatives, noninferiority vs. efficacy design
A priori outcome measures	Extent to which experimental plan captures the relevant changes

PAIN TERMINOLOGY

An extensive language of pain has developed to allow clinicians and scientists to communicate accurately and efficiently about different aspects of pain. The IASP, founded in 1972 by John Bonica, Harold Merskey, and others, has played a major role in developing standardized lexicon and taxonomy of pain.[23,24] Some commonly used pain terms are listed in Table 4.4. Two terms that are especially important in clinical practice are *hyperalgesia* and *allodynia*. Hyperalgesia is the phenomenon of some stimulus that is normally painful being perceived as more painful. This could occur, for example, when a slight burn on the hand or arm while cooking is subsequently exposed to hot steam; the burn will hurt far worse than the discomfort that would have resulted from the exposure of normal skin to hot steam. Allodynia is the phenomenon of some stimulus that is normally not painful now being perceived as painful. This can happen with a blister or abscess exposed to normally nonpainful pressure, a sunburned area of skin, or an inflamed joint that hurts with movement. Hyperalgesia is often observed in neuropathic conditions, allodynia may be observed in neuropathic conditions but is often a hallmark of inflammatory signaling at work to induce nociception.

SUMMARY

In this chapter, we have covered topics relating to definitions of pain and the process of pain assessment. The IASP definition of pain was discussed in detail. The major mechanism-based classification scheme of pain as nociceptive, inflammatory, and neuropathic was presented. A brief history of pain terminology was provided, and the major pain rating scales were introduced, including unidimensional scales such as the NRS and VAS and multidimensional scales such as the MPQ. Principles of pain assessment, organized into physician-, tool- and patient-related principles, were described. The importance of physicians accepting the patient's report of pain was discussed in detail. Critical factors for using pain assessment tools as outcome measures for pain treatment clinical trials were discussed, namely consequences of the placebo effect, the need for randomized controlled trial design, and the necessity of a priori outcome measures. A brief discussion of pain assessment in children, older adults, and nonverbal populations illustrated the utility of alternative assessment tools, such as the Faces Pain Scale. In conclusion, pain assessment is the foundation on which pain

Table 4.4 Pain Terminology: IASP Taxonomy With Selected Examples

Term	IASP Definition	Selected Examples
Pain	An unpleasant sensory and emotional experience associated with actual or potential tissue damage, or described in terms of such damage	
Allodynia	Pain due to a stimulus that does not normally provoke pain	A woman with complex regional pain syndrome screams in pain when you touch her arm with a feather.
Analgesia	Absence of pain in response to stimulation that would normally be painful	A man with a cut on his forehead after a fall receives an intravenous dose of morphine; afterward, an emergency physician sutures this laceration without the man endorsing any pain.
Anesthesia dolorosa	Pain in an area or region that is anesthetic	A woman with meralgia paresthetica—no sensation in the lateral thigh in the distribution of the lateral femoral cutaneous nerve—complains of discomfort in her lateral thigh.
Causalgia	A syndrome of sustained burning pain, allodynia, and hyperpathia after a traumatic nerve lesion, often combined with vasomotor and sudomotor dysfunction and later trophic changes	
Dysesthesia	An unpleasant abnormal sensation, whether spontaneous or evoked	A man with carpal tunnel syndrome complains of an uncomfortable "pins and needles" dysesthesia in his fingers after a day of typing.
Hyperalgesia	Increased pain from a stimulus that normally provokes pain	A man has a laceration on his right arm. When the skin a few inches from this laceration is pricked with a sharp pin, he screams out in pain; when his left arm is pricked, he reports only mild pain.
Hyperesthesia	Increased sensitivity to stimulation, excluding the special senses	
Hyperpathia	A painful syndrome characterized by an abnormally painful reaction to a stimulus, especially a repetitive stimulus, as well as an increased threshold	

Table 4.4 Continued

Term	IASP Definition	Selected Examples
Hypoalgesia	Diminished pain in response to a normally painful stimulus	A man with a cut on his forehead after a fall receives a small intravenous dose of morphine; afterward, an emergency physician sutures this laceration with the man endorsing only mild pain.
Hypoesthesia	Decreased sensitivity to stimulation, excluding the special senses	
Neuralgia	Pain in the distribution of a nerve or nerves	A woman with postherpetic neuralgia complains of pain in her face in the distribution of cranial nerve V; for this neuralgia, her physician prescribes gabapentin.
Neuritis	Inflammation of a nerve or nerves	
Neuropathic pain	Pain caused by a lesion or disease of the somatosensory nervous system	
Central neuropathic pain	Pain caused by a lesion or disease of the central somatosensory nervous system	A herniated disk at L5–S1 results in "lightning-like" shooting pain down the leg.
Peripheral neuropathic pain	Pain caused by a lesion or disease of the peripheral somatosensory nervous system	Compression of the median nerve at the wrist results in carpal tunnel syndrome.
Neuropathy	A disturbance of function or pathologic change in a nerve: in one nerve, mononeuropathy; in several nerves, mononeuropathy multiplex; if diffuse and bilateral, polyneuropathy	A man with poorly controlled diabetes complains of tingling of both his feet; he is diagnosed with diabetic polyneuropathy.
Nociception	The neural process of encoding noxious stimuli	
Nociceptive neuron	A central or peripheral neuron of the somatosensory nervous system that is capable of encoding noxious stimuli	
Nociceptive pain	Pain that arises from actual or threatened damage to non-neural tissue and is due to the activation of nociceptors	
Nociceptive stimulus	An actually or potentially tissue-damaging event transduced and encoded by nociceptors	
Nociceptor	A high-threshold sensory receptor of the peripheral somatosensory nervous system that is capable of transducing and encoding noxious stimuli	

(Continued)

Table 4.4 Continued

Term	IASP Definition	Selected Examples
Noxious stimulus	A stimulus that is damaging or threatens damage to normal tissues	
Pain threshold	The minimum intensity of a stimulus that is perceived as painful	A fingernail is squeezed during a neurologic exam; when enough pressure is applied and the pain threshold has been exceeded, the patient groans in pain.
Pain tolerance level	The maximum intensity of a pain-producing stimulus that a subject is willing to accept in a given situation	
Paresthesia	An abnormal sensation, whether spontaneous or evoked	A woman with herpes simplex virus endorses an odd tingling on her lip; a few hours later, a cold sore forms on her lip.
Sensitization	Increased responsiveness of nociceptive neurons to their normal input and/or recruitment of a response to normally subthreshold inputs	

The IASP definitions listed are reproduced from *Classification of Chronic Pain*, 2nd edition, IASP Task Force on Taxonomy, edited by H. Merskey and N. Bogduk, IASP Press, Seattle, © 1994. The selected examples have been added by this text and are not the property of the IASP. This taxonomy has been reproduced with permission of the International Association for the Study of Pain ® (IASP). The Taxonomy may not be reproduced for any other purpose without permission.

evaluation and treatment stands, it is critically important for clinicians to remain open to increased awareness of the patient's pain experience, only through this understanding do we find the compassion to respond most effectively.

REVIEW QUESTIONS

1. Which of the following are essential aspects of the IASP definition of pain?
   a. Pain is unpleasant.
   b. Pain is a sensory and emotional experience.
   c. Pain is always associated with some tissue damage.
   d. Pain can occur in the absence of actual or impending tissue damage.

2. Which of the following statements about the major mechanism-based classes of pain is not correct?
   a. Nociceptive pain is pain that continues after an injury is healed.
   b. Neuropathic pain includes pain that is associated with abnormalities in the nervous system.

c. Inflammatory pain often involves upregulation of peripheral factors released in response to some insult or injury.
  d. Neuropathic pain does not typically respond to cyclooxygenase inhibitors.

3. Which of the following statements about pain assessment tools is not correct?
   a. The NRS can be used to evaluate pain intensity and is stable over repeated measures.
   b. The NRS is useful only for populations that know how to read.
   c. The VAS is scored by estimating the distance to the zero point on the scale.
   d. The BPI is a multidimensional pain assessment tool that includes information relating to disability associated with pain.

4. Which of the following does not accurately reflect the information about principles of pain assessment presented in this chapter?
   a. The underestimation of pain by physicians and nurses helps prevent abuse of the system by patients who exaggerate their pain in order to obtain medications.
   b. The physician has a responsibility to provide a supportive environment to the patient who is describing pain.
   c. The tools used for pain assessment should be easily understood, sensitive to change, and reliable and reproducible.
   d. Patients have an obligation to learn about basic pain assessment tools, if they are able, in order to report their pain accurately and to record pain at reasonable intervals when requested to do so.

REFERENCES

1. Kuttner L. A Child in Pain: How to Help. What to Do. Vancouver: Hartley & Marks; 1996:76.
2. Murinson BB, Agarwal AK, Haythornthwaite JA. Cognitive expertise, emotional development, and reflective capacity: clinical skills for improved pain care. J Pain. 2008;9:975–983.
3. Merskey H, Bogduk N; IASP Task Force on Taxonomy, eds. Classification of Chronic Pain (2nd ed., pp. 209–214). Seattle: IASP Press; 1994.
4. Vardeh D, Mannion RJ, Woolf CJ. Toward a mechanism-based approach to pain diagnosis. J Pain. 2016;17(9 Suppl):T50–69.
5. Murinson BB. Pain and the humanities: exploring the meaning of pain in medicine through drama, literature, fine arts and philosophy. MedEdPORTAL. 2010;6:8129. doi.org/10.15766/mep_2374-8265.8129.
6. Gold MS, Gebhardt G. Peripheral pain mechanisms and nociceptor sensitization. In Fishman SM, Ballantyne JC, Rathmell JP, eds. Bonica's Management of Pain (4th ed., pp. 24–34). Philadelphia: Lippincott Williams & Williams; 2010.
7. Keele KD. The pain chart. Lancet. 1948;252(6514):6–8.
8. Melzack R. The McGill Pain Questionnaire: major properties and scoring methods. Pain. 1975;1:277–299.
9. Levine JD, Gordon NC, Fields HL. The mechanism of placebo analgesia. Lancet. 1978;2(8091):654–657.

10. Jensen M. Measurement of pain. In Fishman SM, Ballantyne JC, Rathmell JP, eds. Bonica's Management of Pain (4th ed., pp. 252–253). Philadelphia: Lippincott Williams & Williams; 2010.
11. Granovsky Y, Granot M, Nir RR, Yarnitsky D. Objective correlate of subjective pain perception by contact heat-evoked potentials. J Pain. 2008;9(1):53–63.
12. Ferraz MB, Quaresma MR, Aquino LR, et al. Reliability of pain scales in the assessment of literate and illiterate patients with rheumatoid arthritis. J Rheumatol. 1990;17(8):1022–1024.
13. Daut RL, Cleeland CS, Flanery RC. Development of the Wisconsin Brief Pain Questionnaire to assess pain in cancer and other diseases. Pain. 1983;17:197–210.
14. Fishman B, Pasternak S, Wallenstein SL, et al. The Memorial Pain Assessment Card: a valid instrument for the evaluation of cancer pain. Cancer. 1987;60(5):1151–1158.
15. Hicks CL, von Baeyer Cl, Spafford PA, et al. The Faces Pain Scale—Revised: toward a common metric in pediatric pain measurement. Pain. 2001;94:173–183.
16. Merkel SI, Voepel-Lewis T, Shayevitz JR, Malviya S. The FLACC: a behavioural scale for scoring postoperative pain in young children. Pediatr Nurs. 1997;23:293–297.
17. Krechel SW, Bildner J. CRIES: a new neonatal postoperative pain measurement score—initial testing of validity and reliability. Paediatr Anaesth. 1995;5:53–61.
18. Ambuel B, Mamlett KW, Marx CM, Blumer JL. Assessing distress in pediatric intensive care environments: the COMFORT Scale. J Pediatr Psychol. 1992;17:95–109.
19. Breivik EK, Bjornsson GA, Skovlund E. A comparison of pain rating scales by sampling from clinical trial data. Clin J Pain. 2000;16:22–28.
20. The Joint Commission. Pain assessment and management standards for ambulatory care. Accessed February 9, 2019 at: https://www.jointcommission.org/assets/1/18/R3_14_Pain_Assess_Mgmt_AHC_6_20_18_FINAL.pdf.
21. Prkachin KM1, Solomon PE, Ross J. Underestimation of pain by health-care providers: towards a model of the process of inferring pain in others. Can J Nurs Res. 2007;39(2):88–106.
22. Hester NO, Foster RL, Beyer JE. Clinical judgment in assessing children's pain. In Watt-Watson J, Donovan MI, eds. Pain Management: Nursing Perspective (pp. 236–294). St. Louis: Mosby-Year Book; 1992.
23. IASP Task Force on Taxonomy. Part III: pain terms, a current list with definitions and notes on usage. In Merskey H, Bogduk N, eds. Classification of Chronic Pain (2nd ed., pp. 209–214). Seattle: IASP Press; 1994.
24. Turk, DC, Okifuji A. Taxonomies of pain. In Fishman SM, Ballantyne JC, Rathmell JP, eds. Bonica's Management of Pain (4th ed., pp. 14–15). Lippincott Williams & Williams; 2010.

5 Pain Psychology
An Overview of Concepts and Methods

Valerie Jackson

Pain is an opinion on the organism's state of health rather than a mere reflexive response to injury.
—V. S. Ramachandran

LEARNING OBJECTIVES

At the completion of this chapter, the learner should be able to discuss:
  Clinical psychology and the experience of pain, including:

- Psychological factors affecting pain tolerance, thresholds, and behavior
- Different cultures ascribing different meaning to pain
- The association of chronic pain with psychological characteristics of patients
- The impact of chronic, severe pain on psychological functioning
- The significant effects of pain on behavior
- The influence of psychosocial factors and comorbid illness on pain treatment response
- Several clinical psychological methods for the treatment of chronic pain
- Specific clinical psychological treatments that have established efficacy

CASE SCENARIO

A 62-year-old woman with chronic low back pain and scoliosis presents with increased pain in recent months despite taking duloxetine 60 mg daily. She copes with pain by taking ibuprofen and lorazepam as needed, avoiding painful activities, and laying down. Pain is interfering with her ability to work at her desk, play with her grandchildren, and socialize with friends. She is also having difficulty sleeping despite taking tramadol 50 mg and is worried her back pain will continue to worsen.

1. What questions do you have for this patient before making further recommendations?
2. How will you address her worry that her back pain will continue to worsen?
3. Given the patient's use of passive coping methods, how might you encourage more active coping strategies?

INTRODUCTION

Individuals living with chronic pain are likely to experience disruption in multiple areas of life due to pain, including work, social, mood, and other health-associated factors such as sleep and exercise. They are also more likely to experience mental health concerns such as depression, anxiety, and post-traumatic stress disorder (PTSD) than individuals without chronic pain. Furthermore, clinicians caring for patients with chronic pain can struggle at times to help patients manage pain effectively when relying on a medication-centered approach: Side effects can interfere or predominate, medications in general only moderately control pain, and patients may express a preference for medications that can be dangerous at high doses such as opioids and benzodiazepines.

Working with individuals who live with chronic pain requires a paradigm shift from "curing" pain to management of pain over time: aiming for steadily improving function and overall quality of life. Psychological factors play an important role in the patient's responses and reactions to pain, and basic psychoeducation, together with provision of psychological tools, can improve a patient's capacity to cope with pain and to participate in meaningful activities despite pain.

In this chapter, we review psychological concepts associated with pain, assessment tools that can be used in primary care and specialty clinics, pain psychology interventions, and associated psychological conditions and treatment recommendations. Throughout the chapter, a biopsychosocial model of assessment and treatment is utilized to conceptualize the patient and treat appropriately. The goal of psychological approaches is to target improved function and quality of life, which may indirectly improve experience of pain or redirect attention from pain.

A Mind–Body Connection

Historically, the concept of mind–body connection has ebbed and flowed in popularity, with the rise of biological science and research resulting in an initial separation of physiologic and psychological health. In recent decades, there has been a resurgence of conceptualizing health in a more holistic manner, whereby mental health is inextricably related to physical health. One theoretical model commonly used to describe the effects of psychological and environmental factors on pain is the gate control theory.[1] The gate control theory posits that there is both peripheral and central processing of pain information, but that conscious pain experience is moderated by emotion and cognitive appraisal. Various factors besides injury and nerve activity can affect whether the pain gate is "open or closed." For instance, being scratched while hiking by something that looks like a spider will cause increased fear and pain compared with a similar scratch produced while scratching oneself when itchy. The gate control theory first introduced the multidimensional experience of pain. Further theories elaborated on this, including the neuromatrix theory of pain, homeostasis, allostatic load, and hypothalamic-pituitary-adrenal (HPA) axis dysregulation.[2] This chapter focuses more on the diverse pain-influencing factors themselves rather than the proposed mechanisms of their effects on pain.

In the clinical scenario at the beginning of the chapter, a 62-year-old patient with worries about her pain and back getting worse limits her physical activity to avoid experiencing her pain. Factors that affect her pain experience and daily function expand beyond nociception. Such concepts are discussed further throughout this chapter as we learn to understand basic pain psychology concepts and how they may interact with pain management and quality of life.

ASSESSMENT

Chronic pain can affect all areas of life, and thus patients benefit from a holistic understanding of pain, its sources, personal reactions to pain, and consequences. Chronic pain has been shown to cause dysfunction in patients' social lives, relationships with family and friends, work, mood, and daily activities.[3] This widespread area of dysfunction can reduce quality of life as well as overall level of functioning, acting in a cycle to potentially further reduce mood and increase pain. The most universally used model to conceptualize pain from an integrative approach is the biopsychosocial model.[2] This framework and its applications are described next.

Biopsychosocial Model

The biopsychosocial model is used as a theoretical framework to understand the many factors that affect the experience of pain (Figure 5.1). It highlights that pain is more than tissue damage, structural abnormalities, or nerve dysfunction but is in fact affected by psychological factors like depression and social factors like social support.

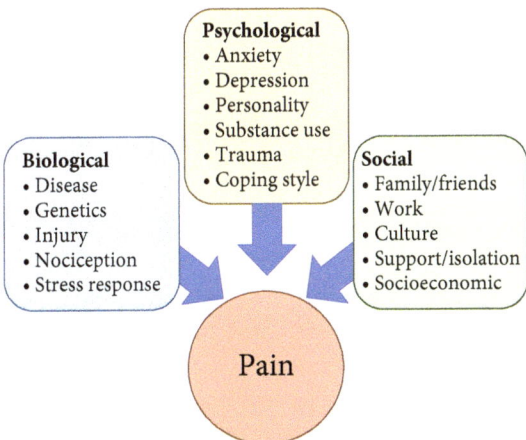

FIGURE 5.1 Biopsychosocial model of pain.

Biological	Psychological	Social
• Scoliosis • Deconditioning • Muscle relaxant • Physiological stress • Other structural dx	• Poor sleep • Pain catastrophizing • Fear avoidance • Passive coping • Sadness • Increased stress	• Less socialization • Low family contact • Reduced activity • Impact on work • Financial worries • Stigma/barriers

FIGURE 5.2 Biopsychosocial conceptualization of clinical vignette.

This chapter focuses on the effects of psychological factors and how they may interact with biological and social factors to influence experience of pain.

For instance, in the clinical vignette of the woman with back pain (Figure 5.2), the patient has a biological source of pain that we know of (scoliosis). She exhibits some psychological factors associated with pain, specifically her worries about pain, sadness about her inability to play with her granddaughter, and poor sleep affecting mental and physical health. She also experiences social impacts of pain, including interference with work (potentially affecting finances) and being less social. Other downstream effects of pain may be assessed, such as deconditioning (biological), history and risk for benzodiazepine misuse (psychological), and cultural factors (social).

Mental Health and Pain

Mental health conditions are significantly correlated with pain. Studies demonstrate higher odds of having comorbid depression, anxiety, PTSD, and substance abuse in individuals with chronic pain. While such cross-sectional studies do not identify cause, there is certainly a bidirectional relationship between mental distress and pain. The bidirectional relationship goes further: Evidence indicates that patients with chronic pain are more likely to develop clinical anxiety, and individuals with preexisting anxiety are more likely to develop chronic pain. There are also many overlapping symptoms associated with pain and various mental health conditions. For instance, social isolation is associated with depression and pain, and when experienced by patients with comorbid physical and mental health challenges, the effects are magnified. In addition, patients with comorbid pain and mental health diagnoses have higher levels of disability than pain patients without mental health conditions. Thus, mental health screening to identify patients in need of psychological services and treatment of mental health problems can reduce pain-related disability. Simple, free tools to evaluate depression (Patient Health Questionnaire-9 [PHQ-9]) and anxiety (Generalized Anxiety Disroder-7 [GAD-7]) can be self-administered by patients and easily interpreted by clinicians.

Social Factors and Pain

A wide range of social factors can affect pain. In the epidemiology of pain, female gender is correlated with both higher risk for chronic pain diagnoses and having comorbid mental health diagnoses such as depression and anxiety. Furthermore, cultural factors can play a role in both the experience and presentation of pain. For instance, research suggests some groups such as East Asian and Latino populations are more likely to report somatic symptoms of emotional distress, such as headache and stomachache, rather than directly reporting anxiety or stress. Specific details are beyond the scope of this chapter and should not be used as an independent predictor of source of pain but rather as a prompt to consider a comprehensive evaluation of pain experience.

Stigma

Stigma associated with pain does exist among providers and in the public, and patients will often describe their stigmatizing experiences or internalize their stigma. This leads to multiple problems, including distrust of providers, reluctance to ask for help from support systems, and anger at being labeled a drug-seeker. Patients may appear defensive that they are not "drug addicts" and "it's not all in my head," but it is likely that they have encountered some form of this message throughout their healthcare experience. To address this concern and build rapport, clinicians seeing patients presenting with pain may begin by noting that they know pain is a challenging experience and believe that their experience of pain is real. Active listening without interrupting the patient's illness narrative is an important tool in establishing rapport at the first visit. Explaining the biopsychosocial model can help patients feel understood and less stigmatized if the clinician suggests nonpharmacologic therapies such as psychology or stress management.

Stress

Stress is a factor that can be considered across the biopsychosocial model. Stress independent of pain and as a result of pain can feed into the cycle of increased pain and disability. Social stressors such as conflict with a spouse may cause emotional feelings of stress and worry, which can trigger a physiologic stress response in the body. Identifying life stressors, individual reactions to stress and emotional coping skills, and physiologic reactivity to stressors can help patients better manage pain and make the connection between the wide variety of factors that amplify pain experience. Stress also has been demonstrated to increase or suppress pain experience, depending on severity of perceived stress. For example, in a life-or-death fight, an individual may experience suppressed pain signals to the brain in order to keep fighting and survive despite injury. By contrast, an anxious individual who receives a stressful phone call from a collections agency may experience increased pain. Understanding the contributions of stress to pain experience, combined with strategies to identify and manage the stressors in patients' lives, can lead to a more effective treatment plan.

To summarize, each of the biopsychosocial variables discussed can worsen pain, and even more so with an interaction effect. For example, depressed mood reduces motivation to participate in healthy activities, leading to further pain disability and low mood. In another example, anxiety increases stress response, which increases sympathetic nervous system activity, leading to increased muscle tension and thereby exacerbating the underlying pain condition. Furthermore, the perception of pain is in fact moderated by the present experience of the individual. For example, if you were to twist your ankle while playing a game of soccer, you might experience a higher level of pain only after the game is over, when endorphins and adrenalin associated with active competition fade. As a whole, there are many factors in addition to biological causes that increase pain and interact with the biology of pain; patients benefit from a thorough assessment of these factors.

PAIN PSYCHOLOGY CONCEPTS

In addition to the biopsychosocial model, some psychological concepts specific to pain psychology can help us further understand a patient's experience and behaviors and thus identify potential additional areas for intervention.

Pain Catastrophizing

Pain catastrophizing is a particular reaction to pain that has been extensively studied and found to be associated with reduced quality of life, increased pain disability, anxiety, depression, pain severity, and even higher level of opioid use. Pain catastrophizing is the negative expectation and reaction to pain or thoughts of pain. It can be understood in three subcategories: magnification of the negative effects of pain, rumination about pain, and feelings of helplessness about pain. High pain catastrophizing has been associated with poor outcomes to medical interventions and can undermine behavioral and medical interventions. For this reason, patients benefit from screening even in medical settings. Pain catastrophizing is also a useful construct in acute pain settings because it is a risk factor for the development of chronic pain. The most common measure used is the Pain Catastrophizing Scale (PCS), a 13-question self-report scale.[4] Higher scores indicate higher levels of pain. Cognitive behavioral therapy (CBT) can reduce the impact of counterproductive pain-associated cognitions and is the most common approach used to reduce pain catastrophizing.

Pain Anxiety

Research has found a significant relationship between fear and avoidance of pain and increased disability from chronic pain. The Pain Anxiety Symptoms Scale (PASS) is a common scale measuring fear and anxiety responses specific to pain, available in validated 40- and 20-item versions.[5] Fear avoidance is a component of pain anxiety in which individuals avoid activities that can increase pain. While this can be protective in many situations (e.g., avoiding touching a hot stove), this can also be unhelpful in cases in which there no significant threat to injury and daily function is affected (e.g., walking increases back pain, so the patient chooses to avoid walking as much as possible and avoids chores such as cooking, getting groceries, or getting the mail). In fact, fear avoidance can be a primary contributor to loss of function and secondary pain effects such as work disability and low mood. Patients may have a mindset that they are waiting for the pain to get better before engaging in daily activities. They may avoid meaningful or pleasurable activities such as going out to dinner or traveling to see family for fear of experiencing increased pain. Confronting the possibility that they can cope with pain and learn to live with pain in this moment can be a difficult but meaningful shift in outlook for patients that allows for increased quality of life. Psychological support can be helpful in this area, particularly in the context of other anxiety disorders. Referral to a psychologist with pain management expertise can dramatically shift the pain experience for a patient with pain anxiety. Some patients have diagnostic conditions that respond well to more psychologically oriented approaches in lieu of aggressive interventional management.

Passive Versus Active Coping

Passive pain coping is coping with pain by accessing treatment modalities in which the patient is a passive recipient of the intervention. This contrasts with active pain coping in which patients take an active role in reacting to and managing their own pain. Passive coping can include pill-taking, reliance on interventional management, multiple surgical procedures, chiropractic, and resting. Active coping can include stretching, participation in physical therapy or regular exercise, self-soothing activities, diaphragmatic breathing, pacing, and cognitive behavioral strategies. Passive coping can reinforce fear and the avoidance of anxiety-provoking stimuli, further enhancing the anxiety response when exposed to the same stimuli in the future. It can also increase pain catastrophizing and lead to further physical deconditioning. Alternatively, individuals with active coping skills feel higher self-efficacy when it comes to living life despite pain. Learning active coping skills empowers patients to take control of their pain and their reactions to pain, which can improve function and quality of life, this is applied in various approaches to therapy, such as cognitive behavioral therapy, see below.

To summarize the assessment section of this chapter, a biopsychosocial model is ideal for understanding the multifactorial factors affecting pain experience. Addressing some specific pain psychology concepts may aid in optimizing treatment outcomes, as may appropriate referrals to psychological treatment if necessary. Screening for common comorbid mental health conditions such as depression and anxiety will better identify appropriate candidates for psychiatric treatment. Most patients will at the least benefit from a discussion about their assessment results and likely have some areas for improvement in their pain management plan.

PAIN PSYCHOLOGY INTERVENTIONS

There is extensive research to show that psychological interventions can improve pain, reduce pain-related disability, help patients achieve functional goals, improve mood, and improve subjective quality of life.[6] The current gold standard for pain psychology interventions is pain CBT, although recent evidence is also suggesting that structured mindfulness approaches like mindfulness-based stress reduction (MBSR) also similarly improve pain-related outcomes compared with treatment as usual.[7] In this section, we introduce the interventions of basic pain psychoeducation, CBT, mindfulness approaches, biofeedback, and relaxation training (Table 5.1).

Psychoeducation

Psychoeducation or providing brief pain science education to patients can actually be quite beneficial to their acceptance of more diverse approaches to pain management (e.g., mindfulness practice). Addressing the "bio" in the biopsychosocial model, clinicians may teach patients about how pain is processed through the nervous system yet is not always an accurate assessment of danger. One useful example is utilizing the

Table 5.1 Evidence-Based Psychological Interventions for Pain

Modality	Description
Cognitive behavioral therapy (CBT)	Applies biopsychosocial approach to pain targeting behavioral and cognitive responses to pain, including cognitive restructuring, behavioral activation, pacing, and psychoeducation about pain and healthy behaviors
Acceptance and commitment therapy (ACT)	Encourages an acceptance-based approach to pain, accompanied by personal awareness and engagement in meaningful activities
Mindfulness-based stress reduction (MBSR)	Utilizes a nonjudgmental approach to pain through daily mindfulness practice intended to increase awareness of the body and breath
Biofeedback (BFB)	Provides immediate feedback through device to show body's response to relaxation exercises or cognitive restructuring

well-known phenomenon of phantom limb pain, which can be a clear way to demonstrate that pain is in fact processed in the brain—sufferers of phantom limb pain continue to experience pain in limbs despite amputation. This example not only is tangible for many patients but also is a non-stigmatizing approach to discussed the role of perception beyond nociception as contributing to the experience of pain. Because of the association of phantom limb pain with veterans, clinicians may convey that this is a phenomenon that certainly doctors and the public do not believe the patients are "faking it" or exaggerating their condition for personal gain and that their pain is in fact real. Nevertheless, traditional approaches such as medication and surgery may be not completely effective in addressing chronic pain because of the complex matrix affecting pain processing and experience of pain. Further education about the gate control theory may be appropriate to elucidate the wide range of factors that can affect an individual's experience of pain.

Cognitive Behavioral Therapy

CBT utilizes the theoretical framework that our thoughts (cogitations), behaviors (action or inaction), and feelings (both emotional and physical) affect each other in a balance such that if one of the three constructs changes, it can affect the others (see Figure 5.3A and B). In this case, the target is to change feelings through adaptations of thoughts or behaviors. Participants learn strategies to identify unhelpful cognitions and behaviors, then methods to challenge these beliefs and/or to change behavior in order to improve emotional and physical functioning. Extensive research shows that CBT is an evidence-based practice for pain management as well as for common correlates like anxiety and depression. Specific "distorted" beliefs, such as pain catastrophizing and pain anxiety, may be challenged, and unhelpful behaviors such as passive coping can be replaced by active coping strategies. Additional pain-specific behaviors targeted include sleep hygiene, pacing for pain, increasing physical activity, and healthy habits such as limiting caffeine and tobacco. During the course of CBT, psychologists may

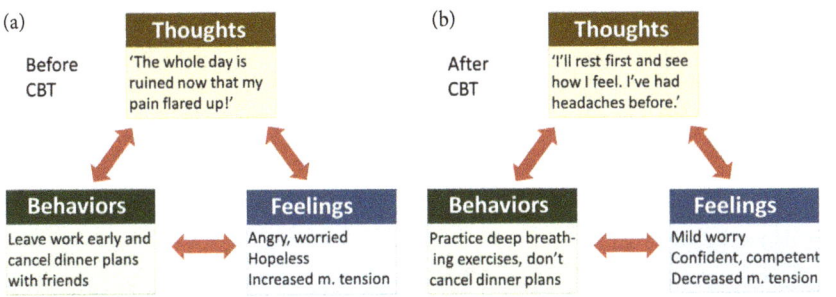

FIGURE 5.3 Cognitive behavioral therapy (CBT) framework—before and after treatment. Example situation: new headache while at work. **A,** Feelings, thoughts, and behaviors before CBT treatment illustrating how these contribute to less effective pain coping. **B,** After CBT treatment, more effective coping strategies reduce the impact of pain altogether as well as the impact of pain on quality of life.

help establish patient goals and, in group or individual settings, provide support throughout treatment to achieve personal goals. Overall goals of pain CBT include improving quality of life, reducing psychological distress, improving coping skills, and improving function.

Acceptance and Commitment Therapy

Acceptance and commitment therapy (ACT) is another psychological intervention that has gained popularity for pain management in recent years. It is a variation of CBT, focusing on accepting rather than challenging unhelpful thoughts and focusing on living a full life despite pain. There is an emphasis on nonjudgment of thoughts and experiences as well as willingness to experience emotional and physical pain rather than struggle to avoid pain.

Mindfulness

Mindfulness strategies are a broad group of skills that have increasing research to show efficacy in pain management and an existing base of evidence for mood, anxiety, and health management. Mindfulness is an awareness of mind and body often learned through movement, meditation, and guided practice. In particular, the 8-week program MBSR has significant research to demonstrate reduction in depression, anxiety, and even pain symptoms in patients with chronic pain conditions, ranging from back pain to fibromyalgia. Importantly, this approach can be effective and useful for many populations, including healthy populations looking for wellness and stress management strategies. Thus, this recommendation is appropriate for most patients, ranging from those with diagnosed mental health disorders to those resistant to or disinterested in other potentially stigmatizing treatments delivered through a mental health setting. Mindfulness-based approaches can also be particularly useful in patients who either are resistant to mental health treatment, do not have access to mental health treatment, or are also looking for strategies they can employ on their own. There are a number of mindfulness tools available in the form of mobile applications, online guided meditations, and a variety of classes and books depending on patient's access and interest level. MBSR has the added benefit of being a structured course that patients can complete in person or online. Patients may be more likely to adhere to this treatment plan, signing up for a course with accountability rather than having the self-motivation to take a one-time recommendation from a clinician to try mindfulness practices.

Relaxation Training

Formal relaxation training teaches individuals to gain control of their autonomic nervous system, primarily through breath and meditation practices. Diaphragmatic breathing is a simple-to-use tool that patients may learn and employ anywhere to reduce sympathetic nervous system activity, thus producing a sense of calm and reducing negative reactions to pain. Other relaxation training can occur through courses, guided meditations, exercises such as progressive muscle relaxation, and hypnosis. Relaxation training can include biofeedback, which has moderate evidence to demonstrate efficacy in pain management, most significantly for migraines.[8]

Biofeedback

Biofeedback is a treatment that helps patients understand and control their physiologic responses across multiple domains, including heart rate, breath, sweat, brainwaves, muscle tension, and peripheral temperature. It utilizes much of the skill development mentioned previously in relaxation training but allows the patient to gain concrete insight to the relationship between mind and body by observing immediate feedback on a device or computer screen. This is often a transformative intervention for patients with chronic pain because it provides visual evidence of how they can consciously control their bodies' reactions (e.g., heart rate, muscle tension) by merely slowing their breath, completing exercises such as progressive muscle relaxation, or thinking of something calming. Biofeedback is sometimes used in conjunction with CBT to demonstrate the effects of thought change on the body. For instance, a patient tells a story of a stressful experience and watches physiologic stress response increase on a computer screen, then discusses coping strategies or alternate perspectives on the problem. The patient then watches a decrease of sympathetic nervous system measures such as decrease in heart rate and sweat. Biofeedback practitioners vary in background and may be difficult to find in some areas.

New approaches to clinical psychological treatments are continuously being developed and applications for pain management are an area of active investigation. Incorporating clinical psychological principles into the practices of other health professionals, e.g., psychologically-informed primary care and physical therapy, is likely to become standard practice.[9] Additional forms of psychological therapy with potential relevance for patients with pain include existential therapy and internal family systems therapy.[10,11]

Aside from psychological interventions mentioned, an essential part of successful pain management is their combination with other treatment modalities. Combining medical interventions with other modalities, such as physical therapy, acupuncture,

CBT, or other diverse approaches, can optimize treatment. In particular, psychological intervention in conjunction with physical therapy can be a powerful combination to address multiple targets, such as physical reconditioning, safe movements/pain anxiety, fear avoidance, behavioral activation for mood, and goal-setting. Overall, emphasizing the role of active pain coping and self-management of pain can empower patients to reframe the role of pain in their lives.

Treatment Response

The response to treatment may be predicted by multiple factors. Ongoing evaluation of self-reported psychological function (e.g., PCS, mood and anxiety measures such as PHQ-9 and GAD-7), as well as pain and disability measures, will help measure whether patients are seeing improvement after treatment. Importantly, in pain management treatment, part of the treatment is to suggest that even in the absence of change in pain intensity, change in level of function or satisfaction with level of function may be included in the definition of "successful treatment." Short-term evaluations may see a regression to the mean; that is, the patient's initial reports on measures are so extreme that the most likely outcome is to appear improved and move toward the mean. Thus, longitudinal measures may help mitigate unclear causes of treatment responses.

SUMMARY

Thinking back to the clinical scenario in the beginning of the chapter, how might you answer the questions differently with the knowledge you have now? Further questions you might ask include whether the patient is worried about potentially damaging her back further through physical activity—this gives an opportunity to clarify to the patient what are safe movements given her medical condition or to make appropriate referrals. It is also an opportunity to educate the patient about the difference between experiencing pain and causing tissue damage through movement. While beyond the scope of this chapter, consideration of healthcare utilization and addressing worries about health are an important component in long-term pain management, and referral to pain psychology may be appropriate if the patient's worries appear to affect her functioning or be disproportionate to her health condition.

In summary, we have reviewed the overlap of biological, psychological, and social interactions on the effects of pain. We also noted the importance of thorough assessment, including pain psychology concepts and basic evaluation of mental health conditions such as depression and anxiety. We then introduced the most commonly used evidence-based psychological practices for pain management. For instance, social isolation and sleep disruption are associated with depression and pain, and when experienced by patients with comorbid physical and mental health challenges, their effects can be magnified; similarly, they can be targeted together through CBT and relaxation strategies. Pain may be increased through physical deconditioning when patients' decreased physical activity is a result of pain, and thus psychoeducation and goal setting within CBT can help patients engage in meaningful physical activities to improve mood and function.

REVIEW QUESTIONS

1. Where does stress fit into the biopsychosocial model of pain?
   a. Biological
   b. Psychological
   c. Social
   d. A and B
   e. All of the above

2. Which pain psychology construct best explains this statement best? *"I've had this pain for years, and I know it's just going to keep getting worse."*
   a. Pain catastrophizing
   b. Fear avoidance
   c. Stress
   d. Pain anxiety

3. Of the following empirically validated pain psychology treatments, which would you recommend first to a patient with chronic migraines and anxiety who does not want mental health treatment?
   a. CBT
   b. MBSR
   c. Biofeedback
   d. ACT

REFERENCES

1. Melzack R, Wall PD. Pain mechanisms: a new theory. Science. 1965;150(3699):971–979.
2. Gatchel R, Peng Y, Peters M, et al. The biopsychosocial approach to chronic pain: scientific advances and future directions. Psychol Bull. 2007;133:581–624.
3. Dueñas M, Ojeda B, Salazar A, et al. A review of chronic pain impact on patients, their social environment and the health care system. J Pain Res. 2016;9:457–467.
4. Sullivan MJ, Bishop SR, Pivik J. The pain catastrophizing scale: development and validation. Psychol Assess. 1995;7(4):524.
5. McCracken L, Dhingra L. (2002). A short version of the Pain Anxiety Symptoms Scale (PASS-20): preliminary development and validity. Pain Res Manage. 2002;7:45–50.
6. Sturgeon JA. (2014). Psychological therapies for the management of chronic pain. Psychol Res Behav Manage. 2014;7:115–124.
7. Cherkin DC, Sherman KJ, Balderson BH, et al. Effect of mindfulness-based stress reduction vs cognitive behavioral therapy or usual care on back pain and functional limitations in adults with chronic low back pain a randomized clinical trial. JAMA. 2016;315(12):1240–1249.
8. Tan G, Sheffer F, Randall L, Teo I, eds. Evidence-Based Practice in Biofeedback and Neurofeedback (3rd ed.). Wheat Ridge, CO: Association for Applied Psychophysiology and Biofeedback; 2016.
9. Miller WR, Rollnick S. *Motivational Interviewing: Helping People Change* (3rd ed.). New York: Guilford Press; 2012.
10. Yalom I. *Existential Psychotherapy*. New York: Basic Books; 1980.
11. Schwartz R. *Internal Family Systems Therapy*. New York: Guilford Press; 1987.

PART II
CLINICAL SKILLS IN THE ASSESSMENT AND CARE OF PAIN

6 Clinical Assessment of Pain
History, Examination, and Clinical Reasoning

Beth B. Hogans

[T]he major complaint encountered among her patients was pain. A patient might be dying of a serious illness, but when asked, "How are you?" would answer, "Well, ok, except I have this terrible pain in my shoulder. I can't sleep. I can't lie on that side."
—David and Lois Simons regarding Dr. Janet Travell

Before you speak, let your words pass through three gates: Is it true? Is it necessary? Is it kind?
—Rumi

LEARNING OBJECTIVES

At the completion of this chapter, the learner should be able to discuss:

- How to structure the interaction into assessment, diagnosis, and treatment
- The elements of a detailed pain history (pain alphabet): Q—quality, R—region, S—severity, T—timing; including the expanded pain alphabet: U—usually associated with, V—very much better with, W—worse with, X—expect to treat
- How patients may have multiple painful conditions and the importance of collecting details for each
- Basic strategies for implementing qualitative scales of pain measurement and how empathetic responses are necessary for obtaining this information
- The primacy of examining the body part that hurts, with awareness of the potential for spontaneous and evoked pain

- How to identify the major examination features that typify painful parts, such as tumor and rubor
- The performance and interpretation of a pain-oriented examination of the head, spine, and extremities, including major landmarks, deformities, features of inflammation or injury, major provocative maneuvers, and basic familiarity with dermatomes, myotomes, and reflexes
- The importance of communication with a patient while examining a painful part
- How to document the examination of a patient with pain
- How to construct a pain differential diagnosis and the relevance of a detailed history

CASE SCENARIO

You are working with a medical student, and your team is called to assess leg pain. The student goes to see the patient and returns quickly, noting that the patient refuses to walk but appears normal. When you go to see the patient, you find an obese man with an arteriovenous fistula. Both legs are edematous with pitting edema, erythema, and atrophic changes and flaking skin. There is a dusky-appearing area on the anterior aspect of the left leg. You suspect the cause may be serious. The student had not inspected the legs and had terminated the encounter when the patient stated he would not allow strength testing.

1. What is your differential diagnosis?
2. How does visual inspection of the limb contribute to this?
3. If it is midway through the rotation for the student and you are to offer some formative feedback about clinical assessment going forward, how will you go about this?

INTRODUCTION

Interview and examination of the patient with pain is a critical skill in clinical care. A large percentage of clinical encounters involve a patient in pain, whether a bothersome sore throat, intractable neuropathic pain, or disabling low back pain, the patient is seeking not only a solution but also a compassionate and concerned professional—someone they can entrust with their fears, vulnerabilities, and hopes; someone who will support and guide them through the myriad of options to the safest, most effective, and most appropriate treatment. Our patients rely on us to be prepared. When 70% of the population experiences low back pain at one time or another and yet less than 0.1% of allopathic medical school curricular content addresses the foundations of pain signaling, the common conditions of the spine, or the assessment and treatment of low back pain, we can almost anticipate failure and disappointment. The unskilled clinician will be eager to end the clinic visit without losing face, and the patient is often desperate for solutions. There are many potential solutions to most pain-associated conditions, and chronic pain especially can be approached from several directions. Because most chronic pain conditions are typically complex in terms of both pathophysiology and psychosocial effects, careful assessment and intermittent reassessment are appropriate. In this chapter, I address the need for comprehensive history-taking, establishment of boundaries, the essential features of the pain-focused examination, and the process of considering diagnostic testing. The processes are often not different from the basics of exceptional patient-focused care in any setting. The difference is in listening and attending to pain, in including pain in the process of developing the differential diagnosis, and in thinking deeply about the multiple routes to further assessing the pain before dismissing the patient with a hasty appraisal and a prescription for pills.

THE PAIN-FOCUSED PATIENT NARRATIVE

"Taking the history," we learn, is an opportunity to engage patients and to establish rapport, building trust. These deeper functions of the clinical interview are explored in Chapter 8. Here we begin by noting that a pain-focused clinical encounter begins with an illness narrative. The illness narrative is the patients' narration of the events of their illness. It is a patient-centered approach to the history of present illness (HPI) or "subjective complaint." The value of the narrative is not only the personal engagement that develops but also the disclosure of key features of the patient's condition. As you listen empathetically to the patient's illness narrative, you will listen closely for the key characteristics of any pain condition.

The key characteristics will guide your development of a differential diagnosis (see the following box).[1] Although much of Chapter 4 was dedicated to an in-depth examination of pain scale selection and use, the pain scale only provides an appraisal of pain intensity. The other key features of pain, classically described in landmark physical diagnosis texts, include "QRST": **q**uality, **r**egion, **s**everity, and **t**iming.[1] It is also valuable to know "UVW": what symptoms **u**sually occur with the pain, what makes the pain **v**ery much better, and what makes the pain **w**orse? To this is added "X": what are the relevant patient factors you need to be apprised of as you e**x**pect to treat pain? All of this information can be extracted from the patient's illness narrative, often without additional questioning. Of course, the expert interviewer may repeat information back to the patient, while checking for understanding and summarizing the narrative.[2] Most patients truly value a clinician who sits on their level and listens without interruption for at least a full 30 seconds. Clinicians who physically sit down when interviewing patients are perceived as having spent more time. The challenge since the advent of the electronic health record (HER) is finding a way to face and listen to patients without attending to the distracting and omnipresent computer. If you can start every visit with at least 30 seconds of undivided attention, intently listening and genuinely observing, your patients will remember you as the one who really listens.

Key Pain Characteristics

Quality: what it feels like (e.g., hot, cold, pressing, throbbing)
Region: where it is located and whether it radiates
Severity: typically measured using a 0–10 scale
Timing: start, timing, constancy, waxing/waning
Usually associated with (associated symptoms)
Very much relieved by (alleviating factors)
Worse with (exacerbating factors)
eXpectation to treat (explore potential patient-related factors that will influence treatment choice

---

The best way to begin a clinical interview is by asking an open-ended question and then listening without interruption as patients explain the circumstances that brought them to seek care. Open-ended questions are those with narrative answers. An open-ended question does not have a yes/no answer. Open-ended starter questions include "What brought you in today?" "How did this pain problem start?" "Can you take me back to the very beginning of the problem?" "When is the last time you remember feeling normal?" For some clinicians, the thought of asking these questions might give them nightmares, but the results of these open-ended queries are never as bad as you might think. The patient's answer will disclose the information you need through this process, and the patient typically will be immensely grateful that someone has taken the time to listen. Some patients will complain that they've "told the story a hundred times already." In this case, gentle encouragement along the lines of, "I can appreciate that this might be difficult but it's really important for me to hear this from you and not take someone else's word for what's going on" is usually enough to indicate your seriousness in being ready to listen.

Some patients who have had pain for a long time will have more than one pain-associated condition to describe. Because of the limitations of clinical scheduling, it is sometimes necessary to detail the characteristics of the most serious of the problems and revisit other, less painful conditions at a subsequent visit. Patients are generally accepting that clinicians have realistic constraints. Make a list of all the pains that the patient wishes to have addressed, characterize the one or more that can be reasonably handled in the first encounter, and make a note to return the rest during a subsequent visit. Conditions that you believe to be outside of your scope of practice may be referred to other providers. Patients may not understand which medical worries are appropriate for specific providers; you can provide guidance in this, especially if you have a reliable network of providers to refer them to and can make a "warm hand-off."

BOUNDARY ISSUES AND THE PAIN-FOCUSED CLINICAL ENCOUNTER

One of the important pearls of clinical wisdom to arise from the efforts at better opioid risk assessment was the broad recognition that early-life sexual abuse may be a risk factor for substance abuse and also for chronic pain.[3] This is important because patients with complex substance use or chronic pain histories may often be living with unaddressed or partially addressed early-life trauma that can color and affect the clinical encounter. This may not be apparent unless (1) you ask about this in an appropriate manner and (2) the patient is willing to share the information. One challenge of addressing trauma is that if the encounter is rushed, patients may feel rejected or that their trust was misplaced. If you are in a practice setting where screening questions or the health record indicates trauma history, you can gently affirm this information and provide an opportunity for elaboration if the patient expresses the capacity to tolerate disclosure. Asking about trauma is especially relevant for patients with conditions that are particularly chronic, disabling, severe, or associated with parts of the body where examination may seem intrusive or where medications such as opioids or antidepressants are being prescribed that carry additional risks for harm.

By the end of the information-gathering phase of the encounter, you should have a sense of what parts of the patient will require examination as you make your physical clinical assessment. It is not uncommon that a patient will feel vulnerable when certain body parts are touched, and some patients are fearful that their pain will be made worse by examination. It is important to explain the plan for examination briefly to patients and to genuinely seek their verbal consent for the planned examination. Because patients with chronic pain and substance abuse have a potential for extra vulnerability and trauma-induced sensitivity, it is especially important to have a low threshold for involving a chaperone or accepting a partial exam based on patient tolerance. It is also important to check back for permission at each stage of the exam and to stop the examination immediately if the patient requests you do so. Always ask permission before moving a drape or article of clothing and before touching, palpating, or manipulating any body part, but especially a potentially painful body part. Sometimes you can ask the patient to outline the painful area or even guide your hand during palpation if they are especially fearful of pain. If a patient has complex regional pain syndrome (CRPS), you must ask about reflex testing because even light pressure on a CRPS-involved limb may be agonizing. In some cases it is necessary to forgo certain exam maneuvers out of consideration for not making a pain problem worse. Patients with suspected sciatica may need deep palpation of the buttock to assess for potential piriformis syndrome; this can be triggering for some trauma survivors, so caution is urged. Every once in a while, a patient with chronic pain will have a strong emotional reaction or pain flare in response to being examined. If you have informed the patient at every step and asked permission before starting and again at every new stage of the exam, you will be glad you did. You can offer support if the patient is tearful or sad, and you should be ready with an ample supply of tissues. Be aware also that some people respond to pain or vulnerability with anger. At times, you may need to increase your distance, and if necessary, you should step out for a minute or two. In the event that you perceive any hint or threat of antagonism, take that feeling very seriously and step back, step out of the room, and seek a chaperone for the rest of the visit.

It is acceptable to encourage most patients to give their best effort during the exam. Because strength testing can require more resistance than the patient is used to giving (e.g., 50 lb), some patients who live with daily pain will have more pain for a couple of days after a formal examination. You may wish to warn your patients that they may feel an increase in stiffness or pain for a couple of days. Anything more than minor muscle pain should be reported back to you. In general, the physical exam maneuvers described here are entirely safe; however, patient factors will predominate in any situation, and this chapter does not represent or supplant formal clinical training.

PAIN-FOCUSED PHYSICAL EXAMINATION

The pain-focused physical examination includes some standardized exam features as well as testing and assessment that are tailored to the patient's specific presentation. You will need to examine the part that hurts; this is described in the next paragraph. In addition to examining the painful part, the screening neurologic exam is immensely helpful in examination of patients with pain. This is because headache, neck pain, and low back pain together make up more pain than all the other conditions together. These conditions, and several others, are most properly assessed through inclusion of a basic screening neurologic exam. First, we address how to focus on and examine a painful part.

Before beginning the exam, make sure to prepare the patient and ask permission. In examining a painful part, it is important to begin with the patient indicating the location of the pain with physical gestures. This will help the provider understand the extent of the problem and possible causes in the differential diagnosis. The next step is to ask permission first and then inspect the painful part. It is critically important to look at areas that patients describe as painful: you will get valuable information if the part appears abnormal and equally valuable information if the part does not look abnormal. Abnormalities on inspection may include changes in coloration, shape, size, angulation, articulation, changes to the skin, and presence of masses.[1] All of these features should be noted. The next phase is palpation, although for a patient with marked pain, palpation or manipulation, whichever is more likely to be painful, is saved for the end of the examination. Palpation should proceed with light palpation followed by deeper palpation until the examiner achieves an adequate assessment of a potential mass.[2] If cancer is suspected, palpation may not be recommended, and it is important to follow local practice in this regard. Findings on palpation may include both the presence of a mass and a deficit in the expected structures (e.g., biceps rupture will leave a gap in the muscle body). Palpation should proceed with clear focus on the patients' tolerance for the pressure and with their explicit permission to continue. If you have knowledge of "effects at a distance," such as trigger points or referred pain patterns, it may be appropriate to palpate the region likely to be contributing to the patient's pain complaint, and you may want to explain that you are trying to better understand the patient's condition by checking for additional exam findings. Next, manipulation or passive range of motion may be appropriate. Support the painful part appropriately as you examine the response to passive movement. Humans have the useful feature of bilateral symmetry in many systems of the body, so side-to-side comparison is often an extremely useful technique in examination. Next, active range of motion and strength testing are performed. In the standard neurologic exam, a general goal of 50 lb of resistance is appropriate for major muscle groups. It is possible to use mechanical factors to advantage; for example, when testing deltoid strength, a provider who is less able to provide good resistance can plant the hands further out toward the patient's elbow, gaining additional leverage to resist the patient's effort. Work carefully and methodically, following the same procedures time and again. Consistency is very important to performing a reproducible and reliable examination and to drawing sound conclusions from your testing. Finally, you may need to perform some "provocative maneuvers." For low back pain, this might include a straight leg raise (SLR); for carpal tunnel syndrome, this might include testing for a Tinel sign.[4]

The remainder of this chapter reviews the principles and details of a screening neurologic exam and then briefly discusses some specific maneuvers relevant to assessment of patients with headache and low back pain.

Screening Neurologic Examination

The screening neurologic exam has six components: mental status, cranial nerves, motor, sensory, coordination, and reflexes. Mental status is assessed through noting the orientation, speech, and basic mental functions of the patient. This can be very simple. Ask patients their name, their location, and the date. If their speech is clear and the patients understand your questions, this will be evident from the interview, and you can note this. More formal testing of speech may not be necessary. Note the patient's level of alertness and whether any drowsiness or sleeping occurs during the visit. Decreased alertness and sleep may be indications of overmedication or substance use. Note the patient's emotional tone: States of aggravation are critical to document because these can support concerns about the patient's goals for the visit and whether a coercive approach is at work.

Cranial nerve testing is especially important for patients with headache or facial pain. You will want to include testing of pupillary light reflex and potentially examine the optic fundus (using a hand-held ophthalmoscope), but warn patients before shining light in their eyes. Room lights should be dimmed for testing the pupillary light reflex. If the patient has marked photophobia, you may want to save this part of the exam for the end because patients find it difficult to cooperate fully with an examiner when pain has occurred early in the exam process. The neurologic exam is dependent on patient cooperation, so sequencing painful exam steps to the end can really help to maintain and build trust with the patient. Brief visual testing involves holding up one or two fingers in various parts of the patient's visual field and asking "how many?" Do not use finger wiggling because motion detection does not necessarily indicate cortical (true) vision; motion can be detected in the brainstem (subcortical levels). Eye movements are next: Have the patient follow your finger through a standard H movement pattern. Any abnormalities that are not well-established should be referred to a neurologist. Ask the patient to close the eyes tightly and then to open the eyes wide open. You are looking for complete symmetry. Touch the patient's face lightly on both sides, once in each of the three dermatomal branches of the fifth cranial nerve (temple, cheek, and jaw); again, symmetry in response is expected and normal. Ask the patient to show the teeth; you may demonstrate this. It is not desirable to ask the patient to smile because smiling recruits an extra set of motor responses from the emotional/affective motor pathways, whereas the purpose of this exam maneuver is to check integrity of the motor cortex–related pathway, that is, volitional control. Ask the patient to open the mouth and say "ahh" as you observe the palate, which should raise symmetrically. Ask the patient to shrug up the shoulders; you may offer resistance to test strength if the patient is not currently experiencing neck or shoulder pain. Finally, ask the patient to stick out the tongue and then move it side to side. It is not necessary to test in more detail for a screening exam; you will refer patients to further evaluation if you detect abnormalities.

The screening motor exam can be limited to a quick test of strength of one proximal and one distal muscle in each arm and each leg. It is preferable not to test the two sides simultaneously but rather to test them separately because simultaneous testing can mask mild weakness due to cortical innervation patterns. A sample muscle pattern would be deltoid, finger extensors, iliopsoas, and tibialis anterior muscles.

Screening sensory testing is focused on just light touch because other modalities can be explore as needed, as in the tests for neuropathy described later. For screening sensation, use your index finger to lightly touch one proximal and one distal site on each limb (i.e., shoulder, hand, thigh, and foot). Any loss of sensation should be recorded.

Coordination may be screened with a finger-to-nose test, having the patient move either index finger from the tip of the nose to your finger held about 2 feet away in three different locations. Coordination may also be screened by observing gait: normal gait, toe gait, and heel gait.

Reflexes should be tested with a reflex hammer. The biceps, patella, and ankle reflexes are appropriate for screening. Asymmetric reflexes in the lower extremity are especially helpful for detecting radiculopathy; however, the ankle reflex is mediated by S1–2 and the patellar reflex by L3–4; therefore, an L5 radiculopathy may not result in obvious reflex loss, and careful interpretation is important. The screening neurologic exam has many parts (see the following box); a template is included in the screening pain exam provided in Appendix I.

Components of the Pain Examination, No Abnormalities Present

Mental Status

Awake and alert
Oriented to place and time
Language: speaks fluently and follows all instructions

Cranial Nerves

Pupils round and reactive to light: ___ => ___ mm
Visual fields: eyes move well together;
Face symmetric to light touch and sharp
Face moves well to eye closure and to show teeth
Palate: elevates symmetrically
Tongue: protrudes midline, moves well
Shoulder shrug: right 5/5; left 5/5

Motor Exam

Deltoid: right 5/5; left 5/5
Hand muscles: right 5/5; left 5/5
Quadriceps: right 5/5; left 5/5
Tibialis anterior: right 5/5; left 5/5

Sensory Exam

Light touch: intact upper and lower extremities
Sharp: normal

Cerebellar

Gait: normal
Toe and heel gait: normal

Reflexes

Right: normal biceps, patella, ankle
Left: normal biceps, patella, ankle

Palpation for Tenderness and Taut Bands

Scalp: none
Scalenes: none
Cervical paraspinals: none
Thoracic paraspinals: none

Lumbar paraspinals: none
Sacroiliac: none
Piriformis: none

Inspection and Palpation

Knee: right normal; left normal
Foot: right normal; left normal; no Tender to pressure from lateral compression/L3–4 intertarsal space

Range of Motion

Straight leg raise: right 90 degrees, no pain; left 90 degrees, no pain
Back: forward flexion; extension
Side bend: right; left
Twist: right; left
Neck: forward flexion; extension
Side bend: right; left
Twist: right; left

Dermatomes and Nerve Root Levels

Dermatomes are patterns of innervation that are observed consistently although not identically based on the nerves from different cranial nerves and spinal nerve roots supplying sensation to the skin over parts of the body. The dermatomes of the body overlap, so most people who lose sensation from just one nerve root level will not have a patch of dense numbness, although some people will be aware of such an area. The dermatomes wrap around the torso from back to front and stream down and around the limbs, reflecting the growth patterns that occur during development. Testing of dermatomes can be especially helpful in distinguishing a nerve root injury (Figure 6.1).

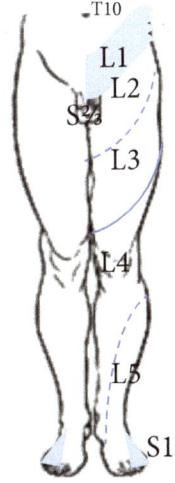

FIGURE 6.1 Illustration of dermatomes of the lower torso and limbs. Landmarks include the L1 dermatome at the inguinal line and the S1 dermatome at the lateral foot. These areas are variable and overlapping, and this figure is a representative composite. © Beth B. Hogans.

Although there is no an exact correspondence, the locations that we use to test muscle reflexes are related (see the following box).

Dermatome Landmarks

Cranial nerve V1: forehead
Cranial nerve V2: cheek
Cranial nerve V3: jaw
Lateral shoulder and thumb: cervical 6
Middle finger: cervical 7
Fifth digit: cervical 8
Nipple line: thoracic 4
Umbilicus: thoracic 10
Lateral hip to medial knee: lumbar 3
Posterior thigh, lateral calf, great toe: lumbar 5
Posterior thigh to lateral aspect of foot: sacral 1
External genitalia: sacral 2–3
Muscle (tendon) reflex levels
Triceps: cranial 7–8
Biceps: cranial 5–6
Patella: lumbar 3–4
Ankle: sacral 1–2
Mnemonic: starting from the ankle: 1–2, 3–4, 5–6, 7–8

SPECIAL PAIN EXAMINATION MANEUVERS

Range of Motion Testing

Range of motion testing is an essential part of the pain-focused exam. Formal range of motion standards exist and are particularly important for disability determination. It is important to be familiar with local practice patterns and to have access to the preferred standards for range of motion testing.[5] Note the presence or absence of pain during testing. More details of range of motion testing are included in the sections describing specific pain-associate conditions.

Palpation for Headache

Palpation of neck and head muscles for patients with headache can help to identify trigger points or other areas of tenderness that may be amenable to treatment and help reduce headache recurrence. Specific muscles can include the trapezius, sternocleidomastoid, cervical strap, temporalis, pterygoid, masseter, and occipitofrontalis muscles.[6] The palpation technique is to use the pads of the fingers to gently apply pressure and move in a circling motion (about 1-cm circles) to perceive the texture and quality of the palpated muscle. Trigger points may be felt as a knot, tender firm nodule, or taut band in the muscle. These are very commonly found in the trapezius, so you can practice on yourself or a friend before attempting this on patients. Some patients with acute and chronic migraine may develop allodynia or pain in response to normally nonpainful touch, so it is important to be aware that patients may experience more pain that might you think usual. This is an important clinical observation and should be recorded.

Palpation for Neck and Back Pain

As with palpation for headache, it is appropriate to palpate the cervical, thoracic, or lumbar paraspinal musculature according to the report of pain.[6,7] Use the same technique applying the pads of the fingers to the skin and pressing in with small circling motions to assess the texture of the muscle. The presence of taut bands or knots in a muscle does not necessarily indicate that that is the primary problem, but it may be an important secondary component that contributes to exacerbating and perpetuating the pain. Especially in the spinal structures where muscle spasm can affect the space between vertebral bones and lead to further painful nerve compression, assessment of muscle tone and quality is important. Patients with disk or nerve injury will often have reflex muscle spasm, the presence of which can help alert the astute clinician to a local problem. Additional guides to the evaluation of low back and spine pain are available from the National Institutes of Health Centers of Excellence in Pain Education program.[7]

Straight Leg Raise Testing

SLR is used to assess the possibility of nerve root compression in the lumbosacral spine. This is performed with the patient recumbent on the back (supine) and the legs extended. Some patients will not tolerate this starting position; an immediate clue that there is low back pain present and likely some spinal degenerative process. When patients are in the starting position, instruct them to let you raise the leg without their assistance. If you can feel that they are helping to raise the leg, remind them that you need to raise the leg without their effort. Raise the leg using your hand under the ankle to keep the knee extended with flexion only at the hip. As the leg is raised from 180 degrees at the hip (extension) to as far at the patient will tolerate, the patient with nerve root tension will begin to experience pain shooting into the leg on the affected side. This can occur at very modest amounts of flexion (10–20 degrees) but may be significant even at 30 to 40 degrees; pain radiating into the leg with modest hip flexion is a positive test, and you should document the site to which radiation occurs and the approximate degree of flexion at which this occurred (i.e., SLR positive, radiating pain to ankle at 20 degrees). Pain localizing only to the back without radiation is not significant, and you should document this as a negative test with pain only in the back. In patients with substantive nerve root compression, the test should be clearly positive on one side. Because there are spinal and local factors that contribute to the pain perception expanding, the patient may have a mildly positive or equivocal result on the contralateral side; this does not invalidate the test. Some clinicians will use a seated SLR, which has some advantages and disadvantages that will not be detailed here.

Peripheral Neuropathy Testing

Peripheral neuropathy testing involves a more detailed assessment of sensory, motor, and reflex responses. In a patient with moderate peripheral neuropathy, it is expected that the ankle reflexes are reduced or absent with relative sparing or more proximal reflexes such as knees and biceps. Motor weakness does not occur in most mild neuropathies, so a finding of motor weakness should precipitate specialist referral or additional testing. The sensory exam is divided into two major categories: large-fiber and small-fiber testing. Large-fiber testing includes vibration and joint position testing. For the purpose of the pain-focused exam, vibration testing may be helpful for detecting vitamin B_{12} deficiency as cause of painful neuropathy, often combined with depression and anemia. Joint position testing may be needed for patients with advancing diabetic neuropathy, but these patients will likely require neurologist and podiatrist involvement. The most relevant sensory test for pain assessment is the evaluation of the small nerve fibers. This is effectively done with a sharp testing instrument. Ordinary safety pins should not be used because these are likely to draw blood. A specialized testing tip (Neurotip) and the sharp broken end of a wooden applicator stick are acceptable alternatives. Because of the C fiber property of wind-up, stressed or dying-back C fibers can be detected by the use of temporal summation testing strategy. The Hogans tapping test (HTT) for small-fiber neuropathy involves taking the sharp testing probe and tapping at a rate of 3 times per second over the legs and feet. There is abundant preclinical evidence that repeated stimulation is a strong stimulus for C fibers, and the HTT is a nonharmful way to elicit evidence of hyperalgesia quickly in a clinic or bedside setting.

Neuroma Testing

A neuroma is a benign enlargement in a nerve or nerve end that becomes highly sensitized as a consequence of the buildup of sodium channels and other stimulus-transducing proteins. Neuromas, when palpated, will elicit painful shocks, jolts, burning sensations, or complex painful dysesthesias (unpleasant sensations). Neuromas can occur at surgical repair sites, injury sites, amputation stumps, and locations of chronic injury. Neuromas in the distal foot (i.e., Morton neuroma) are not uncommon in older adults and can cause chronic foot pain that limits ambulation. A Morton neuroma can be detected by applying pressure from above and below over the spaces between the bones in the forefoot, and also by grasping the forefoot in the hand and applying pressure from medial and lateral sides to push the metatarsal bones together. These maneuvers will elicit reports of marked pain in patients with Morton neuroma. Referral to podiatry can help alleviate this important cause of impaired walking.

Sacroiliac Joint Dysfunction

Testing for sacroiliac (SI) dysfunction is a topic of substantial controversy in the pain literature. About a half-dozen maneuvers are widely used in clinical practice. There is concern about the clinical validity of these maneuvers. More likely than not, the degree of uncertainty about SI joint testing maneuvers reflects the complexity of the SI joint. A compound fibrosynovial joint with multiple planes of constrained movement, the SI joint is active with every step. The SI joint can be dislocated in a number of directions, and detailed testing of the joint is beyond the scope of this text. A simple test is helpful to distinguish likely SI joint dysfunction from Ll5 facet syndrome because the pain associated with these two conditions localizes to the low lateral spine area. The pain associated with SI joint dysfunction most typically localizes to an area 3 cm lateral to the midline at the level of the L5 vertebral body, an area identified by Dr. A. Fortin.[8] The so-called Fortin finger test (FFT) involves asking the patient to place one finger on the area that is most painful. Although patients may initially attempt to indicate a broad area of pain involvement, they should be instructed to place one finger tip on the area that hurts the most. If they place the finger over the area associated with SI joint pain, this is a positive FFT. You may want to meet with a local physical therapist or physiatrist to obtain additional training in SI joint provocative maneuvers if this is of interest in your practice. By contrast, the classic exam finding associated with facet (zygapophyseal) joint dysfunction or Z-joint osteoarthritis is decreased spine extension. The provocative maneuver would be to ask the patient to bend backward as if to look up at the ceiling. Motion is limited by pain in patients with facet joint dysfunction.

A sample pain exam template is provided in Appendix I.

SUMMARY

Interviewing and examining patients with pain is the cornerstone of clinical care. An opportunity to establish trust, build rapport, and learn deeply about your patient all come together to build clinical excellence. Familiarity with the approaches and techniques of pain-focused care will give you the skill set to render aid and apply your knowledge safely and effectively.

REVIEW QUESTIONS

1. Michael is a 57-year-old man who is HIV-positive with an undetectable viral load. He presents with 2 days of painful itching on the right side of his forehead. How will you proceed?
   a. Obtain a detailed history by asking point-by-point questions to obtain key information.
   b. Ask an open-ended question to help the patient start his illness narrative.
   c. Refer the patient immediately to the emergency department.
   d. Fill out a referral slip for dermatology.

2. Gail is a 28-year-old pregnant woman who is expecting her second child. She is in the latter half of the third trimester and presents to her obstetrician's office for an unscheduled appointment. She had a normal obstetrical visit yesterday, and everything with the pregnancy was fine. Today she presents reporting 3 weeks of progressively worsening pelvic pain. After her vital signs are taken and the medical assistant has confirmed there are no signs of threat to the pregnancy, you are asked by the physician on duty to assess the patient. What will you want to know about the pain?
   a. Quality of how the pain feels
   b. Region involved, i.e., where the pain is located and whether it radiates
   c. Source of information about possible causes, e.g., the Internet
   d. Timing of when the pain started and how it has progressed
   e. Worsening factors: what makes the pain worse

3. You are called to evaluate a 68-year-old inpatient with unilateral leg pain following hip surgery. The patient is lucid and mentally intact. You will want to ask the patient about:
   a. Timing of when the pain started and how it has progressed.
   b. Usually associated symptoms, based on a differential diagnosis, e.g., shortness of breath
   c. Things the patient has done that make the pain very much better
   d. What makes the pain worse
   e. The patient's satisfaction with the surgeon who performed the hip replacement

REFERENCES

1. LeBlond R, Brown D, Suneja M, Szot JF. DeGowin's Diagnostic Examination (10th ed.). (Lange). New York: McGraw-Hill Education; 2014.
2. Bickley LS. Bates' Guide to Physical Examination and History Taking (12th ed.). Philadelphia: Lippincott Williams &Wilkins; 2016.
3. Webster LR, Webster RM. Predicting aberrant behaviors in opioid-treated patients: preliminary validation of the Opioid Risk Tool. Pain Med. 2005;6(6):432–442.
4. Orient J. Sapira's Art & Science of Bedside Diagnosis (5th ed., revised reprint). Philadelphia: Lippincott Williams & Wilkins; 2018.
5. Gerhardt J, Cocchiarella L, Lea R. AMA Practical Guide to Range of Motion Assessment. Beverly Farms, MA: OEM Press; 2002.
6. Simons DG, Travell JG, Cummings BD. Travell & Simons' Myofascial Pain and Dysfunction: The Trigger Point Manual (2nd ed.). Philadelphia: Lippincott Williams & Wilkins; 1998.
7. Weiner D, et al. Edna: an older adult with chronic low back pain. Accessed January 31, 2019 at: http://painmeded.com/edna/.
8. Fortin JD1, Falco FJ. The Fortin finger test: an indicator of sacroiliac pain. Am J Orthop (Belle Mead NJ). 1997;26(7):477–480.

7 Diagnostic Reasoning in the Pain-Focused Encounter

Beth B. Hogans

Listen to the patient . . . telling you the diagnosis.[1]
—Sir William Osler

LEARNING OBJECTIVES

At the completion of this chapter, the learner should be able to discuss:

- The role of the pain-focused history and physical exam, including the pain narrative, in providing a foundation for diagnostic reasoning
- The problem list and differential diagnosis, explaining the importance of each in characterizing a patient's clinical state
- The processing of planning and interpreting diagnostic test results
- Common biases that interfere with diagnostic reasoning
- Some approaches for mitigating the impact of biases and preventing diagnostic pitfalls

CASE SCENARIO

A 37-year-old science writer presents for evaluation of headaches. She provides the following description: "I actually have more than one type of headache. One type of headache that I have involves a dull, pressure type pain across the front of my forehead, it feels as though my head is in a vice. When I get this kind of headache, it usually starts in the late morning and progresses so that by late afternoon, I am feeling some stress from the pain. I can usually keep working through this headache, and it will typically go away if I pop a couple of ibuprofen or acetaminophen tablets. If I only had these headaches, I would not come to see you. My second type of headache is more unpredictable. It starts with a mild sense of blurry vision that lasts for about 10 minutes, and a short time after that, I will develop a gradually worsening, pounding pain over the left or right side of my head. If I don't take medicine right away, the headache will get worse pretty quickly until I am just completely overwhelmed. I can get severely nauseous and light sensitive with the headache, and every move I make, especially standing up or sitting down, makes the headache feel like a hot steel hammer pounding on the side of my skull. When the pain is like this, the only thing I can do is lay down in a darkened room and curl up in ball hoping it goes away. Perfume and bright lights seem to set these headaches in motion. Another type of headache that I get is caffeine-withdrawal headache. Especially on days when I skip my morning coffee, I will have a mild dull headache sitting on the top of my head all day. If I don't take some medicine for this, it can turn into a migraine. The reason I came to you today is that I have a new type of pain that has me worried. It is a sharp, shooting pain that's coming over the right side of my head from the back, it shoots forward to my eye at times and seems to be triggered when I am brushing my hair on that side. I sometimes feel like my scalp is tender on that side, but there's no swelling. I wanted to know if you think there's anything that can be done to help make this better.

1. How many headache types does this patient have?
2. What are you going to be looking for on her exam?
3. What findings will trigger you to obtain diagnostic testing?
4. What immediate treatment or treatments would you recommend while this patient is awaiting test results (if any)?

INTRODUCTION

Diagnosis comes primarily from the clinical history. Clinical diagnosis is the cornerstone clinical practice, providing the foundation to reasoned diagnostic testing and rational treatment design. The central question of this chapter is: What is the process by which we move from the pain narrative and clinical exam findings to a valid diagnosis and evidence-based treatment? The process of diagnostic reasoning involves a step-wise extraction of key features, abstraction of the key features, creating of a problem list, elaboration of a differential diagnosis, a plan for diagnostic testing, and a series of defenses against errors and biases. In recent years, the precision of diagnosis in many fields has increased with the advent of molecular medicine, gene sequencing, expression, and transcriptional modulation as well as advances in imaging technology. This is also true in pain care, with the clear advantage that more effective treatment plans result from higher levels of diagnostic precision. The starting point of all differential diagnoses is the patient. Although it may feel frustrating to listen to people describe pain, however, pain is often an exquisitely tuned somatic experience that provides valuable clues to formulating the differential diagnosis. In some areas of clinical practice, such as neurology, it is asserted that history is 90% of the diagnosis and the exam is confirmatory. This is not always true, but the key features of the illness narrative are essential to understanding the potentially relevant conditions and avoiding error.

FOUNDATIONAL ELEMENTS OF DIAGNOSTIC REASONING IN THE PAIN-FOCUSED ENCOUNTER

Characterizing the Chief Complaint From the Pain Narrative

The first step in the diagnostic reasoning process is to obtain a coherent pain narrative from the patient. The process of utilizing the clinical (medical) interview to establish rapport, elicit information, and learn about the patient's values is described in Chapter 6.[2] By posing open-ended questions to start the interview, the clinician is more likely to obtain a fuller illness narrative and also to build more trust with the patient. In listening to the illness narrative, it is important to remain attentive for the principal characteristics of a pain-associated condition (e.g., quality, region; these are listed in Box 7.1), these are listed i. Knowledge of these characteristics, appropriately abstracted, form the foundation of the differential diagnostic process.[3]

Appraising Multiple Pain-Associated Conditions

When a patient presents with a complex pain narrative, such as the patient in the example case at the start of this chapter, it is typically necessary to pull out the features of each of the pain-associated conditions. In the case of the patient here, who as a science writer is quite eloquent and able to describe her conditions succinctly, it may be useful to make or mentally construct a table of the features of each of the conditions (Table 7.1). By doing this, one can readily appreciate that each of the headaches described by the patient is most likely of a particular type, in this case, tension headache, migraine headache, headache secondary to caffeine withdrawal, and occipital neuralgia. Even though over-the-counter analgesia may be partially effective for these headaches, to attain the best results, each of these headaches will require specific management approaches. It is important to characterize the primary pain-associated conditions that are troublesome for the patient. In the setting of time pressures, it may be necessary to prioritize and address problems in sequence; however, the patient with complex, disabling pain will not feel heard if you stop after the first problem. Another reason that it is important to elicit features of multiple problems, if present, is that some pain-associated conditions manifest with multiple pain areas (e.g., rheumatoid arthritis, Lyme disease, physical abuse, peripheral neuropathy, and cancer), illustrating that taking the time to elicit a more comprehensive pain narrative could provide critically important clues to diagnosis.[4]

Box 7.1 Characteristic Features of a Pain-Associated Condition

Quality
Region
Severity
Timing
Usually associated symptoms
Very effective treatments
Worsening factors

Table 7.1 Example of Extracting Characteristic Features From Different Pain Narrative Demonstrating Utility of Key Pain Features in Diagnostic Reasoning

Feature	Headache 1	Headache 2	Headache 3	Headache 4
Quality	Dull pressure	Pounding	Dull	Shooting, stabbing
Region	Bifrontal	Hemicrania	Vertex	Right back of head radiating forward
Severity	Moderate	Severe	Mild	Severe
Timing	Worst in late afternoon	Sporadic, lasting hours to day	Late morning	Short shocks
Usually associated symptoms	None	Visual aura, nausea, photophobia, fatigue	May evolve into migraine	Scalp tenderness
Very effective treatments	Over-the-counter analgesia	Rapid analgesia	Over-the-counter analgesia	To be determined
Worsening factors	Nontreatment	Triggers include perfume and bright lights	Skipping coffee	Provoked by brushing/touch

Attending to Affective Information and Cues in the Encounter

Pain is distinguished by prominent affective impact to the extent that unpleasantness of pain is inseparable from the sensory discriminative dimensions in the absence of mental or pharmacologic manipulations. There are medications and mental states that can produce the phenomenon in which patients will note: "The pain is still there, but it does not bother me as much." With the advent of functional magnetic resonance imaging (MRI), it became clear that pain activates many centers in the brain, but prominently, the rostral anterior cingulate cortex is activated by most painful stimuli. This is valuable clinically because the affective dimensions of pain cause people to seek out clinical care; it also means that failure to attend to a patient's pain will produce unrelieved suffering. When interviewing and examining a patient with pain, it is important to recognize, identify, and respond to affective communication from the patient and any caregivers present.[4] A patient with severe, acute pain may have readily recognizable behaviors such as groaning, wincing, and guarding. It is easy to impute suffering and distress in these circumstances. A patient with severe chronic pain may be experiencing very high levels of pain intensity without the familiar behavioral manifestations we associate with severe acute pain. Nonetheless, distinctive manifestations of chronic pain are often present, so that awareness of chronic pain impacts and interindividual variability, as well as varying disease states, may be necessary to appreciate fully the impact of chronic pain. Especially with chronic pain-associated conditions, it is important to balance patient-centered awareness of the individual's particular experience with clinical knowledge regarding specific pain-associated conditions (Figure 7.1). When addressed in a respectful and empathetic manner, most patients with chronic

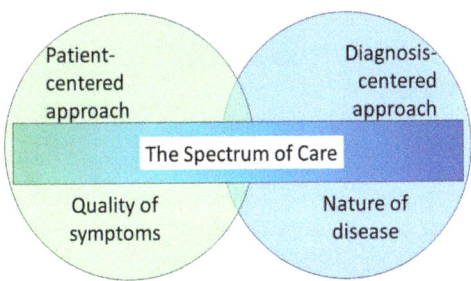

FIGURE 7.1 Patient-centered and diagnosis-centered approaches to clinical decision-making. This figure illustrates a dynamic process in which some clinical encounters predominate, such as emergency care, focus on the disease process, stabilizing the patient, and alleviating threats to life. In other settings, such as management of chronic disease, focusing on the patient's values, beliefs, and motivations is ultimately the most effective route to behavior change and is essential for successful management. In practice, the clinician needs knowledge of the disease and understanding of the patient and must be able to respond dynamically to changing circumstances incorporating awareness of both disease and patient, within a broader biopsychosocial context.

pain are ready to share the experience of their pain as well as the impact that pain has had on their lives. The impact of chronic pain on daily activities and quality of life becomes an important verifiable (objective) feature of chronic pain. It is clearly time to reject the use of the expression that "pain is subjective" and recognize that when one person does not understand another person's pain, it is a failure of intersubjective awareness and particular circumstances that limit mutual understanding. Pain is intersubjective; it is not "subjective." There are always objective manifestations, and we simply may not be able to appreciate or measure them with the tools available to us [Stein]. Avoiding the trap of pain "subjectivity" is very important for maintaining a respectful and empathetic tone toward patients and caregivers. Take the highroad and don't express disdain or disregard for those presenting for care. Affective tone of a clinical encounter has a profound influence on health outcomes, and good tone may be a protective factor for providers as well. It is important to maintain affective accountability toward the patient and endeavor to provide a timely, safe, and humane solution to the problem or problems presented.

Because pain is deeply unpleasant and interferes with productivity and quality of life, it is often necessary to proceed with preliminary treatment to reduce or control pain while diagnostic testing is taking place. It is essential to ensure the patient's safety, so that it is never appropriate to treat pain that might otherwise signal harmful pathology, e.g. cardiac chest pain must be treated with re-vascularization and masking the pain of an acute coronary syndrome could have fatal consequences. But, as long as safety can be assured, it is beneficial to provide pain control measures so that patient's do not suffer needlessly while a diagnostic work up is in progress (Figure 7.2). We use the 'parallel pathway' model to operationalize the balance between symptom-focused treatment decisions and diagnosis-centered testing decisions. Early-stage symptom-focused treatment decisions will typically follow the mechanism-based approach described in Chapter 4 (see Table 4.1), whereas longer-term treatment decisions may include disease-modifying therapies and other treatments tailored to a specific diagnosis.

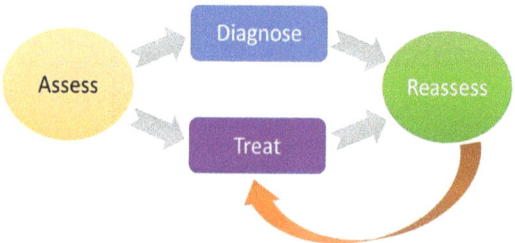

FIGURE 7.2 Parallel pathway model for treatment and diagnosis ensures that treatment is not delayed while diagnostic testing takes place and results in more refined clinical information when pain is moderated. Before rapid computed tomography scanning, acute abdominal pain was managed by withholding pain medication and observing the patient for changes in symptoms to guide diagnostic reasoning. In the modern era, in most situations it is possible to develop a differential diagnosis and diagnostic testing plan based on the presenting symptoms and provide moderate symptom relief while diagnostic testing is in progress. For example, you would advise the patient on conservative measures for ankle pain while awaiting any imaging result that was needed for further treatment.

Integrating Information From the Physical Examination

At the conclusion of the history-taking, the provider should have a mental list of conditions in the differential diagnosis. During the examination, it is important to seek signs and findings that will support or refute prospective diagnoses. For example, if a patient presents with back pain radiating into the back of the leg that has gradually worsened over several days, it is important to check strength, especially foot plantar flexion and dorsiflexion; sensation, especially over the medial, lateral, and dorsal foot; and reflexes, especially at the ankle, and to perform provocative maneuvers such as a straight leg raise (SLR) and spine and hip range of motion. In this focused exam, the provider is searching for information that supports the diagnosis of lumbar radiculopathy and makes other pathology (e.g., piriformis syndrome, sacroiliac dysfunction) less likely. In the case of the middle-aged woman described at the start of the chapter, the provider will be examining for an absence of cranial nerve deficits (e.g., visual loss, sensory loss, acoustic loss); palpating for muscular taut bands (i.e., trigger points); and examining for cervical range of motion. In each case, the provider is seeking to identify any worrisome signs or findings that might necessitate further diagnostic testing and, where possible, to support the most likely elements of the differential diagnosis.

PROBLEM LIST AND DIFFERENTIAL DIAGNOSIS

A problem list is a listing of problems particular to patient utilizing general terms until such time as a more specific diagnosis is established. In the example provided by the case of the science writer with headaches, the problem list might include an entry for frequent headaches, multiple types. This patient may also have entries for other generic problems such as fatigue, stress, low thyroid-stimulating hormone, and family history of migraine. By contrast, the differential diagnosis is a listing of potential specific diagnoses that might pertain given the patient's presenting symptoms. The problem list and differential diagnosis are detailed here.

Creating a Problem List

A problem list should focus on the concerns that the patient has with regard to the provider's practice. If the provider is a primary care provider, then the problem list could be quite broad and include elevate blood pressure, overweight, depressed mood, and other items. If the provider is a pain specialist, the problem list might include items such as headaches of multiple types, frequent headaches, medication overuse, sleep disturbance, and depressed mood. For the pain specialist, the concerns about high blood pressure and low thyroid are concurrent medical conditions, not items to be actively addressed in the pain clinic visit. A problem list aids the provider in addressing the multiplicity of needs that a patient may have in order to receive appropriately coordinated care.

Developing a Differential Diagnosis

The differential diagnosis is one of the core elements of clinical practice. It is an essential task of clinical practice: The patient presents with an illness narrative, and the practitioner elicits symptoms and signs, conducts an examination as appropriate, and assembles this together with the existing diagnostic data (e.g., prior lab work, imaging) and formulates a list of clinical diagnoses that may be reasonably considered. The top of the list is usually the diagnosis that the practitioner considers most likely, although the purpose of the differential diagnosis is to effect a mental discipline compelling practitioners to weigh various alternative explanations for the facts that are before them.[3] In the case of the patient presented at the start of the chapter, the first headache she describes is classic for tension headache; however, it might be reasonable to consider other possibilities, such as medication overuse headache, transformed migraine (if the headache was day after day without interruption), or cervicogenic headache. Given that the headache is bifrontal and is nonpulsatile, it does not present as a classic migraine. The headache is benign, making entities such as tumor, meningitis, or encephalitis unlikely as causes. The second headache is most likely a migraine with aura; however, it is reasonable to consider and weigh other possibilities. This should be accomplished for each of the pain-associated conditions characterized through analysis of the pain narrative, unless there is a unifying diagnosis that seems likely to explain all the symptoms together, in which case a comprehensive differential may be appropriate. The differential diagnosis then guides the determination of whether and what diagnostic testing is appropriate. Typically, a practitioner should be able to entertain three to four possible alternative diagnoses, although in academic medical centers, the differential diagnosis can extend to 20 or more possibilities. A discussion of the differential diagnosis, the relative likelihoods of various items, and the diagnostic testing and initial treatments required often serves as a means to enhance the preparation of a trainee—the process of preparing for rounds or clinical case conference is so central to acquiring and demonstrating knowledge of common disease processes.[5] One framework that can help ensure that potentially serious diagnoses are not missed is to develop a differential diagnosis that include entities that are common as well as those that are potentially catastrophic if overlooked. If one can demonstrate that the potentially catastrophic diagnoses were considered and excluded for specific reasons or explored using a rational approach to testing, this is an important defense against cognitive errors in clinical practice.

Table 7.2 Laboratory Testing and Clinical Rationale in Pain-Associated Conditions

Test	Pain-Associated Condition	Pain Presentation/Features
Lyme	Tick-borne disease more effectively treated if diagnosed early in disease course	Radiculitis, peripheral neuropathy, headache
ANA	Systemic lupus erythematosus	Lupus cerebritis (headache)
Syphilis	Syphilis	Lightning pain
Rheumatoid factor	Rheumatoid may produce vasculitic phenomena in both the central and peripheral nervous systems	Neuropathy, arthritides
HbA_{1C}, 2-hour gtt	Diabetes can produce multiple forms of neuropathy, both focal and diffuse; also susceptibility to infections	Burning feet, mononeuropathy with deep focal thigh or thoracic pain
Hepatitis C	Viremic headache or neuropathy	Persistent headache; burning foot pain with neuropathy
HIV	Multiple if untreated or with elevated viral load: complicated shingles, cytomegalovirus, meningitis (variable forms)	Neuropathic pain focally or more diffuse

FURTHER ASSESSMENT

Laboratory Testing

The pressures on healthcare providers to limiting testing to proper circumstances is increasing, and it is often challenging for new practitioners to recognize the risks associated with alternative diagnoses. In the situation of laboratory testing, there are multiple conditions, the diagnosis of which is often confirmed or refuted by laboratory testing, that may present with persistent pain. These conditions include a number of possibilities, some of which are included in Table 7.2. If there is reason to suspect these conditions, it is important to arrange testing and to follow up on the test results. The information in the table may be helpful in justifying laboratory testing.

Imaging

Imaging is remarkably useful in the diagnosis of acute pain associated with trauma. The choice of imaging modality depends on the primary tissue type that is being inspected. For example, bone is well-visualized by radiography or computed tomography (CT); neural, tendinous, and cartilaginous structures typically require MRI for visualization; and soft tissues may be well-characterized by ultrasound. The modality used for muscle depends on the site and nature of the suspected injury. Persistent pain conditions may or may not require imaging, depending on the clinical context. If a patient has new or worsening pain, or persistent pain that has not been well-characterized but is impairing function and quality of life, perhaps imaging is appropriate. In the

Table 7.3 Features of Various Imaging Modalities

Modality	Especially Useful for	Limitations
Ultrasound	Soft tissue visualization	May be operator dependent; limited spatial resolution
Radiograph	Bone and bony structures	Ultrarapid visualization of bone; radiation limits use to appropriate settings
Computed tomography scan	Bone and bony structures, intracranial blood (SAH, ICH)	Rapid modality; radiation limits use to appropriate settings; although newer machines should use lower amounts of radiation, lifetime exposures accumulate
Magnetic resonance image	High resolution of neural and musculotendinous structures	Time-consuming, claustrophobic reaction; high cost limits access to use in selected patients; safe imaging modality because there is no "radiation"; contrast may remain resident in tissues, a factor that limits contrast use
Positron-emission tomography scan	Cancer staging	Relatively low spatial resolution; radiation is a factor limiting use to selected patients
Bone scan	Regions of bone reconstruction or increased bone metabolism.	Very limited spatial resolution; radiation is a factor limiting use to specially selected patients

realm of low back pain, imaging is a source of considerable controversy. There are strong guidelines directing clinicians not to image acute low back pain, defined as pain of less than 6 weeks duration, unless "red flags" or serious neurologic impairment is present. What happens to the patient if pain persists unresolved and is interfering with work productivity and leisure activity? Imaging is often viewed as the gateway to high healthcare utilization; however, in the hands of all but the most skilled diagnostician, imaging may be a useful adjunct to advance diagnostic thinking and move the patient toward a clearer diagnosis and more appropriate treatment. For most expert diagnosticians, imaging typically is confirmatory. If surgical referral is contemplated, recognize that few surgeons, in the current medicolegal climate, will proceed to surgery without appropriate imaging to visualize and document the relevant pathology. Many surgeons require imaging before the patient's first clinic appointment; local practice patterns will dictate the ordering of testing at the time of referral. Table 7.3 provides basic guidance on selecting imaging modalities in working toward a diagnosis of pain-associated conditions.

Provocative Testing

Testing for specific conditions has variable results, depending on the reliability of the test and the skill of the examiner. Properly conducted, provocative tests such as the

SLR, sacroiliac stress maneuvers, piriformis testing and palpation, examination for taut bands consistent with trigger points, and others pain-associated physical findings, can be helpful for the diagnosis. There are many useful resources on the Internet, such as YouTube videos, that can be very helpful in refreshing and clarifying fine points of the provocative testing maneuvers.

Physical Therapy, Podiatry, and Consultative Assessments

Many pain expert providers embrace the idea that pain is best evaluated and treated in a collaborative environment. At the same time that medical and nursing practice are advancing in terms of technologic, skill-based, and knowledge regarding medical conditions and most effective management, the other allied health fields are advancing. Pharmacists, physical therapists, occupational therapists, speech therapists, psychotherapists, podiatrists, chiropractors, and others have the capacity to contribute meaningfully to advancing the diagnosis of shared patients. Referral to an appropriate professional colleague has the potential to improve care as well as provide insights into diagnostic surety and treatment direction. An example of this is referral of a patient to physical therapy for low back pain radiating to the posterior thigh that the primary care providers does not believe to be radiculopathy but that nonetheless is impairing the patient's function and quality of life. The physical therapist will be able to evaluate and treat this patient, potentially recognizing piriformis syndrome, sacroiliac dysfunction, hamstring strain, or iliotibial band syndrome, which the primary care physician might not have recognized based on their training. Education of most primary care clinicians provides little refinement regarding the differential diagnosis of low back pain with or without radiation, hence the benefit of collaborative care. Both early and late in one's career, there are benefits to self and to patients when appropriate collaboration is pursued.

AVOIDING ERRORS IN DIAGNOSTIC REASONING

Awareness of Diagnostic Reasoning

The process of diagnostic reasoning in pain management may be subject to errors. An important first step in preventing errors in diagnosis and treatment is to recognize the potential for errors to occur. Errors arise from a variety of sources and may be primarily cognitive or derive from affective factors. Box 7.2 summarizes several common errors in diagnostic reasoning. A fuller listing of potential errors is provided by Croskerry.[6] Cognitive errors arise most often from a lack of knowledge; this is especially common in trainees. Cognitive errors can also arise from practice factors such as recent exposure, practicing with settings where certain conditions are seen more frequently, and responding to health system factors such as overreliance on unverified information found in the electronic medical record (propagation of error). Affective errors arise from the emotional or motivational aspects of clinical practice, such as a tendency to take action over observation (commission error), a tendency to want the best for patients (outcome bias), and a tendency to preserve our own reputation (overconfidence bias). In the current clinical environment, there are increasing pressures on clinicians to factor in financial aspects of care, often without sufficient training or resources available to employ knowledge-based decision-making

> **Box 7.2** Biases Arising From Cognitive and Affective Processes in Pain Practice
>
> ### Biases Associated With Cognitive Distortions
>
> Availability bias: decisions reflecting the cognitive availability of a diagnosis, potentially due to recent exposure to one or more patients with that condition
>
> Anchoring bias: tendency to anchor the impression of a patient to first encounter, discounting new relevant information
>
> Base-rate distortion: cognitive habits that inflate or deflate true prevalence of a condition, sometimes used as an ad hoc adjustment for severity of negative outcomes; e.g., syphilis is rare but potentially devastating if undetected
>
> Diagnostic momentum: tendency to stick with a diagnosis
>
> Frequency bias: favoring a common diagnosis
>
> Gambler's fallacy: favoring an alternative diagnosis to "balance out" a more likely diagnosis based on the experience of several recent patients having the latter
>
> Insufficient information bias: clinicians who do not gather a full history may overlook relevant diagnoses
>
> Search satisfying bias: discontinuing diagnostic process after a positive result is returned
>
> Triage cueing bias: decisions influenced by the referral source or route of entry to care
>
> ### Biases Associated With Affective Influences
>
> Commission bias: decisions reflecting the belief that action is more helpful to a patient than (appropriate) inaction
>
> Fundamental attribution bias: decisions reflecting the bias that patients have contributed to their illness; stigmatization of patients with chronic pain, substance use disorder, etc.
>
> Omission bias: decisions reflecting a bias toward inaction deriving from a desire for nonmaleficence (not to expose patient to the risks or harms of treatment)
>
> Outcome bias: favoring diagnostic possibilities associated with more favorable outcomes
>
> Overconfidence bias: reflecting error that the clinician is more knowledgeable or skillful than in actual fact
>
> Sutton's slip: decisions based on pursuing the "obvious" to the exclusion of more thoughtful diagnostic decision-making
>
> Visceral bias: decision-making distorted by emotional arousal, e.g., threat, anger, countertransference
>
> *Adapted from Croskerry P. The importance of cognitive errors in diagnosis and strategies to minimize them. Acad. Med. 2003;78:775–780.*

balancing patients' needs with cost and population health factors; this can lead to the overutilization and underutilization of resources. Another outcome of the complex pressures applied in the absence of sufficient high-quality evidence available at the point of care was the tendency to prescribe opioids and an overreliance on passive strategies for the treatment of pain-associated conditions. There has always been the potential to counterbalance this with an understanding of relevant persistent pain-associated conditions as appropriate to chronic condition strategies (i.e. active self-management strategies, as have gained acceptance in conditions such as diabetes, congestive heart failure, and high blood pressure). However, because clinicians have not been adequately educated about the full range of options available for engaging patients in pain self-management and promoting higher levels of self- efficacy, there is a persistent tendency to favor passive treatment approaches such as surgery and injections over engaging patients in appropriate higher self-efficacy modalities such as physical therapy, home exercise programs, cognitive restructuring, and acceptance commitment therapy–based self-management plans. A final major source of diagnostic error is embodied in the concept of "true-true and unrelated," in which clinical findings that are simultaneously present are incorrectly linked in the provider's mind as both relating to a single diagnosis when in fact one of the findings relates to one relevant diagnosis and the other finding relates to a separate diagnosis. There are circumstances in which a single diagnosis can explain all the relevant findings, but there are also circumstances in which the "parsimonious" explanation is wrong. Especially in the current era when patients are older and often presenting to care with multiple comorbid conditions, it is essential to entertain alternative and sometimes multiple diagnostic possibilities and structure diagnostic evaluations appropriately. Close follow-up is warranted for patients whose clinical response to treatment does not meet expectations.

Disclosure of Errors in Diagnostic Reasoning and Treatment

The consequences of clinical biases and errors are sometimes devastating for patients and families. In the event of clinical error, is it important to be aware of local policies and practices. It is the position of the American Medical Association not only that a physician is ethically bound to "[d]isclose medical errors if they have occurred in the patient's care . . ." but also that information "may be conveyed over time in keeping with the patient's preferences and ability to comprehend . . . sensitively and respectfully."[7] Many have advocated for the fullest possible transparency and disclosure; in doing so, a step-wise approach, preferably that mandated by the relevant healthcare organization, must be followed. The general principles are noted here. First, ensure that supervisory or health systems officers are aware of the error in question as appropriate. Anticipate that there will be procedures to follow. Plan for disclosure as promptly as possible. It is important that disclosure take place in a manner that is comfortable for the patient and as supportive as possible. It is appropriate to introduce the topic in a manner that allows patients to express their own readiness to engage in the topic, potentially using language that invites them to signal their readiness to proceed, such as, "I came across some information that concerned me, that I would like to share with you." Ideally, it is important to sit with your patients and their support persons as appropriate and to maintain open and supportive body language. Sit on the patient's level, ensure privacy, introduce other team members if present, maintain good eye contact and serious demeanor, and allow generous time for questions and for exploring of possibilities. Maintain open lines of communication after the disclosure conversation to the extent allowed by any risk management team guidelines, if relevant. Most important, place the patients at the center of the conversation and endeavor to understand their concerns, anticipate their questions, and support their responses to with direct expressions of empathy and recruitment of support systems as needed. While errors are potentially costly and damaging, the effects of an improperly handled error can be devastating to both patient and provider, and a correctly handled error can lead to more satisfying and effective responses.[8]

SUMMARY

Diagnostic reasoning is a central part of clinical pain care and can be one of the most challenging and rewarding aspects of engaging with patients and their caregivers. We exercise a duty to render care by appropriate preparation of our knowledge, skills, and abilities to provide expert compassionate care to those with pain. Diagnostic reasoning includes bringing together the information gathered from the patient during the diagnostic history-taking and integrating that with the examination findings. Diagnostic testing is often a useful adjunct to the clinical reasoning process and may provide additional insights into a patient's condition. Diagnostic errors are diverse in nature and highly prevalent, but systematic approaches to minimizing these errors holds the promise of a work experience that is subject to less burnout and higher levels of satisfaction while simultaneously increasing patient safety (Box 7.3). It is important to remember that the simplest explanation is not always the most correct: Patients are complex and individual in their presentation and therapeutic needs. Whether errors occur or outcomes reflect our best efforts and those of the patient, we can most genuinely connect with patients through humane, transparent communication about the diagnostic and treatment processes. Through honest alliance with the patient, we can guide all involved toward appropriate levels of pain self-management and higher self-efficacy, typically associated with improved health outcomes.

Box 7.3 Reducing Errors Through Effective Clinical Reasoning (LEADERS LEAD)

Learn about biases
Examine mental processes (metacognition)
Always consider alternatives
Decrease reliance on memory (algorithms, job aids)
Ease task burden
Rehearse and simulate
Structure recall
Look for feedback opportunities
Encourage bias training
Allow sufficient time
Demand accountability

Adapted from Croskerry P. The importance of cognitive errors in diagnosis and strategies to minimize them. Acad. Med. 2003;78:775–780.

REVIEW QUESTIONS

1. A 31-year-old patient presents with an intermittent headache that occurs about every 2 weeks. She notes that the headache is so intense that the only thing she can do is lie down in a darkened room. She notes that the headache at its worst is like a pounding feeling, although times it starts as a pulsating feeling. It can last for up to 3 days if she does not take medicine right away. The headache is usually on the left side, but sometimes it's on the right side instead. Which abstraction of the details of this headache will bring you closest to a clinical diagnosis of this headache?
   a. Throbbing hemicrania, severe intensity, occurs in bouts, female patient, activity worsens pain
   b. Pounding, left- greater than right-sided headache, disabling, patient doesn't always take medicine
   c. Frequent pounding headache, mostly on one side, causes patient to lie down

2. Which of the following is not a correct paring of imaging modality with structure of interest?
   a. Radiograph: bone fracture
   b. MRI: nerves and tendons
   c. Ultrasound: adult brain
   d. CT: complex bony structures

3. Which of the following is not recommended for reducing the negative impact of diagnostic biases?
   a. Reduce task complexity
   b. Learn about biases
   c. Limit time to avoid overthinking
   d. Structure recall

REFERENCES

1. Bliss M. William Osler: A Life in Medicine. Oxford: Oxford University Press; 2007.
2. Cole SA, Byrd J. The Medical Interview: The Three Function Approach (3rd ed.). Philadelphia: Elsevier Saunders; 2013.
3. Nendaz MR, Bordage G. Promoting diagnostic problem representation. Med Educ. 2002;36(8):760–766.
4. Stein E. On the problem of empathy, translated by Waltraut Stein, from The Collected Works of Edith Stein (Vol. 3). Washington, DC: ICS Publications; 1989.
5. Singh H, Thomas EJ, Petersen LA, Studdert DM. Medical errors involving trainees: a study of closed malpractice claims from 5 insurers. Arch Intern Med. 2007;167(19):2030–2036.
6. Croskerry P. The importance of cognitive errors in diagnosis and strategies to minimize them. Acad. Med. 2003;78:775–780.
7. AMA Code of Medical Ethics, Code of Medical Ethics Opinion 2.1.3. Withholding Information from Patients. Withholding information without the patient's knowledge or consent is ethically unacceptable. Accessed July 29, 2018 at: https://www.ama-assn.org/delivering-care/withholding-information-patients.
8. Martinez W1, Hickson GB, Miller BM, et al. Role-modeling and medical error disclosure: a national survey of trainees. Acad Med. 2014;89(3):482–489.

8 Professionalism in Pain Care

Beth B. Hogans

An agony so unbelievable gripped her that her astounded and protesting mind cried out it was impossible such pain should be. . . . [S]he felt tears of failure roll down her face and looked up through them to see the pink nurse looking down at her with unmistakable disappointment.
—Doris Lessing, *A Proper Marriage*

It's been my experience that if a medical person tells you that you're going to feel a little pinch he's really going to hurt you.
—Stephen King, "On Impact"

LEARNING OBJECTIVES

At the completion of this chapter, the learner should be able to discuss:

- The provider's role in the patient's pain narrative, especially the process and value of communicating with compassion and empathy, the characteristics of active listening and its impact on clinician effectiveness, the utility of subjective phenomena and eliciting qualitative descriptors, the process of building rapport, and the development of the therapeutic alliance
- Core concepts in patient-centered care, especially the value and process of shared decision-making, how to incorporate positive lifestyle change into pain management, and the role of self-efficacy in pain-related healthcare outcomes
- Our role as healthcare providers, especially how patient centered-care compares with relationship-centered care, healthcare ethics and its applications to pain practice, how to motivate ourselves to develop a genuine interest in pain mechanisms and relief, and ways to demonstrate interprofessional collaboration
- The components of counseling for collaboration and self-management, especially motivational interviewing and how to apply the stages of change model, coordinate care with other providers, and promote and manage patient choice
- Future directions and trends in pain care professionalism, especially assessment of professionalism skills

CASE SCENARIO

Two high school athletes experience identical ankle fractures. One has a stable home situation and a parent who goes with the student to doctor appointments and therapy sessions. When the doctor offers an opioid medication for pain at the initial appointment, the patient's parent is there offering support and comfort. The student says that it doesn't seem like the pain is all that bad, especially since the air cast was put into place. The student gets home that night and elevates the leg, and the family provides encouragement, bringing food, water to drink, ice packs, and general assistance as needed. Everything goes smoothly, and after a few weeks and some physical therapy (PT), the student is back on two feet; 6 months later, it's as though nothing ever happened.

The other student has no one who can provide transportation to the doctor; in fact, the insurance situation is unstable, so follow-up appointments cannot be made at the time of the acute care appointment. The doctor who sees the student at the first appointment is concerned about the lack of follow-up and provides some extra medication at that first visit; 120 tablets of pain medicine are provided. The student finds that the medication works well for the first night but then while at school, the medication is confiscated and not returned. The student is in a lot of pain and is frustrated; a friend offers to get something to help. The student, who is feeling really stressed about the situation at home where the one remaining parent is recently laid off and has been drinking heavily, agrees to try the pills that the friend offers. The pills help but only for a few hours. A couple of days later, the friend says that no pills were available, but it is possible to get something else which would also help with the pain. The "something else" is an injectable; the student defers because of fear of needles and toughs it out with the pain. Three weeks later, frustrated with the cast. which is bulky and interfering with ease of motion, the student jettisons the cast and feels fine. A month later, the student is playing basketball with friends and reinjures the leg, and the pain is unbelievable. After a radiograph at the urgent care center shows no new fracture, the student is discharged with a prescription for ibuprofen, which is of no help for the pain. The student feels that the provider at the urgent care center was dismissive and shaming. The student feels stigmatized, alone, and angry, compounding the agony of the pain that is much worse than before. The student agrees to try the "something" the friend was offering and dies of an overdose.

IMPACT OF PROFESSIONAL CONDUCT IN PAIN CARE AND THE BIOPSYCHOSOCIAL MODEL
Introduction

A patient comes in for an office visit or awakens from a procedure in pain: she is hurting, limited in what she can do, possibly suffering, and uncertain about the cause of her pain and how long it will continue. You can make all the difference for that patient.

Know how to listen, ask the right questions, and respond with kindness and interest about the patient's condition and explore how it has been approached so far. Then you have a chance to help: You can figure out the problem, order the necessary tests, initiate safe and effective treatment, counsel the patient about your findings and impressions, and motivate the patient to take necessary steps. When the patient returns, you have a chance to help more: to interpret test results in light of the clinical condition, adjust any medications, and motivate the patient toward healthy changes that will foster better long-term outcomes. To work most effectively with patients in pain, it is necessary to understand pain, as you are learning here, and to recognize the essential role of professionalism skills in meeting the special needs of these patients.[1]

As clinicians, we are the "professional in the room" when encountering a patient with pain. Patients rely on us to set the tone, establish useful ground rules for interaction, and provide clinical care that is both competent and considerate of their needs.[2] It is sometimes the case that students may find patients with long-standing pain perplexing or frustrating, and this is where the professionalism skills in pain care are so valuable.[3] By understanding the multiple dimensions of the pain-focused clinical encounter, we can use skills in active listening, establishing rapport, patient-centered care, ethics, shared decision-making together with our genuine interest, compassion, and desire to promote great self-efficacy in our patients to build and manage a comprehensive pain treatment plan that optimizes outcomes and minimizes costs and side effects. This chapter examines the clinician's role in the pain narrative, core concepts in patient-centered care, ethics and the professional role in pain care, and the basics of counseling patients for collaboration and self-management of pain.

Biopsychosocial Model and Safe Pain Care

The foundation of patient-centered pain care is the biopsychosocial model of pain. Applied to pain by Jon Loeser in the 1980s, the biopsychosocial model of pain explains how pain is magnified or reduced by a variety of biological, psychological, and social variables.[4] Still, 35 years later, more than 30,000 people died of opioid overdose in the United States, two-thirds from a prescription opioid. In the scenario that started this chapter, a failure of professionalism skills contributed to a complex problem; most important, the scenario highlights the central role that psychological and social factors play in the development and resolution of pain-associated conditions. A functioning pain system is essential to help us protect our bodies from harm, but the system is prone to many influences, and stressors can lead people to make poor choices such as avoiding activity or choosing risky "treatments."

Communicating Compassion and Empathy

The professional's role in the pain narrative is active listening and compassionate action. In an ideal scenario, the professional's role in the pain narrative is to quickly recognize and address a pain problem, develop a rapid, safe, and fully effective solution, and do so with a respectful and caring manner.[1] In many cases in which pain is secondary to another condition (e.g., strep throat, urinary tract infection), treatment of the primary condition with recommendations for conservative analgesic measures is sufficient. In other cases, the cause of pain is obvious and can be addressed as a component of therapy (e.g., ankle sprain, rotator cuff injury, appendicitis), and outcomes are often quite good. There are other conditions in which the physical findings are subtle or absent (e.g., headache, back pain, diabetic peripheral neuropathy), and in these cases pain treatment can be more challenging. In these situations, having foundational knowledge of common pain syndromes can be helpful because it is then possible to develop a differential diagnosis or diagnostic classification based on the subjective characteristics. As noted by Haythornthwaite and colleagues, having foundational pain knowledge allows a provider to obtain essential information from a patient, and this will ease the patient's sense of isolation and promote an exchange between the patient and provider, at least on a factual basis.[1] Even exchanging information of a factual nature is a start because it will allow the provider to formulate a differential diagnosis, learn about the patient's preferences for treatment, and anticipate some testing and treatment needs. If the provider is able to acknowledge the emotional dimension of pain and provide emotional support to the patient during the clinical encounter, the patient will feel even more understood, and the affective component of pain will be addressed and managed rather than contributing to more pain. An empathetic nod, a reassuring murmur, or a simple expression such as "that must be difficult" will provide a measure of comfort to the patient in pain.

Empathy, Compassion, and Active Listening

It is important to recognize the differences between empathy and compassion and apply each appropriately. Empathy means vicariously understanding the thoughts, feelings, and actions of another. Compassion means being aware of the suffering of another and feeling motivated to relieve that suffering. In contrast to compassion, empathy is not linked to a response per se. If empathy is not linked to a behavioral response, such as an empathetic utterance (e.g., "I'm sorry" or "that sounds difficult") or empathetic action (e.g., "I am ordering this test stat so that we can get this addressed quickly"), empathy is only an internal state that may be passive in nature. Nonetheless, empathy can help us cognitively to understand the details of a pain condition and can lead us toward a diagnosis; empathy can also help the provider approach the emotional tasks of the pain-focused encounter by better appreciating the patient's suffering, potential limitations, and needs. Compassion taps into the fundamental motivation to help others, our awareness of someone else's suffering, and our yearning, desire, interest, or motivation to take action and relieve that suffering. Empathy is useful to the extent that it allows us to connect to the patient's situation, reflect on the patient's feelings, provide affective support, and conceptualize the patient's condition and potential treatment needs. Cole and Bird recommend a three-phase process of empathy, reflection, and legitimation in which the interviewer seeks to understand the patient's experience, reflects on the emotional tone of the patient to explore the feelings expressed, and legitimates the patient's experience as an expression of empathy and first step in building rapport and ultimately a therapeutic alliance (Figures 8.1 and 8.2).[2] One behavioral manifestation of empathy,

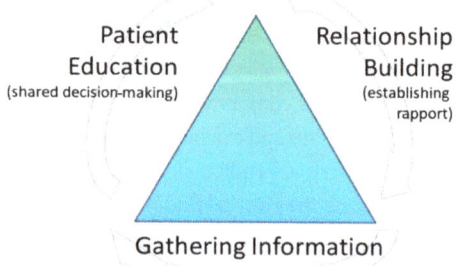

FIGURE 8.1 Traditional three-function model of the patient interview showing information gathering, building rapport, and education of the patient. All components have a positive effect on the relationship and foster trust.

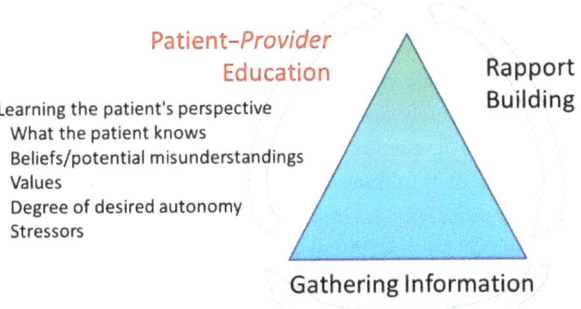

FIGURE 8.2 Updated model of the patient interview showing that the third phase, education, is relevant to both patient and provider. As the patient and provider engage in shared decision-making and the motivational interviewing process, the provider learns more about the patient's healthcare-related values, motivations, and desired degree of autonomy. The provider can then provide better informed suggestions to the patient as the pain self-management plan develops.

compassion, and interest is active listening behavior.[5] Active listening is demonstrated to the patient by several specific behaviors (Box 8.1). Active listening begins with understanding the patient's needs in the encounter, starting with an open-ended question such as, "What brought you to come in today?" and listening when the patient speaks without interrupting. Active listening ultimately results in developing a plan that is responsive to the patient's self-identified needs as well as the clinician's perceived priorities.

Embracing Subjective Phenomena: The Value of Qualitative Descriptors

Sometimes clinicians may feel limited in their ability to understand fully a patient's subjective experiences; however, there is a fundamental value in being able to

---

Box 8.1 Active Listening Behaviors

Seek to optimize patient comfort before starting
Eliminate distractions
Begin with open-ended questions
Do not interrupt; allow the patient to finish the narrative
Encourage the patient to continue
Check for understanding
Elicit essential details
Turn toward the patient while the patient speaks
Maintain culturally appropriate eye contact
Maintain uncrossed limbs and forward-leaning posture

Adapted from Hashim MJ. Patient-centered communication: basic skills. Am Fam Physician. 2017;95(1):29–34.

perceive and interpret what patients can tell us about their conditions. Imagine a patient who cannot speak: We are then left to guess what hurts, how much, and what it feels like. Subjective features of pain, such as severity, regional involvement with radiation, qualitative characteristics, timing, and associated, exacerbating, and alleviating factors, all provide valuable information that lead to forming the differential diagnosis. A moderately severe, band-like, pressure-type headache worsening over the course of the day is a tension headache in all likelihood. A severe, half-head (hemicrania), stabbing or throbbing headache coming on quickly any time of day, associated with light sensitivity, is almost always migraine. In addition, by listening attentively to the subjective description of pain, the patient feels heard, and sometimes believed, and this contributes to fostering rapport, especially when the patient feels understood.

Rapport and Beyond: Building a Therapeutic Alliance

A major goal of our interviewing techniques is not just to gather information but also to build rapport. Rapport is a positive, cooperative relationship between people characterized by harmony, understanding, and empathetic communication. Ultimately, rapport leads to better clinical relations between patient and provider. In clinical studies, when providers and patients demonstrate good rapport, they also report high levels of mutual respect. The goal in all of this is to create a relationship in which patients trust our findings and recommendations and follow through on the necessary parts of the pain treatment plan. As pain treatment moves away from overreliance on opioid medications and other passive strategies, it becomes even more important for us to understand patients, connect with them, and motivate them to follow through with more active treatments, including those that require active patient engagement and effort (Box 8.2).[6]

CORE CONCEPTS IN PATIENT-CENTERED CARE: SHARED DECISION-MAKING, POSITIVE LIFESTYLE CHANGE, AND SELF-EFFICACY
Shared Decision-Making

Following the era of traditional medicine, clinical care has entered a period of major revision and moved toward a focus on patients as the center of clinical practice.[7] Especially as society has diversified, it is more important than ever to understand a patient's preferences, health-related beliefs, values, and motivations.[6] In patient-centered care, there are several guiding principles affecting

---

Box 8.2 Four Ways to Overcome Communication Barriers

Ask–tell–ask (e.g., what do you know about aspirin and heart attacks?)
Tell me more (e.g., tell me more about that episode of dizziness)
Respond to emotion; start by naming the feeling (e.g., you seem sad today)
Assess coping style; patients may be monitors (scan for symptoms) or blunters (deny symptoms)

communication, treatment decisions, and ultimately patient outcomes and satisfaction. Patient-centered care means that one size does not fit all, and we need to tailor treatment plans to the needs of the patient. This is nowhere more relevant than in pain because pain experience varies so widely from one person to the next. Even siblings and twins will have widely different pain experiences under identical circumstances and thus will have very different treatment needs. In addition, each patient carries specific medical comorbidities, cultural habits, and cognitive frameworks (beliefs).

Incorporating Positive Lifestyle Change Into Pain Management

Patients will have widely varying beliefs about the cause of illness and also the path to recovery. Although a small number of patients still express a preference for the doctor to "make decisions" about therapy, many patients appreciate the opportunity to be informed about health and illness and to be involved in the decision-making process.[7] Certainly when it comes to designing lifestyle changes and identifying targets for self-directed behavior change, patients will be much more successful when they are in charge of selecting targets for change.[8]

Role of Self-Efficacy

Although some patients continue to prefer passive treatment strategies such as pills, injections, and surgeries, more and more patients are taking on active approaches to treatment and chronic disease management. The evidence is incontrovertible that exercise and diet are essential to managing and reducing excess weight, hyperglycemia, and muscle deterioration, all associated with chronic pain–associated conditions such as low back pain, arthritis, and neuropathy. We cannot address the epidemic of millions of adults with these chronic conditions without endorsing, encouraging, and supporting more active, healthy lifestyles.[9]

UNDERSTANDING OUR ROLE AS PROVIDERS
Patient-Centered and Relationship-Centered Care

Our role as healthcare providers is to inform patients about potential and real health concerns, explain the available and appropriate treatment options, and with awareness of the patient's values and health-related beliefs, guide the patient through a discussion of selecting the options most appropriate for them and carry out necessary changes through procedures, prescribing, counseling, and guidance. When pain is dismissed or minimized as a subjective complaint, there is a missed opportunity to recognize medical problems and to lead the patient toward healthier lifestyle choices. One important consideration for patient-centered care is that not all providers are identical. Although some pain-associated conditions, such as a fractured ankle, have an established care path (e.g., immobilization and analgesia followed by rehabilitation), other conditions have more options in treatment. Even with the ankle fracture, there is the possibility to reduce reliance on opioid pain control by limiting the timeframe of prescriptions; increasing use of nonpharmacologic pain control strategies, such as elevation, compression, icing, and distraction; and using nonopioid pain medications.

Relationship-centered care acknowledges that providers are different and that there may be variable solutions for many types of pain problems. It might be entirely appropriate for a patient with chronic back pain to pursue interventional pain management; it might also be appropriate for a patient with the same condition to explore integrative medicine or rehabilitative care. Some components of a treatment plan will vary, depending on the provider working with the patient. Ideally, patients should be informed of the scope of practice of the provider and the range of treatments offered before making an appointment.

Ethics in Pain Practice

Ethics are a central part of pain care.[10] The four pillars of healthcare ethics are (1) respect for patient autonomy, which includes honoring patients' right to choose appropriately and direct their own course through the healthcare system; (2) beneficence, which means that a provider will always act in a manner that reflects a positive orientation toward the patient's best interest; (3) nonmaleficence, often based on the maxim, "Primum non nocere" ("first, do no harm"), which means that the provider will never act in a manner that causes harm to the patient; and (4) distributive justice, which addresses the need to be mindful of system factors and resources in making healthcare decisions, balancing costs and benefits of treatment. Clearly, all of these impinge on pain care: Patients have the right to have pain addressed according to their autonomous desire for relief and not to be delegitimized by having pain ignored; patients have the right to expect that healthcare providers will manifest beneficence and work toward relief of their pain; patients have the right to expect that a healthcare provider will not wittingly engage in therapy that provokes pain without addressing it, to knowingly leave them in pain, or to provide treatments that are clearly harmful; and patients have the right to know that consideration of resources may limit their access to treatment and to be advised of potential remedies when this occurs.[10]

Motivating Ourselves: Genuine Interest in Pain Mechanisms and Relief

Perhaps the most important consideration regarding pain as it relates to career longevity and avoidance of burnout is addressing, understanding, and embracing the motivations of providers to assess pain proactively and provide pain relief. People are attracted to healthcare careers for many reasons, but most share a common desire to do good, to utilize aptitudes and talents in a way that affects human well-being.[1,10] This can get lost in the shuffle, and there is strong evidence that self-reported levels of empathy decline as clinical demands increase. It is also the case that so-called reflective practice has a protective effect against burnout. One study found that first- and second-year medical students choosing an enrichment course in pain and the humanities generally demonstrated high levels of reflection with regard to their personal experiences of pain. The impact of high levels of reflection in training are not well established, but medical interns with high levels of reflective practice were motivated to improve their practice and were more aware of empathy.[11] More recently, it has been noted that important sex differences may mean that women are more susceptible to burnout (see Figure 8.3).[12]

Interprofessional Collaboration

Working as part of an effective collaborative team is an important and rewarding way to deliver pain care, especially for complex patients.[13] When patients have been maintained on opioids and a taper is planned, it is far more effective to have an interprofessional team assess and manage decisions about the patient's care. The pharmacist will have special insights into designing a safe and effective opioid-sparing treatment regimen, the physical therapist will bring important energy and ideas for activating endogenous pain protective mechanisms through movement and exercise, the nurse team member will contribute valuable holistic perspectives about the patient's lifestyle factors and barriers to change, and a clinical psychologist can assist by working closely with the patient through the stages of change model, cognitive behavioral therapy models, or acceptance commitment therapy models. Interprofessional education is slowly gaining acceptance in more health professions settings, but ongoing efforts are needed to ensure that when interprofessional education is implemented, the topic of discussion models effective pain care and not failures.[14]

Counseling for Collaboration and Self-Management: Motivational Interviewing and the Stages of Change Model

Knowledge of effective counseling methods and psychological foundations for promoting change is useful in caring for patients with chronic illness and persistent pain. As beautifully described in detail by Miller and Rollnick, some patients are not ready for change (precontemplative), some are deep in the throes of engaging in change talk (action), while still others are maintaining change or dealing with a recurrence of undesirable behaviors.[8] Knowing the stages of change model (Table 8.1) and understanding

Table 8.1 Stages of Change Model and Example Behaviors of Each

Stage	Patient Characteristics	Provider Tasks
Precontemplation	Not thinking about change External locus of control Minimizes negative consequences	Discover and explore patient values Frame benefits and harms in terms of patient's values
Contemplation	Considering costs and benefits of change	Assess commitment to change Assess confidence regarding change
Preparation	Begins to experiment with change	Support steps at change Encourage small steps: build confidence Change talk to build commitment
Action	Changes begins with active steps	Ask about and support change Anticipate and mitigate challenges
Maintenance	Maintaining change behavior	Touch base briefly about behavior Provide support for any stressors
Relapse	Normal but not essential Experiences demoralization	Empathize, highlight gaps between behavior and goals, "roll with resistance," and support self-efficacy

Table 8.2 SMART Goals

S	Specific (e.g., I will walk 1,000 more steps a day next week)
M	Measurable (e.g., I will use my phone to measure my steps each day)
A	Attainable (i.e., within reach)
R	Relevant (e.g., by walking more, I will gain control over my pain)
T	Time-bound (i.e., link the activity to a specific date or time)

that change should be addressed in terms that make it relevant and appealing to the patient are key. A teenager will usually be more concerned about cosmetic effects (e.g., stained teeth), whereas an older patient may be more concerned with preserving lung function or avoiding heart attacks. It is important to explore the patient's health-related values and beliefs in order to interact most effectively with them around behavior change. Finally, goals for change should be "SMART"—**s**pecific, **m**easurable, **a**chievable, **r**esults-focused, and **t**ime-bound (Table 8.2).[15] Start small so that success is likely. For a patient who is sedentary, a SMART goal would be to walk back and forth to the mailbox twice each day until the next appointment. The provider should record specific goals in the medical record and check back with the patient about change at the next visit. Showing interest and follow through regarding behavior change is an important and powerful way to effectuate your compassion for the patient. When successful change occurs, it is essential to pause and appreciate the patient's efforts and accomplishments, taking time to acknowledge the value of the patient's commitment to positive change, savoring the moment. Mindfulness is an essential habit of successful clinicians.

Coordinating With Other Providers, Managing Patient Choice

Finally, clear and courteous communication with colleagues is an important part of professionalism. On occasion, there is reason or opportunity to discuss patients directly with a colleague or colleagues. Often, however, communication is through an electronic note or text. Ideally, these notes are based on a shared biopsychosocial framework.[16] Timely completion of notes is essential, and communication with the patient about the results of each clinical encounter is also necessary. The communication plan for each patient must be tailored to the cognitive capacity; some patients with dementing illness will require simplified treatment plans with steps presented in sequential visits, whereas cognitively intact patients can engage in a multipronged treatment plan depending on temperament and resources of time, cost burdens, and transportation.

Pain Self-Management

Pain self-management is the ultimate goal for many patients with chronic pain. Because optimal management of chronic pain–associated conditions involves many changes to lifestyle, including incorporation of daily exercise, psychological techniques, mind-body practices, complementary therapies, sleep optimization, safe medication use, and improvements to environmental factors, it is critically important that the patient be

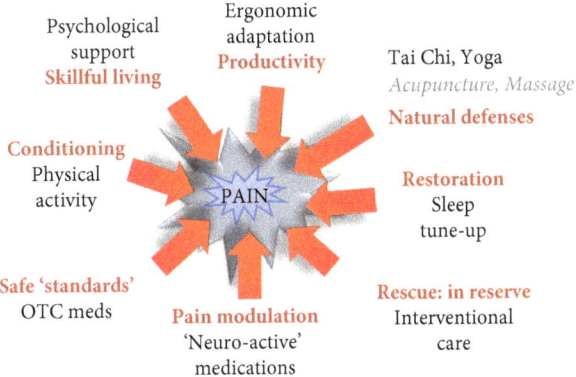

FIGURE 8.3 Interprofessional collaboration involves competency in several domains. These domains include: Communication, Teamwork, Ethics and Values, and Roles and Responsibilities. In the IPEC model, IP collaborative care is patient-centered, as well as community oriented. Also suggested by the model is this figure is a growth in competency as the learner progresses, depicted as the competencies growing in size, moving from left to right.

engaged in the idea of self-management as early as possible. The provider can offer professional expertise, exclude life-limiting and progressive conditions requiring further therapies, and counsel the patient about effective pain self-management approaches, but the provider cannot do it all for the patient. The patient is at the center, and the pain-aware practitioner is "staffing the bench" so that the patient can spend as much time "in the game" as possible. The coordination of provider-directed care and patient self-management is illustrated in Figure 8.4.

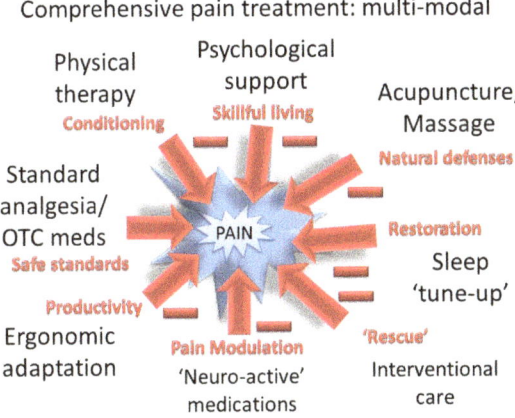

FIGURE 8.4 The coordination of patient self-management and provider-directed pain management activities is illustrated as more effective for most chronic pain conditions. Patients will engage in self-directed activities such as appropriate physical activity, psychological therapies, mind–body practices, sleep hygiene, safe medication use, and optimization of environmental factors, with practitioner support. The healthcare practitioner can direct patients to diagnostic testing and specialty services and introduce new health practices as needed. OTC = over-the-counter.

FUTURE DIRECTIONS

There are several approaches to teaching and assessing the aspects of care described in this chapter. At this time, it appears that no one instrument is widely used as a measure of professionalism in clinical practice; however, patient feedback is often taken as the most important gauge of provider professionalism. It is important to be mindful that patient feedback is likely to be a permanent feature of clinician ratings, and being able to recognize and develop the components of practice that contribute to patient satisfaction and the effectiveness of clinical encounters is important.

SUMMARY

Professionalism process and practice are especially important in pain care due to the profound impacts of pain on subjective experience, quality of life, and productivity as well as the perceived potential for manipulation and secondary gain. Several conceptual models are useful in developing an effective professional perspective on pain, these include the biopsychosocial model, the patient-centered care model, and the stages of change model. Skills in interprofessional collaboration, motivational interviewing, healthcare ethics and foundations of clinical psychology are also essential. Through the application of professionalism skills and concepts, pain care becomes more fulfilling and personally rewarding for clinicians, while patients experience higher levels of satisfaction and better functional outcomes.

REVIEW QUESTIONS

1. A 28-year-old male with a medical history of opioid dependence and active heroin use presents for follow-up of right ankle pain. He reports that the pain is worse after a day at work, the pain is unbearably intense at night, and he is back to using heroin, after a stint at rehab, in order to control his ankle pain. After you interview him and examine the ankle, you believe that he has chronic musculoskeletal ankle pain that is made worse by muscle atrophy and some mild contractures that are restricting the ankle from a normal range of motion. You believe that the patient would benefit from a course of PT. The patient states that PT has not helped in the past. Of the following, what is your best next step?
   a. Refer him for an pain injection to reduce the pain immediately
   b. Try to elicit his specific concerns about the prior PT experience
   c. Prescribe a limited number of opioid pain pills so that he can premedicate before PT
   d. Recommend a surgical consultation
   e. Write a prescription for PT and tell him to come back after the treatment is completed

2. Active listening behaviors can include the following:
   a. Making sure the patient is as comfortable as possible at the beginning
   b. Focusing the interview through carefully targeted questions that show you're listening
   c. Turning away from patients when they speak so that they can speak freely

d. Staring wide-eyed at patients so that they know you are paying attention
   e. Interrupting frequently to confirm important details

3. SMART goals are the following, *except*:
   a. Specific
   b. Measurable
   c. Ambitious
   d. Relevant
   e. Time-bound

REFERENCES

1. Murinson BB, Agarwal AK, Haythornthwaite JA. Cognitive expertise, emotional development, and reflective capacity: clinical skills for improved pain care. J Pain. 2008;9:975–983.
2. Cole SA, Byrd J. The Medical Interview: The Three Function Approach (3rd ed.). Philadelphia: Elsevier Saunders; 2013.
3. Bair M. Learning from our learners: implications for pain management education in medical schools. Pain Med. 2011;12:1139–1141.
4. Loeser JD. Perspectives on pain. In: Turner P, ed. Proceedings of the First World Congress on Clinical Pharmacology and Therapeutics (pp. 313–316). London: Macmillan; 1980.
5. Hashim MJ. Patient-centered communication: basic skills. Am Fam Physician. 2017;95(1):29–34.
6. Agarwal AK, Murinson BB. New dimensions in patient-physician interaction: values, autonomy, and medical information in the patient-centered clinical encounter. Rambam Maimonides Med J. 2012;3(3):e0017.
7. Emanuel EJ, Emanuel LL. Four models of the physician-patient relationship. JAMA. 1992;267:2221–2226.
8. Miller WR, Rollnick S. Motivational Interviewing: Helping People Change (3rd ed.). New York: Guilford Press; 2012.
9. Seligman ME, Railton P, Baumeister RF, Sripada C. Navigating into the future or driven by the past. Perspect Psychol Sci. 2013;8(2):119–141.
10. Giordano J. Moral agency in pain medicine: philosophy, practice and virtue. Pain Physician. 2006;9(1):41–46.
11. Levine RB, Kern DE, Wright SM. The impact of prompted narrative writing during internship on reflective practice: a qualitative study. Adv Health Sci Educ Theory Pract. 2008;13(5):723–733.
12. Spataro BM, Tilstra SA, Rubio DM, McNeil MA. The toxicity of self-blame: sex differences in burnout and coping in internal medicine trainees. J Womens Health (Larchmt). 2016;25(11):1147–1152.
13. Gordon DB, Watt-Watson J, Hogans BB. Interprofessional pain education: with, from, and about competent, collaborative practice teams to transform pain care. Pain Rep. 2018;3(3):e663.
14. Fishman SM, Young HM, Lucas Arwood E, et al. Core competencies for pain management: results of an interprofessional consensus summit. Pain Med. 2013;14(7):971–981.
15. Siegert RJ, Taylor WJ. Theoretical aspects of goal-setting and motivation in rehabilitation. Disabil Rehabil. 2004;26(1):1–8.
16. Smith RC, Fortin AH, Dwamena F, Frankel RM. An evidence-based patient-centered method makes the biopsychosocial model scientific. Patient Educ Couns. 2013;91(3):265–270.

PART III
PAIN TREATMENTS AND APPROACHES TO MANAGEMENT

9 Standard Systemic Analgesic Agents

Acetaminophen, Nonsteroidal Anti-Inflammatory Drugs, and Opioids

Michele L. Matthews and
Benjamin S. Kematick

The medicines of today are based upon thousands of years of knowledge accumulated from folklore, serendipity and scientific discovery. The new medicines of tomorrow will be based on the discoveries that are being made now, arising from basic research in laboratories around the world.
—Sir John Robert Vane (1927–2004)*

LEARNING OBJECTIVES

At the completion of this chapter, the learner should be able to discuss:

- Nonopioid analgesics, including their mechanism of action, place in therapy, dosing, and adverse effect
- Opioids, including their receptor activity, place in therapy, dosing, and adverse effects
- The role of short-acting and extended-release (ER) or long-acting opioid formulations, including situations when combined use may be indicated
- How to calculate appropriate equianalgesic doses of opioids when given patient-specific information

* English pharmacologist and recipient of the Nobel Prize in Physiology or Medicine in 1982 for his work in the understanding of how aspirin produced pain relief and anti-inflammatory effects.

CASE SCENARIO

A 49-year-old male with pancreatic cancer presents with pain in his abdomen radiating to his back. He has been prescribed morphine 15-mg tablets, 2 tablets every 4 hours as needed, and is taking his dose approximately four times per day, and his pain is now well controlled. He would like to switch to a regimen that allows him to take fewer opioids per day.

1. How do you convert the patient to ER 12-hour morphine tablets (available in 15-, 30-, 60-, and 100-mg tablets)?
2. If the ER morphine is not providing sufficient pain relief for acute pain flares, how will you treat his breakthrough pain? What opioid might you use?

The patient's pancreatic cancer has progressed, with new metastases to bone and lung. His pain is no longer well controlled on ER morphine 60 mg twice daily and morphine 15 mg every 4 hours as needed. When asked, he says that he has been taking 6 immediate-release (IR) morphine tablets daily. He is not experiencing any fatigue, nausea, or trouble breathing. Because of a new insurance restriction, he must be converted to IR and ER oxycodone for his long-acting baseline pain regimen. In this example, use a 33% reduction for incomplete cross-tolerance. IR oxycodone is available in 5-, 10-, 15-, 20-, and 30-mg tablets. ER oxycodone is available in 10-, 20-, 40-, 60-, and 80-mg tablets.

3. How will you convert his morphine to IR and ER oxycodone? What dose and frequency will you prescribe for him?

See the Case Scenario Revisited at end of the chapter for a detailed discussion on opioid dose conversions and appropriate calculations for the patient.

INTRODUCTION

Drugs used for pain management are categorized as standard systemic analgesic agents, including nonopioid and opioid analgesics, and other, neuromodulating, agents that are addressed in subsequent chapters. There is significant variability in individual response to analgesics, and choice of therapy should foremost include patient-specific consideration of balancing efficacy with tolerability. Combining analgesics with different mechanisms of action as a multimodal approach to therapy may result in enhanced analgesia while limiting dose-related toxicities due to the synergistic properties of the regimen. This chapter will focus on the role of nonopioid and opioid analgesics for the management of pain.

The next chapter will address neuromodulating agents, formerly referred to as "adjuvant analgesics." The term *adjuvant* was used historically to describe the neuromodulating agents, a misleading term for patients and others, implying that the neuromodulating class of agents is less effective or only utilized secondary to standard systemic analgesia—yet there are many circumstances in which this does not pertain. In many situations calling for immediate procedural pain control, so-called adjuvant analgesics (i.e., benzocaine or lidocaine) may be the only pain-relieving medication used during the procedure (e.g., suturing, dental work). This may be followed by treatment with a standard systemic analgesic to provide postprocedural pain relief as needed, but in this case, the neuromodulating agent is clearly the primary pain-relieving drug, and not an adjuvant.

NONOPIOID ANALGESICS

Acetaminophen

Acetaminophen is widely utilized for its analgesic and antipyretic properties. It is approved by the US Food and Drug Administration (FDA) as safe and effective when used appropriately. The exact mechanism by which acetaminophen exerts its analgesic effect is unclear but is likely related to inhibition of the cyclooxygenase-3 (COX-3) enzyme resulting in the inhibition of central prostaglandin synthesis and elevation of the pain threshold. However, it has no clinically significant anti-inflammatory effect at therapeutic doses. When administered orally, acetaminophen reaches maximum plasma concentrations within 1 hour in adults and has an oral bioavailability of 85 to 98%. In healthy adults, acetaminophen has a half-life of approximately 2.4 hours.

Acetaminophen is available in various formulations, including tablets and capsules (80 mg, 325 mg, 500 mg, or 650 mg), oral suspension (160 mg/5 mL), rectal suppositories (80 mg), and intravenous (IV) solution (10 mg/mL).

The recommended oral dose for infants and children is 10 to 15 mg/kg/dose. It is the most widely used antipyretic and pain reliever in children. For many, myalgias and skin allodynia will accompany fever, so treatment of fever with acetaminophen or nonsteroidal anti-inflammatory drugs (NSAIDs) provides important symptomatic relief. It is possible to develop an allergy to acetaminophen, and the medication should be held if a rash or other symptoms of allergy develop. Although there has been some question about the development of asthma, this remains controversial and is not viewed as a contraindication to use of acetaminophen in infants and children. By contrast, aspirin has been associated with Reye syndrome in adolescents and teens and should be avoided in those with any possibility of chickenpox, so acetaminophen has an important role as a safe alternative for management of fever and minor pain in children. Nonaspirin NSAIDs are also used for pediatric pain and fever.

The recommended oral dose for mild to moderate pain in adults is 500 to 650 mg every 4 hours. A maximum single dose of no more than 1,000 mg can also be used utilized. Acetaminophen IV solution can be used adjunctively with opioids in patients with moderate to severe pain. Dosing of the IV solution in patients who weigh more than 50 kg is 1,000 mg IV every 6 hours or 650 mg IV every 4 hours. Because of the high oral bioavailability of acetaminophen, no dose adjustment is necessary when converting from an oral to IV dose. Dosing intervals should be extended to every 6 or 8 hours in patients with renal impairment (glomerular filtration rate <50 mL/min). The maximum daily dose of acetaminophen should not exceed 4,000 mg/day in the absence of hepatic or renal disease, concomitant hepatotoxic drugs, malnutrition (due to lack of glutathione stores), or alcohol use. The use of acetaminophen should be limited to less than 2,000 mg/day in hepatic disease, and liver function should be monitored closely.

Acetaminophen is widely recommended for various acute and chronic pain syndromes. Tension headache is the most common form of headache and may respond especially well to acetaminophen; doses of 1,000 mg were comparable to 400 mg of ibuprofen, and caffeine-aspirin-acetaminophen combination products demonstrate more efficacy than acetaminophen alone. Extended periods of daily dosing with acetaminophen (or NSAIDs) may lead to chronic daily headache. For acute low back pain, however, acetaminophen was not different from placebo.[1] Although recommended for arthritis pain, there is no evidence to support the use of acetaminophen alone for the management of chronic low back pain.[1] The efficacy of both oral and IV acetaminophen for perioperative pain management has been demonstrated in studies involving orthopedic surgeries, and use as a component of multimodal analgesia may reduce postoperative opioid requirements.[2]

Acetaminophen is generally considered safe when taken within therapeutic doses. It is largely metabolized by the liver through conjugation with glucuronide or sulfate or through oxidation by the cytochrome P450 (CYP) 2E1 enzyme. Oxidation by the CYP2E1 pathway produces the hepatotoxic metabolite, *N*-acetyl-*p*-benzoquinone imine (NAPQI), which is then conjugated with glutathione to produce nontoxic metabolites. Patients with liver damage are at an increased risk for acetaminophen toxicity, particularly due to NAPQI accumulation. Adverse effects may include nausea, vomiting, or mild and reversible elevation in liver function tests. At higher doses or when used in patients with risk factors, hepatotoxicity can develop, leading to an increased risk for death. Acute overdoses can be treated with *N*-acetylcysteine. In general, there is minimal risk for drug–drug interactions with acetaminophen use. Coadministration with isoniazid can increase the risk for hepatotoxicity due to inhibition of CYP2E1-mediated metabolism of acetaminophen, and when used with warfarin, acetaminophen may inhibit warfarin metabolism or interfere with clotting factor formation, resulting in an increased risk for bleeding. Carbamazepine, an anticonvulsant used for trigeminal neuralgia, can increase acetaminophen metabolism, resulting in abnormally high levels of hepatotoxic metabolites.

NONSTEROIDAL ANTI-INFLAMMATORY DRUGS

NSAIDs are versatile analgesics. They are commonly utilized for general mild to moderate pain as well as pain that is associated with osteoarthritis, rheumatoid arthritis, bursitis, tendonitis, ankylosing spondylosis, gout, migraine, menorrhagia, pericarditis, and bone pain. They are also available in numerous formulations, including oral tablets, capsules, and suspensions, IV solutions (e.g., ketorolac and ibuprofen), and commercially available topical gel, patch, and solution (e.g., diclofenac). NSAIDs can also be compounded alone or in combination with other analgesics (e.g., ketamine, lidocaine) for topical use. An advantage of topical NSAIDs is limited systemic absorption, which ranges from 3 to 10%; therefore, these formulations may be ideal for patients at risk for adverse events. IV ibuprofen is also indicated for the management of moderate to severe pain as an adjunct to opioid analgesics in adults and children 6 months and older. Parenteral and intranasal ketorolac can also be used for moderate to severe acute pain as an alternative to an opioid, but this use is limited to no more than 5 consecutive days. Select NSAIDs are marketed in combination with gastroprotective agents (e.g., proton pump inhibitors, misoprostol) to improve tolerability, and naproxen is available in combination with sumatriptan for the acute treatment of migraine attacks. Nano-formulated NSAIDs are manufactured through a process that can produce drug particles that are approximately 10 times smaller than conventional drug particles, thereby increasing the total surface area of the particle, which allows for faster dissolution of the drug and achievement of analgesia at lower doses.

Ibuprofen is most commonly formulated as a free acid but can be prepared in a ionylated salt form in combination with sodium, lysine, or arginine. Clinical trials have demonstrated that these alternative formulations have faster absorption times and higher peak plasma concentrations, and they are associated with greater likelihood of pain relief and longer pain-free periods. Currently, these salted formulations are not widely available, but in the United States, ibuprofen-sodium may be purchased over-the-counter as Advil Filmtabs. Clinical trials of dental pain indicate that 200-mg (equivalent) doses of ibuprofen-sodium were comparable to 400-mg doses of standard ibuprofen.

COX isoenzymes are responsible for various physiologic responses, some of which are directly related to the pathophysiology of pain. The COX-1 isoenzyme is expressed in most tissues and is responsible for prostaglandin synthesis and maintenance of normal renal function, gastric mucosal integrity, and hemostasis, while the COX-2 isoenzyme is mostly expressed in the brain, kidney, bones, and reproductive organs and is inducible in response to inflammatory mediators. NSAIDs produce anti-inflammatory, antipyretic, and analgesic effects without steroidal activity by decreasing the production of prostaglandins through the inhibition of the COX-1 and COX-2 isoenzymes. NSAID use is associated with reversible inhibition of these isoenzymes, with the exception of aspirin, which causes irreversible inhibition, most notably within platelets. NSAIDs differ based on their chemical structure (Table 9.1), selectivity for these COX isoenzymes (Table 9.2), and pharmacokinetic profile, specifically with regard to plasma half-life and dosing (Table 9.3).[3,4] Selective inhibitors of COX-2 were developed to provide similar efficacy to traditional NSAIDs with improved gastrointestinal (GI) tolerability. Most of these agents, with the exception of celecoxib, are no longer on the US market because of their adverse cardiovascular profile.

Table 9.1 Chemical Classes of Nonsteroidal Anti-Inflammatory Drugs

Acetic acids	Etodolac, indomethacin, ketorolac, nabumetone, sulindac, tolmetin
Diarylheterocyclics	Celecoxib, valdecoxib
Enolic acids	Meloxicam, piroxicam
Fenamic acids	Meclofenamate
Phenylacetic acids	Diclofenac, lumiracoxib
Propionic acids	Fenoprofen, flurbiprofen, ibuprofen, ketoprofen, naproxen, oxaprozin
Salicylates	Aspirin, choline magnesium trisalicylate, diflunisal, magnesium salicylate, salsalate
Sulfones	Etoricoxib, rofecoxib

From Brunton LL, Hilal-Dandan R, Knollmann BC. Goodman & Gilman's: The Pharmacological Basis of Therapeutics (13th ed.; 2017). Available at: http://accesspharmacy.mhmedical.com/content.aspx?sectionid=170271972&bookid=2189&jumpsectionID=172480663&Resultclick=2.

Table 9.2 Nonsteroidal Anti-Inflammatory Drug and Cyclooxygenase Isoenzyme Selectivity

COX-1 Selective[a]	Nonselective	COX-2 Selective[b]
Ketorolac	Ibuprofen	Lumiracoxib
Flurbiprofen	Diflunisal	Etoricoxib
Ketoprofen		Rofecoxib
Indomethacin		Etodolac
Tolmetin		Valdecoxib
Aspirin		Celecoxib
Nabumetone		Diclofenac
Fenoprofen		Meloxicam
Meclofenamate		
Sulindac		
Naproxen		
Piroxicam		

[a]Listed in order of decreasing COX-1 selectivity.
[b]Listed in order of decreasing COX-2 selectivity.
From Brunton LL, Hilal-Dandan R, Knollmann BC. Goodman & Gilman's: The Pharmacological Basis of Therapeutics (13th ed.; 2017). Available at: http://accesspharmacy.mhmedical.com/content.aspx?sectionid=170271972&bookid=2189&jumpsectionID=172480663&Resultclick=2.

With numerous NSAIDs available, it is important to note that there is significant interpatient variability with regard to efficacy and safety between these drugs. This is presumed to be related to aforementioned differences, including varying chemical structures. Therefore, treatment failure with one NSAID may not preclude the use of an alternative NSAID if chosen from a different chemical class. Furthermore, the lowest effective dose of an NSAID should be used for the shortest amount of time, especially in older adults because of increased sensitivity to adverse effects.

Adverse events associated with NSAIDs affect several systems, including the GI tract, cardiovascular system, kidneys, and liver. Common GI-related adverse effects include dyspepsia and nausea; however, serious complications can occur, including gastric or duodenal ulcers with bleeding or perforation. Risk factors include alcohol use, *Helicobacter pylori* infection, smoking, and concomitant use of drugs that confer GI risks (e.g., corticosteroids). COX-2 inhibitors are less likely to cause gastric ulcers compared with equivalent doses of nonselective NSAIDs, and the rate of developing ulcers is reduced with coadministration of a gastroprotective agent such as a proton pump inhibitor.

NSAIDs can increase blood pressure as well as the risk for heart failure and serious cardiovascular thrombotic events, including myocardial infarction and stroke. This risk can occur early in treatment and may increase with duration of use. The risk for cardiovascular events from NSAID use is influenced by dose, half-life, degree of COX-2 selectivity, potency, and treatment duration. Use of COX-2 selective inhibitors,

Table 9.3 Comparison of Nonsteroidal Anti-Inflammatory Drugs Based on Half-Life and Dosing

NSAID	Half-Life (hr)	Initial Oral Adult Dose for Pain	Maximum Daily Dose
Meclofenamate	0.8–2.1	50 to 100 mg every 4 to 6 hours	400 mg
Diclofenac	1–2	50 mg 3 times daily	NA
Ibuprofen	~2	400 mg every 4 to 6 hours	3,200 mg
Ketoprofen	2–4	25 to 50 mg every 6 to 8 hours	300 mg
Fenoprofen	~3	200 mg every 4 to 6 hours	3,200 mg
Indomethacin	2.6–11.2	20 mg 3 times daily or 40 mg 2 or 3 times daily	200 mg
Aspirin	3–6	325 to 650 mg as needed every 4 hours	4,000 mg
Tolmetin	1–5	400 mg 3 times daily	1,800 mg
Ketorolac[a]	~5	10 mg every 4 to 6 hours	40 mg
Flurbiprofen	4.7–5.7	200 to 300 mg/day in 2 to 4 divided doses	NA
Etodolac	6.4	200 to 400 mg every 6 to 8 hours	1,000 mg
Sulindac	7.8	150 mg twice daily	400 mg
Celecoxib	~11	200 mg once daily or 100 mg twice daily	NA
Diflunisal	8–12	1,000 mg followed by 500 mg every 12 hours	1,500 mg
Naproxen	12–17	500 mg every 12 hours or 250 mg every 6 to 8 hours	~1,000 mg
Meloxicam	15–22	5 mg once daily	15 mg (tablets) 10 mg (capsules)
Nabumetone	~24	1.000 mg once daily	NA
Piroxicam	50	20 mg once daily	NA
Oxaprozin	41–55	1,200 mg once daily	1,800 mg or 26 mg/kg

[a]Maintenance dosing following intravenous or intramuscular use; should not be used for more than 5 consecutive days, including all routes of administration.

NA = not available.

From Nonsteroidal anti-inflammatory drugs. Drug Facts and Comparisons. Facts & Comparisons [database online]. St. Louis: Wolters Kluwer Health; May 2017. Accessed December 14, 2017

including diclofenac, should be reserved for patients without cardiac risk factors who are at risk for GI adverse effects. NSAIDs are contraindicated for the treatment of perioperative pain in the setting of coronary artery bypass graft surgery.

NSAID-induced impairment of renal function may result from inhibition of renal prostaglandin synthesis, which may cause renal insufficiency and nephrotic syndrome. Elevated hepatic enzymes occur in up to 15% of patients receiving systemic NSAIDs.

Chronic use of diclofenac is associated with a higher rate of hepatic injury compared with other NSAIDs. It is recommended that NSAIDs be avoided in advanced hepatic or renal disease.

There are several drug interactions to consider with the use of NSAIDs. The combination of an NSAID with an angiotensin-converting enzyme inhibitor can reduce renal function and cause significant hyperkalemia, resulting in a cardiac arrhythmia in patients with risk factors. Corticosteroids and serotonergic medications (e.g., selective serotonin reuptake inhibitors [SSRIs]) can increase the risk for GI-related adverse events. Coadministration with warfarin can result in altered bleeding risk, which is variable based on which NSAID is used. NSAIDs can reduce renal clearance of lithium, leading to toxicity. Finally, NSAIDs are highly protein bound, and when combined with other drugs with similar protein binding, this could lead to drug displacement, higher concentrations of free drug, and an increased risk for toxicity.

OPIOIDS

Opioids have been used for thousands of years for pain management; however, their place in therapy remains controversial, especially for the management of chronic pain. Following several decades during which opioids were prescribed for only patients with severe pain in the setting of life-limiting illness, increased opioid utilization for chronic noncancer pain occurred in the early 2000s. A dramatic rise in opioid overdose deaths led the Centers for Disease Control and Prevention to declare an opioid crisis and issue stringent new guidelines for prescription of opioids.[5] Recognizing both the potential benefits and risks of opioid therapy in the treatment of acute and chronic pain is essential for the clinician to treat patients in pain effectively with or intentionally without opioid therapy. In the absence of comprehensive pain management incorporating self-management approaches, psychological involvement, and physical therapies, opioids may not be appropriate for treatment of chronic noncancer pain. Even in acute care settings, where opioids remain a central component of perioperative and periprocedural pain management, assessment and mitigation of opioid risks are necessary before initiating therapy.

Opioids act on the mu, kappa, and delta receptors. These opioid receptors normally bind to endogenous ligands, including enkephalins, endorphins, and dynorphins. All opioid receptors are G protein coupled and are found in the central nervous system, where they can affect the descending modulation of pain signals. Opioid receptors are also located in the GI tract, cardiac tissue, immune system, vas deferens, and limbs. Agonist activity at the μ-opioid receptor is primarily associated with the analgesic effect observed by opioids, while action at delta and kappa receptors contributes to the analgesic effect to a lesser degree. Opioids are thought to be most effective for moderate to severe nociceptive pain, such as pain from acute trauma, postsurgical pain, and cancer pain. When used appropriately, opioids can have dramatic benefits, including reduction in pain intensity, increased function, and improved quality of life. Opioids can be delivered to patients enterally by the mouth or rectum, or parentally though the IV, subcutaneous, transdermal, epidural, intrathecal, sublingual, intra-articular, intranasal, and inhaled routes of administration. This means that without regard to a patient's medical condition, there is likely

Table 9.4 Classification of Opioids

Phenanthrenes	Diphenylheptanes	Phenylpiperidines	Miscellaneous
Full agonists			
Morphine	Propoxyphene[a]	Fentanyl	Levorphanol[b]
Codeine	Methadone[b,c]	Meperidine[c]	Tapentadol[c]
Hydromorphone		Sufentanil	**Weak agonists**
Hydrocodone		Alfentanil	Tramadol[c]
Oxymorphone		Loperamide[d]	**Mixed/partial agonists**
Oxycodone		Diphenoxylate[d]	Butorphanol
Mixed/partial agonists			
Buprenorphine			
Nalbuphine			
Antagonists			
Naloxone			
Naltrexone			

[a]No longer on the market in the United States.
[b]Also has effects as an NMDA receptor antagonist.
[c]Also a monoamine reuptake inhibitor.
[d]Do not cross the blood–brain barrier or provide analgesia at therapeutic doses; are used to treat diarrhea.
From Drewes AM, Jensen RD, Nielsen LM, et al. Differences between opioids: pharmacological, experimental, clinical and economical perspectives. Br J Clin Pharmacol. 2013;75(1):60–78.

to be an effective way of providing analgesia with an opioid, which may not be available with other analgesics.

Opioids are categorized by chemical structure or action at the opioid receptors (Table 9.4).[6,7] There are three major chemical classes of opioids: phenanthrenes, diphenylheptanes, and phenylpiperidines. This can be clinically relevant when discussing patient allergies to medications; for example, if a patient is truly allergic to a phenanthrene opioid (e.g., morphine), a phenylpiperidine opioid or diphenylheptane opioid may provide a safer alternative. Opioids also vary based on receptor activity, that is, agonism (Table 9.5).[8] An opioid may be an agonist at one receptor while simultaneously being an antagonist at another receptor. For example, butorphanol is a kappa receptor agonist and a partial agonist or a mixed agonist–antagonist with low activity at the μ-opioid receptor. Additionally, because butorphanol produces less effect at the μ-opioid receptor, it may produce less respiratory depression than morphine at equivalent doses.

Class Effects of Opioids

All opioids are known to cause sedation, constipation, nausea, somnolence, respiratory depression, dizziness, vomiting, delirium, physical dependence, and withdrawal.[9] Other potential adverse effects include euphoria, dysphoria, pruritus, hypogonadism, sexual dysfunction, urinary retention, and anxiety. Potential signs of opioid intoxication include respiratory depression, sedation, unresponsiveness, and miosis. Opioid intoxication can lead to death from respiratory suppression. Opioid

Table 9.5 Opioid Agonist Receptor Adverse Effects

Mu	Kappa	Delta
Physical dependence	Sedation	Physical dependence
Respiratory depression	Miosis	Antidepressant effects
Miosis	Dysphoria	
Euphoria	Cough suppression	
Reduced gastrointestinal motility		
Cough suppression		

From Fine PG, Portenoy RK. A Clinical Guide to Opioid Analgesia. Minneapolis: Healthcare Information Programs; 2004; Stein C, et al. Nature 2003.

intoxication and overdose are more likely to occur in the presence of drug interactions, especially with additionally sedating medications such as benzodiazepines, but they can also occur when illicit sources surreptitiously supply higher potency opioids. Opioid overdose is considered a medical emergency and should be reversed with an opiate antagonist such as naloxone, described in detail later.

Patients typically develop physical dependence to opioids with chronic opioid dosing. Abrupt withdrawal of opioid medications in these patients causes intense pain, restlessness, sweating, hypertension, insomnia, diarrhea, and anxiety. Nonetheless, withdrawal from opioids alone in an otherwise healthy patient is not fatal. For this reason, full reversal of opioid agonists with an opioid antagonist in an emergency situation is the most prudent action to take. Paradoxically, chronic opioid use has been observed to cause hyperalgesia and is associated with reduced pain thresholds and tolerance; the exact mechanisms accounting for these changes are unknown.

Tolerance and physical dependence are expected with continuous opioid dosing. Repeated doses of opioids may lead to tolerance, which means that increased doses would be needed to produce stable levels of analgesia. However, with dose escalation, the likelihood of serious adverse events such as misuse or respiratory depression may occur. Therefore, a risk–benefit assessment is important before initiation and then continuously throughout therapy. Opioid misuse is defined as taking more medication than prescribed, which may lead to the precipitation of withdrawal. Misuse can increase the risk for abuse. Common methods of opioid abuse include altering the route of administration (i.e., insufflation or injection of an oral tablet), altering the dosage form (e.g., manipulating an ER formulation to release over a shorter period of time, causing higher drug levels in the body), or obtaining drug from other sources, including other providers and nonmedical sources. Aberrant behaviors exist on a spectrum, and it can be difficult for clinicians to objectively determine the risk for misuse and abuse. There are a number of tools aimed to help clinicians screen patients before therapy or to screen for misuse during therapy (see Chapter 20 for details).

Phenanthrenes

The oldest form of exogenous opioid was derived from the opium plant *Papaver somniferum* and the naturally occurring opioid alkaloid morphine, which was isolated from the opium poppy in 1806.[10] Other naturally occurring opioids include codeine, thebaine, and papaverine. Subsequent chemical manipulations of morphine yielded a variety of other opioids, such as hydrocodone, oxycodone, oxymorphone, and hydromorphone. The class of opioids that are chemically related to morphine is called phenanthrenes.

Full Agonists

Morphine Morphine is a full agonist at the μ-opioid receptor that is responsible for its analgesic effect. Morphine is approved for use in the management of moderate to severe acute and chronic pain and is available in a number of formulations and various strengths for oral, rectal, topical, IV, and neuraxial administration. Appropriate dosing of IR oral morphine for acute pain in an opioid-naïve patient is 7.5 to15 mg every 4 hours. The usual starting IV dose is three times less than that of oral dosing because of greater bioavailability (e.g., 2.5 to 5 mg IV every 4 hours). Morphine is well absorbed from the GI tract with an oral bioavailability of 40%. The maximum analgesic effect of morphine occurs approximately 15 minutes after IV administration, with 80% of its analgesic effect observed after 6 minutes. Maximum analgesic effect occurs approximately 60 minutes after oral ingestion. Specific plasma levels of morphine (and other opioids) do not correlate with interpatient safety or efficacy and can vary widely. Morphine undergoes phase II metabolism in the liver by the uridine diphosphate glucuronosyltransferase system (UGT), in particular UGT 2B7, primarily to active metabolites morphine-3-glucuronide (M3G) and morphine-6-glucuronide (M6G), and to a lesser extent hydromorphone. M3G and M6G are excreted in urine. The elimination half-life of morphine is approximately 2 hours. In patients with renal impairment, morphine has been associated with increased risk for toxicity due to reduced clearance of active metabolites.[11]

Codeine Codeine is a natural phenanthrene opioid isolated from the opium poppy. Codeine itself has no analgesic activity in vivo and must be converted to an active form primarily through CYP2D6-mediated metabolism to morphine. Codeine metabolism is highly variable and subject to both decreased and increased metabolism; this variable metabolism can affect certain ethnic groups more prominently. The FDA has issued a contraindication for use of codeine for children 12 years and younger and a warning regarding the use of codeine for those age 12 to 18 years with conditions that increase risk for serious breathing problems as well as a warning for mothers against breastfeeding while taking codeine.

Hydromorphone Hydromorphone is a semisynthetic derivative of morphine, first developed in 1926, and has commonly been used as an alternative to morphine. Hydromorphone has a similar chemical structure to morphine but is more lipophilic, lipid soluble, and potent. This allows for a smaller overall dose of hydromorphone to produce the same analgesic effect. However, the most common adverse effects (e.g., constipation, nausea) still occur at therapeutic doses. Hydromorphone is well absorbed after oral administration with a bioavailability of 60%. Onset of analgesia is approximately 30 minutes after oral administration, and peak analgesic effect occurs within 1 hour. Hydromorphone primarily undergoes phase II metabolism to inactive metabolites, including hydromorphone-3-glucuronide (H3G). These metabolites are primarily excreted in the urine with a terminal half-life of 2 to 3 hours. Appropriate oral dosing of hydromorphone for moderate to severe pain in an opioid-naïve patient is 2 to 4 mg every 4 hours as needed. Hydromorphone is available in IR oral tablets and liquid, rectal suppository, solution for injection, and a once-daily ER oral tablets.

Hydrocodone Hydrocodone is a semisynthetic derivative of codeine and is partially active at the μ-opioid receptors. Hydrocodone is also metabolized in the body to hydromorphone, which is expected to contribute to some of its analgesic effect. When administered orally, hydrocodone has approximately the same analgesic potency of morphine. Compared with codeine, hydrocodone crosses the blood–brain barrier more rapidly, relating to a higher potential for abuse. Hydrocodone is commonly formulated with other analgesics such as acetaminophen or ibuprofen and is well-absorbed after oral administration. Analgesic effect is expected 30 minutes after oral administration, with peak effect expected within approximately 90 minutes. Hydrocodone is metabolized by CYP3A4 to an inactive metabolite (norhydrocodone) and by CYP2D6 to an active metabolite (hydromorphone). Inactive metabolites of hydrocodone are excreted through urine with a terminal half-life between 3 and 4 hours. Appropriate oral dosing of IR hydrocodone combination tablets in an opiate-naïve patient is 5 to 10 mg every 4 hours as needed. Hydrocodone is available in a number of combination tablets, combination liquids, and ER capsules and tablets.

Oxymorphone Oxymorphone is a semisynthetic derivative of morphine and is a full agonist at μ-opioid receptors. Oxymorphone is more lipid soluble than morphine or oxycodone and crosses the blood–brain barrier more quickly. Oxymorphone is metabolized extensively through first-pass metabolism and has an oral bioavailability of approximately 10%. Despite low oral bioavailability, oxymorphone is expected to be approximately three times more potent than morphine at a given dose level. Onset of analgesia occurs approximately 15 to 30 minutes after ingestion, and peak analgesia occurs after 30 to 60 minutes. Oxymorphone is metabolized extensively by the UGT system primarily to oxymorphone-3-glucuronide, which has an unknown analgesic activity. The elimination half-life of oxymorphone is approximately 8 hours, leading to an expected analgesic effect window of 4 to 6 hours. An appropriate starting dose of oxymorphone in an opioid-naïve patient is 5 mg every 4 to 6 hours as needed. Oxymorphone is available as IR tablets, solution for injection, and ER tablets. ER oxymorphone was originally approved for use in 2006 for the management of moderate to severe pain around the clock. In 2012, oxymorphone ER was reformulated in an attempt to make the medication resistant to physical and chemical manipulation. This reformulation was approved by the FDA; however, the FDA determined that the data on the reformulation did not show that the reformulation could be expected to meaningfully reduce abuse. In 2017, after reports of IV abuse of the reformulation of oxymorphone ER being associated with a serious outbreak of HIV and hepatitis C as well as thrombotic microangiopathy, the FDA asked the manufacturer to remove the reformulation of oxymorphone ER tablets from the market.[13] The original oxymorphone ER tablet formulation is still available for use.

Oxycodone Oxycodone is a semisynthetic derivative of thebaine. Like hydrocodone, oxycodone is also metabolized in vivo to an active metabolite (oxymorphone); however, the clinical significance of this reaction is controversial. When given orally, it has a similar analgesic effect to morphine; however, when given neuraxially, it seems to be far less potent. Noroxycodone, a primary metabolite of oxycodone, does seem to have analgesic effect, but only at extremely high concentrations. Noroxycodone has the potential to be a neurotoxic metabolite that can accumulate in renal dysfunction at high doses. Oxycodone is well-absorbed after oral administration and has a bioavailability for IR formulations between 60 and 80%. Onset of analgesia occurs 15 minutes after oral administration, with maximal analgesic effect seen after approximately 60 minutes. Oxycodone is metabolized to oxymorphone by CYP2D6 and to noroxycodone by CYP3A4. Oxycodone and its metabolites are primarily excreted in the urine and have an elimination half-life of about 3 to 5 hours and an expected analgesic efficacy of 4 to 6 hours. An appropriate starting dose of oxycodone in an opiate-naïve patient would be 5 to 10 mg every 4 to 6 hours as needed. Oxycodone is available in IR tablets and liquids, combination tablets with acetaminophen or aspirin, ER tablets and capsules (as oxycodone base), and ER combination tablets and capsules formulated with an opioid antagonist intended to deter abuse.

Mixed Agonist–Antagonists

Buprenorphine Buprenorphine is a semisynthetic mixed opioid agonist–antagonist, with activity as a partial μ-opioid receptor agonist and an antagonist at the kappa- and delta-opioid receptors. Buprenorphine, in most formulations, is FDA approved for the treatment of opioid use disorder and is used off-label for pain. There is a transbuccal formulation of buprenorphine that is approved for chronic pain, but as noted in the package insert, it is "[t]o be prescribed only by health care providers knowledgeable in use of potent opioids for management of chronic pain." Buprenorphine binds more tightly to μ-opioid receptors than other opioid agonists, which has important clinical implications. At low doses, buprenorphine acts as a potent μ-opioid receptor agonist, effective for the treatment of pain. However, because it is a partial μ-opioid receptor agonist at higher doses, its agonist activity has a ceiling effect, particularly on respiratory depression. Therefore, buprenorphine at higher doses can be given with a lower likelihood of fatal respiratory events, while still occupying opioid receptors and potentially reducing cravings. Nonetheless, buprenorphine carries black box warnings for respiratory suppression and addiction and additional education (Risk Evaluation and Mitigation Strategies [REMS]) is required in order to prescribe this medication. The analgesic ceiling for buprenorphine occurs between 8 and 16 mg daily; the doses used for opioid use disorder are typically insufficient for severe, around-the-clock pain. Buprenorphine is extensively metabolized through first-pass metabolism when absorbed by the oral route but is highly lipophilic and readily absorbed when given sublingually and transdermally. Buprenorphine is metabolized to norbuprenorphine by CYP3A4 and other metabolites that are primarily excreted in the feces. Buprenorphine and norbuprenorphine have long half-lives (up to 26 hours). Low-dose buprenorphine for pain is administered by transdermal patches, IV injection, or sublingual tablets. Transdermal buprenorphine patches are applied once weekly and take approximately 24 hours to deliver a significant amount of buprenorphine, reaching steady state 3 days after application. Low-dose buprenorphine for chronic pain should only be initiated for patients requiring around-the-clock opioid analgesia of less than 80 daily oral morphine equivalents (OMEs). An appropriate starting dose of the transdermal patch in an opioid-naïve patient may be 5 μg/hour applied once weekly, or for the sublingual tablet, 75 μg twice daily.

Treatment of acute pain in patients maintained on high-dose buprenorphine may be challenging because of the long duration of action and receptor occupancy. If prescribed for pain, it is recommended that patients who are to undergo elective surgery be titrated off of buprenorphine 24 to 48 hours before the procedure and transitioned to an alternate opioid. If, however, buprenorphine is prescribed for addiction, the risk for a potential setback may be great, and continuing the buprenorphine may be indicated. Medication decisions should be individualized and coordinated with the prescriber. If buprenorphine is continued, nonopioid, interventional, and nonpharmacologic strategies should be maximized because pain can be difficult to manage with opioids. Patients may require higher doses of full opioid agonists in the postoperative period. In the case of low-dose buprenorphine, short-acting full opioid agonists can still be given to patients requiring medication for breakthrough pain as long as monitoring for respiratory suppression is available.

Antagonists

Naloxone Naloxone is a semisynthetic opioid receptor antagonist, structurally similar to oxymorphone. Naloxone can rapidly reverse the effects of opioid intoxication and is the drug of choice for reversal of opioid overdose by police and first responders. While naloxone can bind and quickly reverse the effect of an opioid overdose, its duration of action lasts only minutes, meaning that in the cases of an opioid overdose with an ER or long-acting opioid (e.g., methadone), multiple doses or a continuous infusion may be required. There are many state regulations making naloxone available without a prescription under a standing order between a local physician and a pharmacy. Naloxone itself cannot be misused or abused and will have minimal effect if given to a person not on an opioid. If given to a patient on chronic opioid therapy for pain, naloxone will reverse the analgesic effect as well as precipitate withdrawal. In most cases, opioid withdrawal is not fatal, but severe withdrawal may require intensive supportive care. In the event of an opioid overdose, intranasal, IV, or intramuscular naloxone should be administered, with a repeat dose within 2 to 3 minutes (Table 9.6).[9] Emergency services should be contacted at the time of naloxone administration. Naloxone can also be used to reverse suspected opioid intoxication (e.g., respiratory rate <8 breaths/min or O_2 sat <90% or Richmond Agitation and Sedation Scale (RASS) score of –4 or –5) in an acute care setting because of iatrogenic opioid escalation. In this case, 0.04 mg IV should be administered every 3 to 5 minutes until the patient recovers. Naloxone is formulated with a number of full agonists in ER formulations to discourage abuse. When taken orally as formulated in a combination tablet, naloxone has poor bioavailability and will not precipitate withdrawal when administered with an opioid agonist.

Naltrexone Naltrexone is a semisynthetic opioid receptor antagonist derived from thebaine that is structurally similar to oxymorphone, like naloxone. Unlike naloxone, naltrexone has better oral bioavailability and a longer duration of action. This is due to its relatively longer elimination half-life of 6 to 14 hours when given orally and 5 to 10 days when given intramuscularly. Naltrexone is generally not used in emergency situations to reverse an opioid overdose, owing to its long onset of action compared with naloxone. Like naloxone, it is sometimes formulated with ER opioid formulations to deter abuse. In such formulations, the naltrexone dose is not high enough to cause withdrawal when administered orally with an agonist, but is high enough to discourage

Table 9.6 Naloxone for Reversal of Opioid Overdose

Formulation	1 mg/mL needleless syringe (with nasal mucosal atomizer device)	4 mg/0.1 mL Nasal spray (Narcan)	0.4 mg/0.4 mL intramuscular injection (Evzio)	0.4 mg/mL intravenous solution
Route	Intranasal	Intranasal	Intramuscular (autoinjector)	Intravenous
Administration	Spray 1 mL in each nostril, may repeat after 2–3 minutes	Spray contents of entire syringe into one nostril, may repeat after 2–3 minutes	Inject into anterolateral aspect of thigh per audio directions, can repeat after 2–3 minutes	Inject 0.4 mg IV, may repeat after 2–3 minutes. Lower doses (0.04 mg) may be administered every 3–5 minutes for suspected intoxication

Clinical Pharmacology. Tampa: Elsevier; 2018. (Updated April 2018.) Available at: http://www.clinicalpharmacology-ip.com.

abuse by intranasal or IV routes. Naltrexone is indicated for the maintenance treatment of alcohol dependence and for the prevention of relapse of opioid use disorder following complete detoxification. It is available as an oral tablet that can be taken once daily or once every 3 days. It can also be given as a monthly intramuscular injection to aid with compliance. Patients should be off of opioids for at least 7 days before the administration of naltrexone to avoid precipitating withdrawal. Patients who have opioid use disorder must be counseled on the risk for fatal overdose in the event of resuming opioid agonist use. This can occur as the result of reduced tolerance and loss of naltrexone occupancy on opioid receptors.

Phenylpiperidines

Phenylpiperidine-type opioids refer to the synthetic opioids, which are structurally similar to meperidine. This class contains opioids that are important to the management of pain (fentanyl) as well as opioids that are of critical importance in anesthesia (sufentanil, remifentanil, and alfentanil). Additionally, the phenylpiperidines include peripherally acting loperamide and diphenoxylate, which have no analgesic effect because they lack the ability to cross the blood–brain barrier and are used in the treatment of diarrhea.

Meperidine

Meperidine was the first wholly synthetic opioid, and it is still used for the treatment of infusion-related rigors of amphotericin B and for postoperative shivering. Meperidine inhibits dopamine and norepinephrine transporters, similarly to cocaine, which may be responsible for greater euphoric effect and negative effects on cognition. Meperidine also acts as a serotonin reuptake inhibitor and can increase the risk for serotonin syndrome, especially when used in combination with other serotonergic drugs, especially monoamine oxidase (MAO) inhibitors. The primary metabolite (normeperidine) has an extremely long half-life, is neurotoxic, and can accumulate in renal dysfunction. In addition, meperidine neurotoxicity can manifest as hallucinations, myoclonus, and seizures. Its use is limited. Meperidine is available as an oral liquid, oral tablets, and solution for injection.

Fentanyl

Fentanyl is a synthetic opioid that was introduced in the late 1960s in an effort to replace morphine during cardiac surgery. Fentanyl is 75 to 100 times more potent than morphine and is much more lipophilic. When given parenterally, fentanyl has a rapid onset of action and reaches peak analgesic effect within minutes. Analgesia from a parenteral dose of fentanyl typically only lasts 1 hour. It can cross the blood–brain barrier rapidly, exert its action quickly, and therefore pose a higher risk for abuse. Fentanyl is not administered through the oral route because of extensive first-pass metabolism; however, it is readily absorbed into subcutaneous tissue from the skin. When given transdermally, fentanyl provides potent around-the-clock opioid analgesia. Transdermal fentanyl delivers medication to the subcutaneous fat of a patient at a constant rate, which is then released into the bloodstream at a steady rate. Transdermal fentanyl patches are replaced every 3 days, and steady state is achieved after 6 days at a specific dose level. Transdermal fentanyl should not be initiated in an opioid-naïve patient because of risks for sedation, respiratory depression, and overdose. Fentanyl is metabolized primarily by CYP3A4 to norfentanyl, an inactive metabolite. Potent CYP3A4 inhibitors like azole antifungals and nondihydropyridine calcium channel blockers can drastically affect the plasma levels of fentanyl. Any patients maintained on a transdermal fentanyl patch should have any changes to their medication regimen routinely assessed to identify drug interactions that could lead to opioid intoxication. Because fentanyl is primarily metabolized by the liver to inactive metabolites, it can be an appealing choice to use in patients with renal dysfunction. There are also a number of transmucosal immediate-release fentanyl (TIRF) products available to treat acute severe breakthrough pain in opioid-tolerant patients with cancer pain. TIRF products mimic the rapid onset of action of IV fentanyl; however, dosing between TIRF products is not equivalent to IV dosing, and there is no equivalency among the products. Therefore, prescribers are required to use product-specific prescribing information for dosing and titration. TIRF medications require enrollment into a REMS program before prescribing. TIRF medications should only be prescribed to patients who are opioid tolerant, are taking an ER or long-acting opioid, and have cancer pain.

Diphenylheptanes

The diphenylheptane opioids are the last major class of opioids. There remains only one diphenylheptane (methadone) still on the market after the removal of propoxyphene because of increased cardiotoxicity.

Methadone

Methadone is a synthetic, long-acting opioid agonist developed in Germany in the 1940s; for decades, it has been used for the treatment of chronic pain and opioid use disorder. Respiratory suppression is a major side effect that can result in death. Methadone has characteristics that can make it useful for pain management; however, it is a challenging drug because of safety concerns. Methadone has a dual mechanism of action as a full μ-opioid receptor agonist and an N-methyl-D-aspartate (NMDA) receptor antagonist, which makes methadone an appealing option to treat complex pain with mixed etiology (e.g., presence of both neuropathic and nociceptive pain). Methadone is a racemic mixture of both R- and S-methadone. The R-stereo isomer is responsible for the μ-opioid receptor actions, while the S-stereo isomer is responsible for the NMDA receptor antagonism and QTc-prolongation effects by action on the human ether-a-go-go (HERG) potassium channel. Methadone has a unique pharmacokinetic profile owing to its biphasic elimination by CYP3A4 and CYP2D6. Methadone is highly lipophilic and widely distributes in fat stores. The terminal half-life of methadone ranges from 6 to 150 hours, while the analgesic effect lasts for only 4 to 12 hours. Accumulation of the methadone will occur after repeated doses, making titration to effect a much slower process, ranging from days to weeks. Changes in methadone dosing should not occur more frequently than once every 5 to 7 days because attempts at more rapid titration can lead to fatal effects as doses accumulate and respiratory failure occurs. Methadone is not easily converted from other opioids because of the NMDA receptor antagonism, which can reverse opioid tolerance. As such, there is no linear conversion from other opioids to methadone, and at higher doses of other opioids, this conversion factor greatly increases. The nonlinear conversion, in addition to the cardiac conduction properties and numerous drug interactions, has resulted in deaths from methadone use to increase at a faster rate than any other drug-related fatality. Therefore, electrocardiographic (ECG) monitoring should be initiated with the use of methadone for chronic pain, and changes to the ECG should be monitored with dose increases and with the initiation of any medication that may interact with methadone. The long duration of action of methadone also makes it an appealing choice for opioid use disorder. For this indication, methadone is dosed once daily and must be dispensed from licensed methadone maintenance clinics. When patients on methadone maintenance therapy are admitted to an acute care setting, it is important to continue their daily methadone dose. If additional opioids are required to treat pain in a patient on methadone maintenance, short-acting full μ-opioid agonists are used. When initiating methadone in an opioid-naïve patient, an appropriate oral dose is 2.5 mg two or three times daily. Methadone is available in oral tablets, oral liquid, and solution for injection.

Miscellaneous

Tapentadol

Tapentadol is a synthetic centrally acting opioid analgesic originally approved by the FDA for the treatment of pain in 2008. In addition to action at the μ-opioid receptor, tapentadol is also a norepinephrine reuptake inhibitor, making it an appealing option for the treatment of both nociceptive and neuropathic pain. Tapentadol primarily undergoes metabolism to inactive metabolites by the UGT system, with contributions by CYP2C9, CYP2C19, and CYP2D6. Peak analgesia after oral tapentadol administration occurs after 60 to 90 minutes, with analgesic effect expected to last 4 to 6 hours. Tapentadol should be used with caution with other serotonergic agents, including SSRIs, selective serotonin/norepinephrine reuptake inhibitors (SNRIs), and MAO inhibitors. A typical starting dose of tapentadol in an opioid-naïve patient is 50 mg every 6 hours as needed. Tapentadol is also available in ER formulation, which is dosed every 12 hours. Unlike other opioids, tapentadol has a maximum daily dose of 600 mg for IR formulations and 500 mg for ER formulations, owing to toxicity from norepinephrine reuptake inhibition.

Tramadol

Tramadol is a synthetic opioid agonist with weak action at the μ-opioid receptor and also acts as an SNRI. Tramadol itself exerts very weak affinity for the μ-opioid receptor, while its metabolite, O-desmethyltramadol, is a more potent μ-opioid agonist. The majority of the analgesic effect of tramadol is derived primarily from the SNRI properties. Like tapentadol, tramadol must be used with caution with concomitant serotonergic agents, including other SSRIs and MAO inhibitors. Tramadol may be most useful in patients with mild to moderate pain, and patients with moderate to severe pain should be treated with more potent opioid analgesics like morphine. Like tapentadol, tramadol has a maximum daily dose of 400 mg per day for IR formulations and 300 mg per day for ER formulations. Tramadol is available as IR tablets, ER tablets, and IR combination tablets with acetaminophen.

Levorphanol

Levorphanol is a semisynthetic μ-opioid agonist that is structurally similar to dextromethorphan and has many unique properties compared with other phenanthrene opioids. Levorphanol exhibits strong NMDA receptor antagonism and weak monoamine reuptake inhibition, which may be useful in the treatment of neuropathic pain. Levorphanol also demonstrates a long duration of action, ranging from 6 to 15 hours. Unlike methadone, levorphanol does not act on the HERG potassium channel in cardiac tissue, resulting in a lower risk for QTc prolongation. Levorphanol undergoes phase II metabolism by the UGT system to an active metabolite (levorphanol-3-glucuronide) and is excreted in the urine with an elimination half-life of 11 to 16 hours, which increases up to 30 hours in the setting of chronic dosing, After oral dosing, the peak analgesic effect is observed approximately within 1 hour. Because of NMDA receptor antagonism, conversion from other opioids must be done with caution owing to potential for reversal of opioid tolerance. Despite the potential utility in complex pain syndromes, levorphanol has been available in limited supply, resulting in higher costs and lower clinical utilization. An appropriate oral dose for pain requiring around-the-clock opioid therapy in an opioid-naïve patient is 2 mg every 12 hours. Levorphanol is available as oral tablets and solution for injection.

Principles of Around-the-Clock Opioid Dosing and a Primer on Opioid Conversion

Patients with moderate to severe around-the-clock pain (e.g., cancer pain) may require an analgesic regimen that provides adequate pain relief and restoration of function.

Long-acting and ER opioids provide a way for patients to take medication less often while achieving adequate pain relief. Long-acting and ER opioids should (1) not be prescribed by providers who have not completed the required REMS training, and (2) not be started in opioid-naïve patients except under special circumstances, such as the initiation of methadone or levorphanol in a complex pain state with nociceptive and neuropathic characteristics. After a patient has been titrated to the lowest effective dose of a short-acting opioid, it may be appropriate to convert most of the patient's opioid requirement into an ER or long-acting opioid to provide around-the-clock analgesia. Most short-acting opioids are also available in ER formulations; therefore, conversions between these two formulations are generally straightforward. For example, if a patient is taking oxycodone IR 5 mg every 4 hours, the total daily dose of oxycodone is calculated as 30 mg. ER oxycodone is available in numerous strengths and is dosed to be taken every 12 hours; therefore, in this scenario, the new regimen would be oxycodone ER 15 mg every 12 hours. However, often because of price or insurance coverage issues, short-acting strong opioids may need to be converted to a different opioid agonist. As such, it is necessary to convert one opioid to another based on analgesic potency. Through years of clinical experience, animal models, and single-dose human studies, many opioid conversion tables have been developed to help guide clinicians; however, these tables are not infallible and are often used as a starting point when discussing opioid conversions. Equianalgesic doses of opioids are included in Tables 9.7–9.10.[14]

Opioid conversion tables provide the equianalgesic doses of different opioids and at a variety of routes. For example, 30 mg of oral morphine is equianalgesic to 10 mg of parenteral morphine and 20 mg of oral oxycodone. This provides a clinician with a reasonable starting point to convert between the various opioids. With chronic opioid dosing, tolerance develops, which results in a higher dose of an opioid to achieve the same analgesic effect. However, when converting between different opioid analgesics, the tolerance obtained to one agent does not completely occur with others, a phenomenon called *incomplete cross-tolerance*. Therefore, a dose reduction is often necessary to ensure that the new opioid regimen will not precipitate opioid intoxication or overdose. While there are no specific guidelines, it is generally recommended to reduce the dose by 25 to 50% or more based on patient-specific factors, including current level of analgesia, adverse effects, and medical comorbidities. In patients who are experiencing inadequate analgesia before conversion, a conservative reduction would be warranted. In patients with adequate pain relief who are experiencing opioid-related

Table 9.7 Equianalgesic Doses for Select Opioids

Drug	Oral/Rectal (mg)	Parenteral (mg)
Morphine	30	10
Oxycodone HCl	20	—
Hydrocodone	30	—
Hydromorphone	7.5	1.5
Fentanyl	—	0.1 (100 µg)
Oxymorphone	10	1

Table 9.8 Equianalgesic Conversion Table for Opioids

Oral/Rectal Dose (mg)	Opioid Analgesic	Parenteral Dose (mg)
30	Morphine	10
0.4 (sublingual)	Buprenorphine	0.3
200	Codeine	100
—	Fentanyl	0.1
30	Hydrocodone	—
7.5	Hydromorphone	1.5
20	Oxycodone	—
10	Oxymorphone	1
50–75	Tapentadol	—
120	Tramadol	—

adverse effects like nausea or somnolence, a more aggressive dose reduction should be considered.

The use of an opioid around the clock for persistent pain is often sufficient to provide adequate analgesia. However, some patients may experience breakthrough pain, which is a phenomenon of predictable or unpredictable pain that can occur with or without physical activity or other voluntary or involuntary movements (e.g., sneezing). It is best described in cancer pain syndromes but can also occur in noncancer pain syndromes. In these cases, it may be necessary to provide access to a short-acting opioid to manage acute pain flares on an as-needed basis. If the short-acting opioid is used at the maximum allowed frequency for an extended period of time, the dosing of the ER or long-acting formulation should be adjusted. No specific guidelines for the management of breakthrough pain exist, but it is generally recommended that a single breakthrough dose should be 10 to 15% of the total daily dose of the ER or long-acting opioid. Examples of various opioid equianalgesic conversions are shown in the Case Scenario Revisited at the end of this chapter.

Table 9.9 Equianalgesic Conversion for Transdermal Fentanyl

Oral 24-Hour Morphine Equivalent (mg/day)	Transdermal Fentanyl Dose (mcg/hour)
60–134	25
135–224	50
225–314	75
315–404	100
405–494	125
495–584	150
585–674	175
675–764	200
765–854	225
855–944	250
945–1034	275
1035–1124	300

Table 9.10 Equianalgesic Conversion for Methadone

Oral 24-Hour Morphine Equivalent (mg/day)	Dose Ratio (Morphine:Methadone)
<100	4:1
101–300	8:1
301–600	10:1
601–800	12:1
801–1000	15:1
≥1001	20:1

SUMMARY

The approach to pain management should be individualized and should integrate the use of multimodal analgesia whenever possible. Nonopioid analgesics can be used in combination with opioid therapy to minimize adverse effects and facilitate achievement of therapeutic goals that are appropriate for the patient and the clinical scenario. When used appropriately, opioids can be an effective treatment modality for acute or chronic pain because of the availability of various agents with differing pharmacologic profiles and routes of administration. The use of an opioid should be considered when benefits outweigh the potential risks and should be used at the lowest dose for the shortest duration of time when possible. Continuation of therapy without a corresponding benefit can lead to severe long-term consequences such as misuse, addiction, overdose, and death.

REVIEW QUESTIONS

1. Which one of the following statements regarding NSAIDs for pain management is/are TRUE? Select all that apply.
   a. There is significant interpatient variability with regard to their efficacy.
   b. There is significant interpatient variability with regard to their safety.
   c. They are only available in oral formulations.
   d. They are effective alone for severe acute and chronic pain.

2. A 41-year-old man with acute shoulder pain presents to the ambulatory care clinic after taking over-the-counter ibuprofen for 2 weeks with no relief. He reports that his pain is of moderate intensity and is intermittent. The pain has not limited his function or ability to work. He is requesting an analgesic to take as needed. His past medical history is noncontributory. He is allergic to sulfa drugs (anaphylaxis). Which of the following is the *most* appropriate analgesic option for this patient?
   a. Acetaminophen 1,000 mg given orally every 4 hours around the clock
   b. Celecoxib 200 mg given orally every 12 hours around the clock
   c. Meloxicam 7.5 mg given orally once daily as needed
   d. Hydrocodone/acetaminophen 5 mg given orally every 4 hours as needed

3. A 59-year-old patient is experiencing acute pain in the knees due to osteoarthritis. Past medical history is significant for hypertension,

renal impairment, and coronary artery disease. Which of the following nonopioid analgesics is most appropriate for acute pain management?
a. Ibuprofen
b. Indomethacin
c. Ketorolac
d. Topical diclofenac

4. Which one of the following nonopioid analgesics should be avoided in a patient with chronic pain from osteoarthritis?
a. Acetaminophen
b. Ketorolac
c. Ibuprofen
d. Celecoxib

5. Which of the following is a potential pharmacologic effect of an opioid on the μ-opioid receptor?
a. Hypertension
b. Constipation
c. Tachypnea
d. Mydriasis

6. Which of the following statements regarding opioid therapy is correct?
a. Opioid analgesics are similar in their affinity for the μ-, δ-, and κ-opioid receptors, and action at different opioid receptors can produces similar clinical effects.
b. In patients who are opioid tolerant and experiencing opioid intoxication withdrawal can be fatal, so reversal agents must be administered with caution.
c. In chronic opioid dosing a tolerance can build, requiring higher doses to achieve the same clinical effect.
d. Methadone and levorphanol antagonize gamma-aminobutyric acid (GABA) receptors, potentially altering opioid tolerance and making linear conversions impossible

7. Which of the following is an appropriate dose of IR morphine for breakthrough pain in a patient who is taking ER hydromorphone 32 mg once daily?
a. 20 mg IR oxycodone tablet every 4 hours as needed
b. 15 mg IR morphine tablet every 4 hours as needed
c. 5 mg IR oxymorphone tablet every 12 hours as needed
d. 8 mg IR hydromorphone tablet every 6 hours as needed

CASE SCENARIO REVISITED

A 49-year-old male with pancreatic cancer presents with pain in his abdomen radiating to his back. He has been prescribed morphine 15-mg tablets, 2 tablets every 4 hours as needed and is taking his dose approximately four times per day; his pain is now well controlled. He would like to switch to a regimen that allows him to take fewer opioids per day. Convert the patient to ER 12-hour morphine tablets (available in 15-, 30-, 60-, and 100-mg tablets).

Since the patient's pain is currently controlled while taking 2 tablets of morphine 15 mg four times daily, we should convert that dose to an extended release formulation.

2 tabs/dose × 15 mg morphine/tab × 4 dose/day = 120 mg mophine/day

120 mg morphine/day × 1 day/2 dose = 60 mg morphine/dose (every 12 hours)

An appropriate new regimen for the patient would be 60 mg morphine sulfate ER tablets every 12 hours.

The patient is worried that when he works around the house, his pain may be out of control. Choose an appropriate breakthrough pain regimen for him with IR oral morphine sulfate (available as 15- and 30-mg tablets).

An appropriate breakthrough pain dose would be a single dose that is 10 to 15% of the total daily dose of baseline opioid given on an as-needed basis.

60 mg morphine/dose × 2 dose/day = 120 mg morphine/day

120 mg morphine × 10% = 12 mg morphine

120 mg morphine × 15% = 18 mg morphine

Since morphine is available in 15- and 30-mg tablets, choose 15 mg as a breakthrough dose.
  An appropriate breakthrough regimen for the patient would be 15 mg morphine sulfate IR tablets every 4 hours as needed.

The patient's pancreatic cancer has progressed, with new metastases to bone and lung. His pain is no longer well controlled on morphine ER 60 mg twice daily and morphine 15 mg every 4 hours as needed. When asked, he says that he has been taking six IR morphine tablets daily. He is not experiencing any fatigue, nausea, or trouble breathing. Because of a new insurance restriction, he must be converted to IR and ER oxycodone for his long-acting baseline pain regimen. In this example, use a 33% reduction for incomplete cross-tolerance. IR oxycodone is available in 5-, 10-, 15-, 20-, and 30-mg tablets. ER oxycodone is available in 10-, 20-, 40-, 60-, and 80-mg tablets.

When calculating his total opioid use to convert to a new regimen, both long-acting and short-acting opioid must be accounted for.

60 mg morphine/dose × 2 dose/day = 120 mg morphine/day from long acting

15 mg morphine/dose × 6 dose/day = 90 mg morphine/day from short acting

120 mg morphine/day + 90 mg morphine/day = 210 mg morphine/day total

210 mg morphine × 20 mg oral oxycodone/30 mg orl morphine
 = 140 mg oxycodone

140 mg oxycodone − 33% = 94 mg morphine daily

94 mg oxycodone/day × 1 day/2 dose = 47 mg oxycodone/dose (every 12 hours)

The closest dose that we can make using available tablets is 40 mg every 12 hours. Now we need to calculate a new dose of breakthrough medication.

40 mg oxycodone/dose × 2 dose/day = 80 mg oxycodone/day

80 mg oxycodone × 10% = 8 mg oxycodone

80 mg oxycodone × 15% = 12 mg oxycodone

Since we had to reduce the patient's baseline dose because of product availability, it would be appropriate to choose either 10 mg oxycodone by mouth every 4 hours as needed or 15 mg by mouth every 4 hours as needed.

An appropriate new regimen for the patient would be ER oxycodone 40 mg every 12 hours and IR oxycodone 15 mg every 4 hours as needed for pain.

Caution: ER oxycodone and ER or long-acting opioids are not appropriate for opioid-naïve patients.

REFERENCES

1. Chou R, Deyo R, Friedly J, et al. Systemic pharmacologic therapies for low back pain: a systematic review for an American College of Physicians clinical practice guideline. Ann Intern Med. 2017;166(7):480–492.
2. Sinatra RS, Jahr JS, Reynolds L, et al. Intravenous acetaminophen for pain after major orthopedic surgery: an expanded analysis. Pain Pract. 2012;12(5):357–365.
3. Brunton LL, Hilal-Dandan R, Knollmann BC. Goodman & Gilman's: The Pharmacological Basis of Therapeutics (13th ed., 2017). Accessed: February 10, 2018 at: http://accesspharmacy.mhmedical.com/content.aspx?sectionid=170271972&bookid=2189&jumpsectionID=172480663&Resultclick=2.
4. Nonsteroidal anti-inflammatory drugs. Drug Facts and Comparisons. Facts & Comparisons [database online]. St. Louis: Wolters Kluwer Health, Inc; May 2017. Accessed December 14, 2017.
5. Frieden TR, Houry D. Reducing the risks of relief: the CDC opioid-prescribing guideline. N Engl J Med. 2016;374(16):1501–1504.
6. Drewes AM, Jensen RD, Nielsen LM, et al. Differences between opioids: pharmacological, experimental, clinical and economical perspectives. Br J Clin Pharmacol. 2013;75(1):60–78.

7. Cox BM, Christie MJ, Devi L, Toll L, Traynor JR. Challenges for opioid receptor nomenclature: IUPHAR Review 9. Br J Pharmacol. 2015;172(2):317–323.
8. Fine PG, Portenoy RK. A Clinical Guide to Opioid Analgesia. Minneapolis: Healthcare Information Programs; 2004.
9. Clinical Pharmacology [database online]. Tampa, FL: Gold Standard; 2017. Accessed at: http://www.clinicalpharmacology.com.
10. Schmitz R. Friedrich Wilhelm Sertürner and the discovery of morphine. Pharm Hist. 1985;27(2):61–74.
11. Lee KA, Ganta N, Horton JR, Chai E. Evidence for neurotoxicity due to morphine or hydromorphone use in renal impairment: a systematic review. J Palliat Med. 2016;19(11):1179–1187.
12. Madadi P, Koren G, Cairns J, et al. Safety of codeine during breastfeeding: fatal morphine poisoning in the breastfed neonate of a mother prescribed codeine. Can Fam Physician. 2007;53(1):33–35.
13. FDA News Release. FDA requests removal of Opana ER for risks related to abuse. June 8 2017. Accessed April 25, 2018 at: https://www.fda.gov/NewsEvents/Newsroom/PressAnnouncements/ucm562401.htm.
14. McPherson ML. Demystifying Opioid Conversion Calculations: A Guide for Effective Dosing. Bethesda, MD: American Society of Health-System Pharmacists; 2010.

ADDITIONAL READING

Moore RA, Derry S, Straube S, et al. Faster, higher, stronger? Evidence for formulation and efficacy for ibuprofen in acute pain. Pain. 2014;155(1):14–21.

Stephens G, Derry S, Moore RA. Paracetamol (acetaminophen) for acute treatment of episodic tension-type headache in adults. Cochrane Database Syst Rev. 2016;(6):CD011889.

10 Neuromodulating Agents

Beth B. Hogans

If my Sun is cured from the fire that burns his feet, I will give a golden cup with a handle of lapis lazuli to Goddess Ningal.
—Queen Putuhepa, Hittite tablets (c. 1250 B.C.E.)*

LEARNING OBJECTIVES

At the completion of this chapter, the learner should be able to discuss:

- How neuromodulating agents may be effective in chronic and neuropathic pain conditions but multiple agents may be necessary
- Which anticonvulsants are used in therapy of chronic pain states and how major side effects may require active monitoring
- Tricyclic antidepressants have, for several decades, been effective for neuropathic pain, but black box suicide warnings and cardiac risks necessitate precautions
- Most newer generation antidepressants do not relieve pain, but some selective serotonin/norepinephrine reuptake inhibitors (SNRIs) may be effective for neuropathic pain
- Local anesthetics and other ion channel–specific agents can be effective against both acute and chronic pain
- Additional agents that may be of use, including clonidine, baclofen, and prednisone, and routes of application may include topical

CASE SCENARIO

A 54-year-old diabetic patient in your longitudinal clinic developed annoying burning pain in the feet at night. You diagnosed neuropathy, optimized diabetes control, and

---

* The great antiquity and poignancy of this quote is testimony to the persistence and intractability of neuropathic pain.

ruled out other causes of neuropathy. At first, a bedtime dose of amitriptyline was helpful with the pain, but the burning is now deeply bothersome both day and night, and drowsiness from the amitriptyline is interfering with work.

1. Your patient asks, "Why did you prescribe an antidepressant? Depression is not my problem." What will you tell the patient?
2. Given the oversedation with amitriptyline, you decide to try another medication. How will you explain the alternatives to the patient?
3. If you need to add a second or third medication to help control this pain, what are your choices and how will you decide among them?
4. How important are nonpharmacologic approaches, and what would you include?

INTRODUCTION

Some forms of pain are not adequately managed with standard analgesic agents. When this is the case, neuromodulating agents may prove useful. The term *neuromodulating agent* describes drugs from a wide variety of medication classes that modify neuronal activity as a principle mechanism of action. This chapter explores an array of diverse agents, all with demonstrated efficacy against certain forms of pain. These agents are categorized in the following classes: anticonvulsants, antidepressants, ion channel–selective agents, and other agents. Recognizing these classes has important clinical significance, as illustrated by the patient who wonders why an antidepressant is prescribed when depression is not the problem. Friends, family, and even pharmacists may unwittingly ask these same questions and prompt the patient to noncompliance. Taking time to explain the therapy using the information in this chapter can prevent treatment delays. In patients with chronic and neuropathic pain, these medications can and do serve as *the primary medications with efficacy against pain*, so these medications would be incorrectly referred to as "adjuvant" medications. An adjuvant is a substance used as an adjunct to another, principle treatment. For neuropathic pain, in particular, so-called standard nonopioid analgesic agents (e.g., ibuprofen) will have little to no efficacy, whereas the anticonvulsant and pain-active antidepressant medications described here are proven to provide benefit to many patients (see the following boxes).

Why Do We Use Anticonvulsants to Treat Pain?

The principal reason that is put forth to explain the use of anticonvulsants in the treatment of pain relates to the idea that chronic pain often results from increased activity by the pain-sensing pathways of the body. This nociceptive processing system comprises neurons, axons, and synapses; similarly to epilepsy, the defect lies in activity of the nervous system. Although the anticonvulsants work by several different mechanisms, such as decreasing Na^+ channel excitability (phenytoin), increasing GABAergic signaling (topiramate), and blocking presynaptic Ca^{++} entry (gabapentin), these same mechanisms are believed to be helpful in alleviating certain forms of chronic pain. It may be helpful to explain to your patient that the drugs in this class are not only used to treat epilepsy and that you are prescribing the medication because of its proven track record for helping patients with pain.]

How Do Antidepressants Work Against Pain?

The specific mechanisms by which antidepressants work in the treatment of pain is still an area of active research, and the precise reasons that these medications work as they do are not known. Importantly, monoamine oxidase inhibitors and SSRIs are not effective against pain, strongly suggesting that pain relief is not a byproduct of treating underlying depression in patients with chronic pain. Although there is an association between chronic pain and depression, it is not believed that antidepressants make pain better by alleviating depression. Interestingly, the TCAs and those newer generation antidepressants (SNRIs) that are effective against pain have NE reuptake inhibition capability.[4] In some forms of pain, it is clear that there is a derangement of the sympathetic nervous system, but although clonidine is helpful for some patients with pain, blocking NE is not widely effective against pain.

Forms of pain responding to neuromodulating agents include chronic pain and neuropathic pain.[1] Chronic pain can require years of treatment, in contrast to acute pain, which can often be controlled with a short course of a cyclooxygenase (COX) inhibitor. Thus, the medications chosen for chronic pain treatment should exhibit minimal or no long-term side effects and avoid negative potential consequences of prolonged use, such as tolerance and dependence. Neuropathic pain conditions, as a group, simply don't respond to COX inhibitors. In addition, neuropathic pain conditions tend to be persistent, thereby making alternatives to opioid analgesia essential. For these reasons, neuromodulating agents play a major role in neuropathic pain treatment. An example is trigeminal neuralgia, a condition that is completely resistant to treatment with COX inhibitors but responds very well to carbamazepine or oxcarbazepine, medications originally developed as anticonvulsants.

Multiple Mechanisms, Multiple Agents

Throughout this chapter, there is an emphasis on the proposed mechanisms associated with each medication, using words and illustrations; this is to enhance understanding of the agents, recognize the mechanisms of pain, and facilitate planning if more than one drug is needed (Figure 10.1). In fact, it is fairly typical of neuromodulating drugs

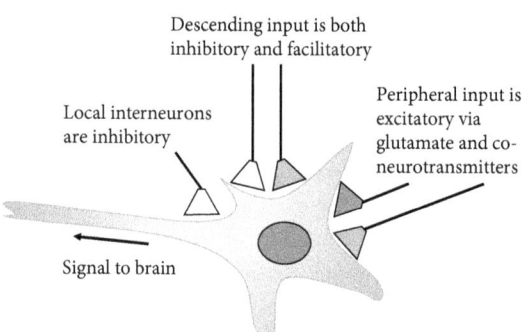

FIGURE 10.1 Dorsal horn neurons receive synaptic input from primary afferents, descending projections, and interneurons.

that they have only partial efficacy in alleviating pain, and there are several drugs in this chapter that are considered efficacious even though they *reduce but do not eliminate pain*. Because of this, it is often the case that multiple neuromodulating agents may be used in combination. What are the best guidelines for the use of multiple agents for the management of pain? Here, the categorization of neuromodulating agents by drug class is helpful. As a general rule: drugs from separate classes may potentially be used in combination, but it is less advisable to combine two drugs from a single class (e.g., two antidepressants). As always, it is recommended that prescribing physicians perform a drug interaction profile before initiating multidrug treatment; by contrast, within-class drug combinations must be approached with exceptional caution. Clinicians-in-training should consult an experienced clinician, or perhaps a pharmacist, to obtain appropriate guidance. How do we know that the use of multiple agents is more help than harm? Although the rationale for combining drugs with complementary mechanisms is sound, at present there is very limited clinical evidence to support most multidrug combinations. In the case example, the 54 year-old patient with diabetic neuropathy may require an anticonvulsant and an antidepressant for her ongoing pain as well as a more aggressive coordinated non-pharmacological plan, potentially including formal clinical psychology involvement. The use of anti-convulsants and anti-depressants is discussed here, the elements of clinical psychological pain treatments are discussed in the latter part of Chapter 5, and diabetic peripheral neuropathy specifically is addressed in Chapter 16. For the structure of the agents in this chapter, see Appendix II.

As a rule, the neuromodulating agents have effects on neurological function, including drowsiness, dizziness, and mild cognitive slowing; patients should be advised to refrain from driving and other high risk activities during initiation and titration of therapy.

ANTICONVULSANTS
Gabapentin

Gabapentin was originally developed and introduced in 1993 as an anticonvulsant. It was approved for adjunct therapy for seizures and subsequently for postherpetic neuralgia. A "designer drug," gabapentin shares structural homology with gamma-aminobutyric acid (GABA). Originally approved as adjunctive therapy for partial complex epilepsy, as patients co-diagnosed with epilepsy and neuropathic pain reported dramatic pain relief, gabapentin rapidly found use as an adjunctive agent for the treatment of pain. Although initially thought to act by a variety of mechanisms, including effects on GABA processing, the primary mechanism of action is currently believed to be by inhibiting calcium entry, through $\alpha_2\delta$ calcium channels, into the presynaptic nerve terminal of dorsal horn neurons (Figure 10.2). This mechanism of action distinguishes gabapentin from the older generation anticonvulsants and may illuminate the anecdotal reports from patients that this medication *seems to decrease the intensity of pain but not take it away*. Sometimes, patients will comment that they are not sure the medication is really helping until they attempt discontinuation and the pain is suddenly worse. The precise mechanism of action is not known.

Gabapentin is available in capsules with strengths ranging from 100 and 300 mg to 800 mg, including extended-release (ER) and liquid formulations.[2] Dosing strategies include beginning with a dose of 300 mg at bedtime (100 mg for older patients)

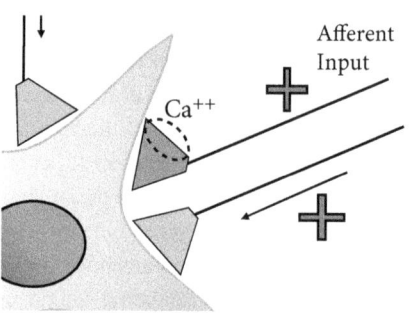

FIGURE 10.2 Gabapentin reduces presynaptic calcium influx through $\alpha_2\delta$-subunit–containing calcium channels.

and increasing by 300 mg (100 mg) increments as tolerated, not to exceed 3,600 mg. The half-life of gabapentin is such that most patients will need to take gabapentin three times (every 8 hours) a day. When gabapentin (immediate-release formulation) is taken as a twice-daily dose, the drug levels fall at the end of the dosing interval, and the patient may actually experience worsened pain, so dosing three times daily is preferred.

The drug is minimally metabolized and is eliminated largely intact through urine (about 80%) and stool. Gabapentin has minimal protein binding and does not substantively induce or inhibit liver enzymes; thus, there are few drug–drug interactions. Gabapentin is generally well tolerated; has a good safety profile, especially when compared to alternatives; can be combined with other neuromodulating agents; and may work especially well in combination with a pain-active antidepressant.

Side effects that may limit use of gabapentin include sedation, cognitive impairment, dizziness, and gastrointestinal upset. Dizziness or wooziness is especially concerning in older adults, and cautions should be given and precautions taken (e.g., physical therapy referral for balance training). Clinical examination findings of poor balance, unsteady gait, or orthostatic hypotension may signal increased risk. Unusual symptoms such as a profound worsening of pain or suicidal ideation have been noted, but the most common complaint is a difficulty with concentrating or multitasking. These cognitive effects are generally mild but may limit the use of the medication for daytime pain; patients of late-middle age may be especially sensitive to these effects, which include impairments in multitasking and short-term memory. Serious adverse reactions with gabapentin have been reported and included rash (Stevens-Johnson syndrome) and hematologic effects.

Pregabalin

Pregabalin was released for use in treatment of diabetic peripheral neuropathy, postherpetic neuralgia, and partial-onset seizures beginning in 2005. Developed based on structural homology to gabapentin, pregabalin is more potent, and the effective doses range from 150 to 300 mg per day, doses of up to 600 mg per day have been studied but may not provide additional efficacy.

Pregabalin is available in capsules ranging from 25 to 300 mg and a liquid solution.[2] Dosing strategies include beginning with 50 or 75 mg one to three times per day and increasing every 5 to 7 days. The half-life of pregabalin is slightly longer than that of gabapentin, which means that patients may be able to take pregabalin twice daily; this dosing regimen can be much preferred by patients who are working. By contrast, gabapentin usually requires a midday or afternoon dose, which may be inconvenient in a work context and may result in late afternoon sleepiness that can interfere with commuting.

Side effects of pregabalin have included dizziness, somnolence, and peripheral edema. Other cholinergic-type side effects have been reported. Serious adverse effects may occur, but experience thus far is limited. The drug, largely unmetabolized, is excreted by the kidneys. Like gabapentin, pregabalin has few drug–drug interactions.

Carbamazepine and Oxcarbazepine

Carbamazepine was developed in the mid-20th century as a compound structurally related to the tricyclic antidepressants (TCAs). Initially tested for antidepressant activity, carbamazepine was subsequently found to alleviate trigeminal neuralgia. It is highly effective against partial and secondary generalized tonic-clonic epilepsy. The response rate for patients with trigeminal neuralgia approaches 70%. Clinical trials indicate that carbamazepine is partially effective against painful peripheral neuropathy; however, these benefits may be outweighed by the adverse effects. Pain that is lancinating or shock-like may be especially responsive. Oxcarbazepine is a related compound with similar action.

Carbamazepine is available in ER tablets ranging from 100 to 400 mg.[2] Dosing strategies for treatment of trigeminal neuralgia include beginning with a dose of 200 mg (ER) per day and increasing by 200-mg increments every 3 days as tolerated to a dose of 600 to 800 mg daily. The drug is metabolized by the liver and induces hepatic microsomal enzymes; thus, there are significant drug–drug interactions. Carbamazepine reduces levels of oral contraceptives, antidepressants, benzodiazepines, and other medications. Physicians should perform a drug interaction profile before initiating treatment with this medication. Carbamazepine levels should be monitored during medication changes.

Serious adverse reactions to carbamazepine are known, and an active monitoring program is necessary. Serious adverse reactions include rash (life-threatening), hyponatremia, elevated liver enzymes, leukopenia, thrombocytopenia, Stevens-Johnson syndrome, and aplastic anemia. Appropriate monitoring includes measurement of complete blood count with platelets, liver enzymes, and serum sodium at baseline, 1 and 3 months, and subsequent intervals. Other side effects limiting carbamazepine use include, dizziness, double vision, and gastrointestinal upset.

Lamotrigine

Lamotrigine is an anticonvulsant medication, approved by the US Food and Drug Administration (FDA) in 1994, that has found use in the management of peripheral neuropathy (Figure 10.3). Initially developed as an inhibitor of folic acid metabolism, lamotrigine prolongs the refractory period following an action potential, perhaps through an interaction with voltage-dependent sodium channels. Lamotrigine inhibits glutamate release but does not affect other major neurotransmitter systems. Although

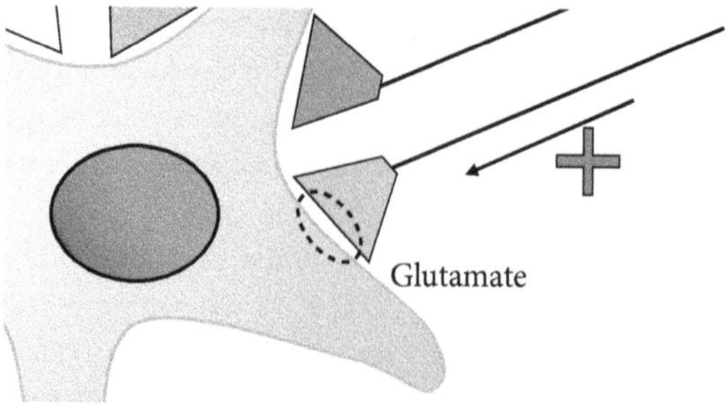

FIGURE 10.3 Lamotrigine reduces ion flux through glutamate channels.

lamotrigine has not been universally effective in clinical trials against pain, it has been shown to be of benefit in HIV peripheral neuropathy.

Lamotrigine is available in 25-, 100-, 150-, and 200-mg tablets.[2] Because of the potential for a serious rash, treatment with lamotrigine requires gradual introduction. It is possible to begin with 25 mg/day and increase by 25 mg increments every 14 days as tolerated to 100 to 200 mg/day. The drug is metabolized by the liver and excreted in the urine. Significant drug–drug interactions include reduced lamotrigine levels during coadministration of enzyme-inducing drugs such as carbamazepine. Physicians should perform a drug interaction profile before combining other drugs with this medication.

Serious adverse reactions with lamotrigine are reported, and slow upward dose tapering and an active monitoring program are necessary. Serious adverse reactions have included a potentially life-threatening rash, hepatotoxicity, and hematologic effects. The patient must be instructed about monitoring for rashes while on this medication. The potential for rash is reduced when the medication is started at low dose and increased slowly.

Topiramate

Topiramate is an anticonvulsant medication, approved by the FDA in 1996, that has found use in the management of some pain conditions, including FDA-approved use in migraine headache (Figure 10.4). The response rate for patients with migraine is said to be comparable to or better than that of other prophylactic agents. Although the use of topiramate in other pain conditions is more limited, there is some evidence that this medication is useful for conditions with neuropathic-type pain. Although topiramate is an inhibitor of carbonic anhydrase, the important proposed mechanisms of action include an increase in GABA-mediated chloride ion flux and inhibitory

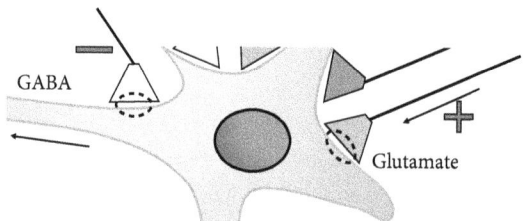

FIGURE 10.4 Topiramate, mechanisms of action.

effects on α-amino-3-hydroxy-5-methyl-4-isoxazolepropionic acid (AMPA)-kainate glutamate receptors.

Topiramate is available in 25-, 50-, 100-, and 200-mg tablets and in other formulations including sprinkle capsules and ER capsules.[2] Effective dosing strategies for treatment of migraine include a total dose of 100 or 200 mg/day. The side effects of topiramate are better tolerated with gradual introduction of medication, so one strategy would be to introduce 25 or 50 mg at bedtime and increase by 25 or 50 mg after 7 days, titrated for effect to a dose of 200 mg twice daily. Topiramate is metabolized minimally by liver, but most topiramate is excreted intact in the urine. Carbamazepine and phenytoin alter the metabolism of topiramate, resulting in lower blood levels.

The side effects of topiramate are primarily cognitive and worsen with increasing doses or rapid dose escalation. Serious adverse reactions include hepatotoxicity, pancreatitis, and hematologic effects. Mental slowing, word-finding difficulty, and dysgeusia may limit tolerability of topiramate. In contrast to most other anticonvulsants and other neuromodulating medications, topiramate does not appear to be associated with weight gain, and many patients experience modest weight loss while on this medication.

Phenytoin, Valproic Acid, and Others

Other anticonvulsants such as phenytoin and valproic acid have been used for the treatment of peripheral neuropathy, headache, and other forms of pain. These older anticonvulsants are associated with potentially serious adverse effects, such as gingival hyperplasia (phenytoin) and hepatotoxicity (valproic acid), that limit their usefulness in clinical practice.

ANTIDEPRESSANTS

Tricyclic Antidepressants

TCAs were first synthesized as phenothiazine derivatives valued for their antihistamine activity (Figure 10.5). Clinical use soon demonstrated that these agents were effective against depression, and they have had widespread use for this. Beginning in the 1970s, evidence accumulated that these agents were effective for the treatment of chronic pain, and ensuing clinical trials have demonstrated that these agents are effective against many forms of chronic pain, including postherpetic neuralgia, headache, and peripheral neuropathy.[3,4] The agents described in this chapter are all effective against chronic pain, and they are distinguished by the extent of their anticholinergic activity. The side effects of TCAs are often more profound in older patients, and careful titration is necessary in these patients. It is currently recommended, because of the potential for prolongation of cardiac repolarization, that all patients older than 40 years have a normal electrocardiogram (ECG) confirmed before the initiation of therapy with TCAs.[5] Suicidal ideation may occur; patients should be warned to report this to their healthcare providers immediately. Patients must be counseled about suicide risks before prescribing, consistent with the black box warnings for these and all antidepressants.

Amitriptyline is effective and widely used in the treatment of neuropathic pain; however, it is strongly anticholinergic and produces dry mouth, sedation, and postural

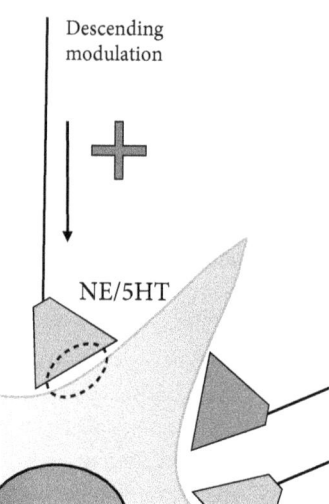

FIGURE 10.5 Antidepressants, mechanism of action.

hypotension. The strongly sedating effects of amitriptyline are helpful in those patients for whom night pain is particularly bothersome. It inhibits reuptake of 5-HT and also somewhat norepinephrine (NE). In addition, amitriptyline can block sodium channels. Starting doses of 5 or 10 mg at bedtime may result in sedation and pain relief, with cautious upward titration to 50 mg nightly as necessitated by symptoms, if tolerated. Amitriptyline is supplied as tablets of 10 and 25 mg and higher doses. The medication is available in higher strength tablets that are not generally appropriate for use in the context of chronic pain because it was originally used as an antidepressant and in that context was prescribed at higher doses. For chronic pain use, lower doses, starting with 5 or 10 mg at bedtime, are appropriate. Screening ECG is needed for those older than 40 years to ensure no antecedent QT prolongation. It is essential to counsel patients and caregivers about the black box warnings for amitriptyline and all antidepressants regarding increasing risks and rates of suicide. Patients should be advised to call immediately and stop the medication for suicidal ideation.

Nortriptyline is a popular TCA for the treatment of neuropathic pain. The anticholinergic effects of nortriptyline are intermediate. Starting doses of 5 or 10 mg at bedtime may appropriate. Doses for management of chronic pain may generally not exceed 75 mg daily, although when used as monotherapy for post-herpetic neuralgia, higher doses, not to exceed 150 mg daily may be necessary; caution and close monitoring are urged. Nortriptyline is supplied as capsules of 10 and 25 mg and higher doses; it is also available as a solution that can be used to titrate very low doses for sensitive patients. The side effects include urinary retention and constipation. Amitriptyline is metabolized in the body to form nortriptyline. It inhibits NE reuptake and only weakly inhibits 5-HT reuptake. Screening ECG and black box warnings pertain.

Desipramine is a less sedating alternative; it is the least anticholinergic of the three TCAs described here and can be well tolerated for daytime use, although dose-limiting tachycardia is common. A nonsedating TCA can be helpful for patients who are employed. Desipramine is supplied as tablets of 10 and 25 mg and higher doses, but doses higher than 25 mg daily should be avoided. Tachycardia is a serious dose-related side effect, and patients must be prescreened and monitored closely. It strongly inhibits

NE reuptake and only weakly inhibits 5-HT reuptake. Screening ECG and black box warnings pertain.

Newer Antidepressants: SSRIs and SNRIs

Newer antidepressants are characterized by increased selectivity of effects on neurotransmitter reuptake. Importantly, most of the newer antidepressants are *not* effective against pain, and as a group, the selective serotonin reuptake inhibitors (SSRIs), including fluoxetine and paroxetine, are not useful in pain treatment. Two newer antidepressants that are effective, venlafaxine and duloxetine, are distinguished by inhibiting reuptake of NE as well as serotonin (SNRIs).

Venlafaxine was developed as an antidepressant and has a unique chemical structure. It strongly inhibits the reuptake of serotonin and has more moderate effects on NE reuptake; the effects on NE are more pronounced at higher concentrations. Venlafaxine is available in 25-, 37.5-, 50-, 75-, and 150-mg scored tablets and as ER capsules of 37.5, 75, 150, and 225 mg.[2] One clinical trial showed that 75 mg was not better than placebo but that a dose of 150 to 225 mg was beneficial. Dosing should not exceed 225 mg daily. Comparison with imipramine showed similar efficacy. Careful titration may be necessary because higher doses can produce increases in heart rate and blood pressure. Venlafaxine should be avoided in patients with high blood pressure at baseline. Some patients have experienced an unpleasant withdrawal syndrome while discontinuing this medication, and as with all the antidepressants described in this chapter, gradual discontinuation (as well as gradual tapering up) is recommended unless circumstances dictate otherwise. Serious adverse effects include hypertension, which, if preexisting, precludes use of this medication and suicidality in common with all antidepressants. Black box warnings pertain.

Duloxetine is approved for use as an antidepressant for the treatment of painful diabetic peripheral neuropathy, fibromyalgia, and chronic musculoskeletal pain. Duloxetine is an inhibitor of serotonin and NE reuptake. It has been demonstrated to be effective in painful diabetic neuropathy; in two 12-week trials, effects were evident within 1 week of beginning treatment. In clinical practice, after a period of initial benefit at 60 mg daily, it is sometimes necessary to adjust the dosage upward in order to obtain a persistent effect. Duloxetine is available in 20-, 30-, and 60-mg capsules that must be swallowed whole. In most patients it is preferable to begin therapy gradually.[2] Dosing strategies include beginning with 20 or 30 mg daily and increasing to a maximum of 90 mg daily, lower for smaller people. Side effects include nausea and somnolence; irritability, hyperhidrosis, constipation, and vomiting are also reported. Suicidal ideation may occur; patients should be warned to report this to their healthcare providers immediately. Black box warnings pertain.

Milnacipran is an SNRI approved for the treatment of fibromyalgia. It is also used as an antidepressant in Europe and elsewhere. It has significant interactions with monoamine oxidase inhibitors and triptans to produce serotonin syndrome. Potential side effects include headache, nausea, constipation, and dizziness. The efficacy of milnacipran for fibromyalgia is considered to be moderate. Clinical trials have indicated that the side-effect profile may be more tolerable than that of the TCAs, but individualization of therapy is always appropriate and necessary. The medication is usually titrated from 12.5 mg daily to a target of 50 mg twice daily depending on therapeutic response. The maximum dose is 200 mg daily. Black box warnings pertain.

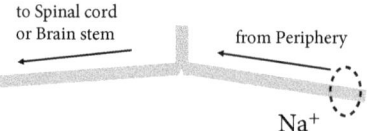

FIGURE 10.6 Local anesthetics, mechanism of action.

ION CHANNEL–SELECTIVE AGENTS
Lidocaine

Lidocaine, synthesized in 1943, acts by use-dependent blockade of sodium channels (Figure 10.6). Because lidocaine consists of a hydrophobic aromatic ring attached to a weakly basic tertiary amine, the properties of lidocaine depend strongly on pH. At neutral pH, lidocaine is charged, and although it can bind well to the sodium channel, it cannot permeate cell membranes to access the intracellular binding site. A pH near 9 allows neutralization of the charge on the amine and promotes tissue access; infected tissues with low pH may be more resistant to effects of local anesthetic. Nonetheless, lidocaine can be used to help manage nociceptive, inflammatory, and neuropathic pain. It works directly on the sensory axons and nerve endings that signal pain. A small percentage of patients have demonstrated rashes in response to patch application of lidocaine. Significant systemic concentrations that would result in cardiac and other effects rarely result from appropriate topical application or infiltration analgesia with lidocaine. Nonetheless, patients should be instructed not to exceed the dosage instructions, e.g., apply a chick-pea sized amount, and to carefully follow instructions for application of patches and topical preparations. Use of lidocaine intravenously has been studied for some severe pain conditions but is not generally relevant to outpatient primary care management of pain-associated conditions. Over-the-counter topical formulations, most 5%, are available and may be a useful part of managing focal neuropathic or other pain.

Ziconotide

Ziconotide is a synthesized analogue of a recently identified component of snail venom that acts by blocking N-type calcium channels (Figure 10.7). N-type calcium

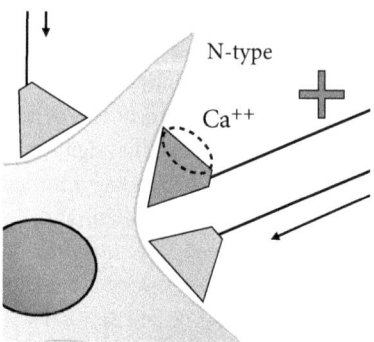

FIGURE 10.7 Ziconotide, mechanism of action.

channels are important for the presynaptic influx of Ca⁺⁺ required for release of neurotransmitter from the central terminals of primary afferent nociceptive neurons in the dorsal horn.[6] It has been demonstrated that there is a high concentration of N-type calcium channels in laminae I and II of the spinal cord. (These channels are also present on presynaptic sympathetics that release NE; thus, intravenous ziconotide leads to hypotension and is not clinically useful.) Ziconotide is a 25-amino acid peptide with six cysteines and is part of a larger family of omega-conopeptides that all block neuronal voltage-gated calcium channels. Although this peptide in the active configuration (three disulfide bonds) is hydrophilic, it does not penetrate membranes and must be delivered intrathecally to work against chronic pain. This is a specialty medication that is delivered through a catheter.

Ketamine

Ketamine is an *N*-methyl-D-aspartate (NMDA) receptor antagonist that blocks the excitatory effects of glutamate on the second-order sensory neuron (Figure 10.8). Ketamine acts as a noncompetitive antagonist by blocking the channel of the NMDA ionotropic glutamate receptor. Widely used as an anesthetic agent in veterinary medicine, its use in humans has been limited by the phenomenon of dissociation and unpleasant hallucinations that occur in some adults treated with this medication. It is frequently used successfully with midazolam for pediatric sedation. Uses for ketamine in the treatment of chronic pain are constrained by low parenteral availability; ketamine can be used in intravenous formulation for acute treatment; given intravenously, it is a specialty medication not utilized in a primary care context. Topical formulations are available as well, but caution and careful patient selection are warranted.

Capsaicin

Capsaicin, a derivative of hot chili peppers, is a TRPV1 agonist (Figure 10.9). TRPV1 is a prototypical member of the supergene family identified as *TRP* for transient receptor potential, described in Chapter 2.[7] The TRP gene products are involved in signal transduction in peripheral afferent terminals, and TRPV1 transduces painful heat in that when exposed to an appropriate degree of heat, the channel opens and permits the flow of cations across the cell membrane, resulting in a transient depolarization of the peripheral nerve terminal. This leads to the initiation of an action potential in a heat-sensing nociceptive neuron. Capsaicin, as an agonist of the TRPV1

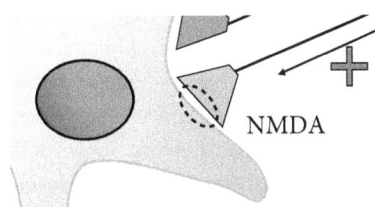

FIGURE 10.8 Ketamine, mechanism of action.

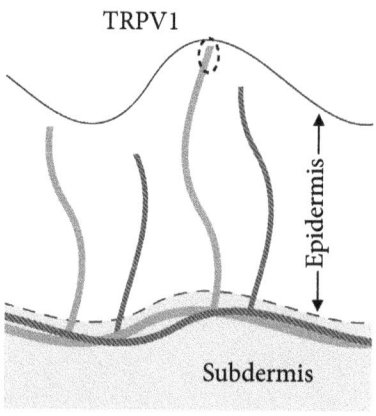

FIGURE 10.9 Capsaicin is a TRPV1 agonist. Topical application leads to activation followed by inactivation of epidermal nerve fibers and to dying back of these fibers due to calcium-mediated toxicity leading to decreased pain sensation.

channel, thus leads to depolarization and activation of the heat nociceptors. Repeated or sustained application of capsaicin results in a downregulation of this class of heat-sensing fibers and, at higher concentrations, may lead to transient destruction of nociceptive nerve endings. The psychophysical consequence of this mechanism of action is that application of capsaicin initially produces a strong burning sensation in normal people and may be intolerably painful in patients with peripheral neuropathy. Repeated application can lead to an area of anesthesia and a decrease in spontaneous burning pain. Capsaicin produces severe persistent burning in contact with mucous membranes and can cause severe pain with accidental introduction into the eye. The agent in topical form must be applied five times daily to attain efficacy, which is characterized as a state of numbness or decreased pain that is only attained after the initial pain-provoking phase is endured. It is generally not helpful for patients with peripheral neuropathy and may make their pain much worse. Pragmatic experience suggests that potential uses may include knee or shoulder arthritis, settings where activated nerve fibers are close to the skin. Capsaicin is most useful in highly motivated patients who don't mind donning gloves and frequent reapplication procedures required for efficacy.

OTHER AGENTS
Clonidine

Clonidine is an α_2-adrenergic agonist that has multiple applications: as an antihypertensive, for the treatment of drug withdrawal, and as a neuromodulating treatment for chronic pain. In treatment of hypertension, clonidine acts as a central NE agonist that results in a reduction of peripheral NE. In the setting of sympathetically mediated chronic pain, it is proposed that clonidine acts at α_2-noradrenergic receptors to result in a long-term downregulation of these receptors. Shown at the right in Figure 10.10, the formation of aberrant sympathetic sprouts into the dorsal root ganglion is postulated; the presence of these aberrant sprouts has been demonstrated in some animal models of neuropathic pain.

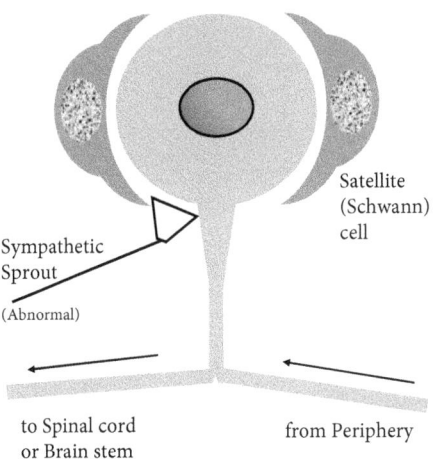

FIGURE 10.10 Primary afferent neuron (medium gray) with supporting satellite cells and aberrant sympathetic sprout.

Prednisone

Prednisone is unique among the neuromodulating agents described in this chapter in that it does not have a direct effect on transmission of neuronal signals at the level of the axon or synapse. Nonetheless, it has been observed that prednisone and other steroids have profound effects on pain processing, clearly in inflammatory pain but also in other pain conditions. In addition, it has been observed in some patients chronically treated with steroids that during the tapering of medications, there is a phenomenon of idiopathic pain; this pain can take a variety of forms, including diffuse musculoskeletal aches or a sudden worsening of prior neuropathic pain. Prednisone pulse dosing can be useful in the treatment of migraine status or severe persistent headache. Prednisone is used in the treatment of various painful rheumatologic conditions, and high doses of prednisone remain first-line treatment for painful conditions such as polymyositis and temporal arteritis after the diagnosis is established. The presumed sites of action are multiple. *It is very important to stringently avoid the use of chronic steroids, even at low dose, for treatment of undefined chronic pain.* The effects of long-term steroids are deleterious and include increasing hypertension, hyperlipidemia, diabetes, osteoporosis, muscle deterioration, skin thinning, and other serious health harms. Although patients may report relief of pain with steroid treatment, at present there is no basis for chronic steroid treatment without a concomitant, serologic, or biopsy-proved disease-based diagnosis. Importantly, although some practitioners continue to utilize prednisone tapers for acute musculoskeletal pain, there is no evidence-based support for the use of steroids in the treatment of low back pain.[8]

Baclofen

Baclofen is a GABA-B agonist that plays an important role in treatment of muscle spasm and spasticity; it may also have a role in modulating pain pathways, but this is not completely established (Figure 10.11). Baclofen is available as 10- and 20-mg

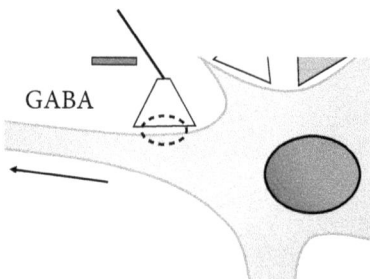

FIGURE 10.11 Baclofen, mechanism of action.

tablets.[2] Dose-limiting side effects include sedation, dizziness, and poor muscle tone. As with essentially all of the neuromodulating agents, patients should be advised to avoid driving during initiation and titration of therapy; with time, the medication effects on alertness may lessen. Serious adverse effects, including respiratory suppression, potentially fatal seizures, and muscle spasms, have occurred with rapid withdrawal.

Diazepam

Diazepam is a frequently prescribed benzodiazepine (Figure 10.12). First developed in the late 1950s and introduced into clinical use in the 1960s, benzodiazepines act on the GABA-A receptor to potentiate the influx of chloride ions by binding to an allosteric site on the receptor and increasing the frequency of channel opening events in the presence of GABA. Diazepam is useful as a muscle relaxant and an anxiolytic, but *benzodiazepines are not effective for the modulation of pain.* As a class, benzodiazepines are limited in their utility as adjunctive agents in treating pain because of the tolerance that develops to the desired effects. In an appropriate setting, diazepam can be useful for the treatment of musculoskeletal pain or pain relating to muscle spasms. In some settings such as headache related to muscle spasms or treatment of subacute pain resulting from a strain or sprain injury, it can be beneficial to prescribe a 2-week course of diazepam with an NSAID for muscle relaxation and anti-inflammatory effects, but patient selection is very important because diazepam can be abused. A small oral dose of diazepam may be offered as premedication for management of anxiety related to having a magnetic resonance imaging procedure

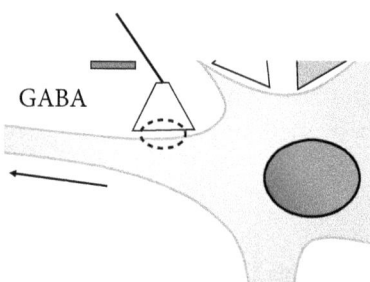

FIGURE 10.12 Diazepam, mechanism of action.

performed. When benzodiazepines are chronically administered (months to years), there is a risk for seizure resulting from abrupt withdrawal, and these drugs are listed as Drug Enforcement Administration scheduled drugs because of their abuse potential. Diazepam is metabolized by the liver and has several active metabolites. Excretion is by the kidney. Drug–drug interactions include the potential for excessive sedation when diazepam is combined with many other medications described in this chapter, including anticonvulsants and TCAs as well as opioid analgesics, antihistamines, and antihypertensives. Alcohol greatly potentiates the risk for fatal overdose and should be strictly avoided.

TOPICAL AGENTS

Many neuromodulating agents described in this chapter are available in topical formulations. Commonly used and widely available topical agents include lidocaine and capsaicin; however, other agents such as amitriptyline, baclofen, ketamine, gabapentin, prednisone, and ketoprofen (an NSAID) are among those available for topical formulation through special, compounding pharmacies. Compounding pharmacists can prepare solutions, sprays, creams, and ointments for topical application, based on detailed instructions. The properties of the topical carrier agent have an impact on the absorption of the agent, and newer formulations involve the use of lipid micelles to improve drug penetration. Multiple neuromodulating agents can be combined in a single preparation. Topical treatments offer the advantage of focal drug delivery to a painful area with lower systemic drug levels (Figure 10.13). Patients are often very interested in ways to treat a painful area without ingesting drugs, and topical agents represent an important method of drug delivery whose promise remains to be explored further. Because of health system factors, topical preparations have not generally undergone extensive clinical testing. There are a limited number of clinical trials supporting the use of topical agents, but this remains an area of future research. Trainees and new practitioners should consult with a health professional experienced in pain medicine and the use of these preparations before prescribing these to patients. Patients should be instructed not to exceed the prescribed dosage and to refrain from the use of occlusive dressings and heating pads with these agents.

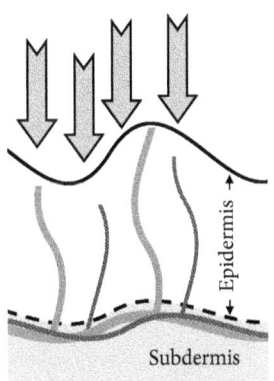

FIGURE 10.13 Primary afferent nerve terminals in skin. Use of topical agent: *gray arrows*.

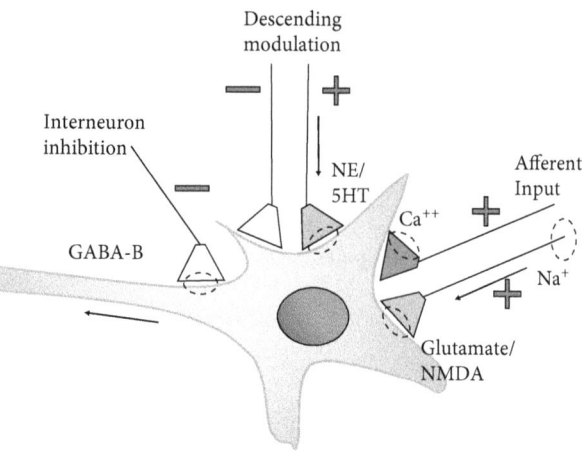

FIGURE 10.14 Schematic of spinal dorsal horn with multiple proposed sites of drug action.

SUMMARY

In this chapter the effects of a wide diversity of neuromodulating agents are described. The various classes include antidepressants, anticonvulsants, ion channel–specific agents, and others. The classification by agent is important for patient education and rational therapeutic decision-making. It is important to be aware of side-effect profiles because some of these medications can produce serious adverse reactions. The pain-active anticonvulsants include gabapentin, pregabalin, carbamazepine, lamotrigine, and topiramate. The pain-active antidepressants include amitriptyline, nortriptyline, desipramine, venlafaxine, and duloxetine. The ion channel–specific agents that are useful for pain include lidocaine, ziconotide, ketamine, and capsaicin. The other pain-active neuromodulating agents discussed in this chapter include baclofen, prednisone, clonidine, and diazepam. These agents can be applied through various routes; topical application is an important route of administration for which further research is needed (Figure 10.14). Because many of the neuromodulating agents are only partially effective in alleviating pain, combinations of drugs are often needed, so understanding the mechanisms of action can aid in the construction of a rational polypharmaceutical regimen.

REVIEW QUESTIONS

1. Which of the following are correct regarding the use of anticonvulsants for treatment of pain (choose all that are correct):
    a. Carbamazepine is especially useful for the treatment of trigeminal neuralgia, and monitoring for serious adverse effects such as hyponatremia and bone marrow suppression is a necessary part of the treatment plan.
    b. Gabapentin is only useful as an adjunctive agent in the treatment of pain, but it is known to have interactions with many other medications.
    c. Lamotrigine may be effective in treating some forms of pain, but it is associated with a potentially life-threatening rash and treatment must be introduced gradually.
    d. Topiramate has been shown to be of benefit in the treatment of migraine headache.

2. Which of the following statements about the use of antidepressants for the treatment of pain is not correct?
   a. Desipramine is a TCA with relatively few anticholinergic effects and strongly inhibits NE reuptake.
   b. Nortriptyline is classified as an SSRI and is not effective against the treatment of pain.
   c. Amitriptyline is a strongly sedating TCA with strong anticholinergic effects. It is useful for the treatment of neuropathic pain that impairs sleep and is an inhibitor of serotonin and NE reuptake.
   d. TCA overdoses are associated with toxicities such as tachycardia, QT prolongation, and life-threatening arrhythmias. Screening before TCAs includes a normal baseline ECG in all patients older than 40 years before treatment.

3. Which of these statements about newer antidepressants (SSRIs and SNRIs) is not correct?
   a. Most SSRIs are not effective in the treatment of pain, and the effects of these medications in pain treatment trials may be confounded by the complex interactions between pain and depression.
   b. Venlafaxine is effective for some patients in the treatment of neuropathic pain.
   c. In discontinuing the use of SNRIs such as venlafaxine, it is advisable to taper the medication slowly to avoid precipitating a flu-like withdrawal syndrome.
   d. Duloxetine is an SNRI that has been shown to be effective in the treatment of pain associated with diabetic neuropathy.

REFERENCES

1. Merskey H, Bogduk N; IASP Task Force on Taxonomy. Classification of Chronic Pain (2nd ed.) Seattle: IASP Press; 1994:209–214.
2. Skidmore-Roth L. Mosby's Nursing Drug Reference 2019 (32nd ed.). St. Louis: Elsevier; 2019.
3. Taub A. Relief of postherpetic neuralgia with psychotropic drugs. J Neurosurg. 1973;39:235–239.
4. Egbuniki I, Chaffee B. Antidepressants in the management of chronic pain syndromes. Pharmacotherapy. 1990;10(4):262–270.
5. Murinson B. The role of antidepressants in the treatment of chronic pain. In Deer T, ed. Treatment of Chronic Pain by Medical Approaches (pp. 43–50). New York: Springer; 2015.
6. Miljanich GP. Ziconotide: neuronal calcium channel blocker for treating severe chronic pain. Curr Med Chem. 2004;11(23):3029–3040.
7. Caterina MJ, Schumacher MA, Tominaga M, et al. The capsaicin receptor: a heat-activated ion channel in the pain pathway. Nature. 1997;389(6653):816–824.
8. Chou R, Qaseem A, Snow V, et al. Diagnosis and treatment of low back pain: a joint clinical practice guideline from the American College of Physicians and the American Pain Society. Ann Intern Med. 2007;147(7):478–491.

11 Interventional Techniques and Surgical Management of Pain

Mark Young, Andrew Rubens, and Antje M. Barreveld

Pain medicine as a discipline has struggled with the creation of scientific evidence regarding the usefulness of many of the techniques we employ. In this, the new era of evidence-based medicine, it is crucial that we all understand the level of evidence that exists for the treatments we employ.... [W]ith more consistent methodology, we can continue the work of assembling scientific trials to determine which among these techniques are most useful in aiding our patients suffering with pain.
—James P. Rathmell, MD (July 2011)[1]

LEARNING OBJECTIVES

At the completion of this chapter, the learner should be able to discuss:

- The indications for and benefits of various interventional pain management techniques for treating pain
- Peripheral nerve, muscle, joint, and spinal interventional targets
- Potential risks of interventional procedures

CASE SCENARIO

A 43-year-old woman has had more than 2 months of low back pain radiating into her right leg and foot. She has been unable to be physically active like she used to be and enjoys biking and running. She denies any bowel or bladder symptoms and is able to go to work. She completed 6 weeks of physical therapy and continues to have pain. Magnetic resonance imaging (MRI) demonstrates a right paracentral L4–5 disk herniation with nerve impingement.

1. What interventional options could she try? How long can she expect relief from an injection therapy? What are the risks of the injection?
2. Should she see a surgeon first?

INTRODUCTION

Interventional and surgical procedures can be an important component of multimodal care for diagnosing and treating chronic pain.[1,2] Diagnostic nerve blocks with local anesthetic alone can help localize pain to the region of a single nerve by temporarily numbing the putatively symptomatic nerve. Conversely, therapeutic procedures involve injections of medication mixtures that often include steroids to antagonize inflammatory processes. In general, injections that include steroid appear to be most beneficial in treating acute to subacute pain when inflammatory processes are active. For chronic pain, steroid injections may provide a temporary functional benefit, such as making it possible to initiate participation in physical activity, but relief beyond 6 weeks has not been shown to be statistically significant in most clinical studies. Sensory nerve ablation can interrupt pain signaling from painful sites of the body. This can be achieved chemically with neuroablative agents such as ethanol or thermally with radiofrequency ablation (RFA). In contrast to steroid injections, neuroablative techniques may provide relief that can last for many months. Electrical stimulation of the neuraxis can reduce chronic pain through a mechanism termed neuromodulation, wherein ascending and descending pain signals are altered.

Interventions are performed by experienced and formally trained proceduralists and can be guided by surface landmarks, fluoroscopy (radiography), computed tomography (CT), or ultrasound. Landmark technique relies on surface anatomy and palpation. It can be appropriate for superficial procedures such as pericranial nerve blocks and trigger point injections to muscles. Fluoroscopy is utilized for interventions that use bony targets for procedural endpoints. A radiography machine that rotates on a semicircular track in multiple dimensions, fluoroscopy can help interventionalists guide needles safely and accurately to deep bony structures. CT guidance permits visualization of bone and soft tissues such as internal organs. It is used more frequently by interventional radiologists. Radiation safety issues are also important factors to consider when choosing an image guidance modality. Ultrasound can guide procedures with soft tissue targets because different tissues such as muscles, blood vessels, and nerves can be identified and differentiated from one another. This chapter aims to introduce you to various interventional procedures for providing diagnostic and therapeutic pain relief. Additional detailed descriptions of indications, evidence, risks, benefits, and images can be explored in numerous other interventional chapters and texts.[1-7]

HEAD AND FACE PROCEDURES

Peripheral Cranial Nerve Blocks
Indications

We perform peripheral nerve blocks of the scalp to treat cephalalgia related to occipital neuralgia or neuralgias of the auriculotemporal nerve and supraorbital nerve, either unilateral or bilateral.[7] Blockade of these nerves can be done safely in a serial fashion, utilizing local anesthetic with or without steroid, to provide ongoing relief to patients suffering from head pain that is refractory to medications and behavioral methods of pain control. If steroid is used, careful attention must be paid to limit the total accumulated dose that a patient receives in order to minimize the risk for adverse effects.

The primary peripheral nerves that provide innervation to the scalp include four branches of the trigeminal nerve (cranial nerve V) and two branches of the cervical nerve roots C2 and C3. The supraorbital and supratrochlear nerves, branches of V1, innervate the forehead and upper portion of the eyelids. They exit the skull through small foramina above the superomedial aspect of the bony orbit of each eye. The auriculotemporal nerve, a branch of V3, innervates the region of the scalp anterior and superior to each ear. The greater occipital nerves, branches of the dorsal ramus of C2 on each side, travel medial to the occipital arteries to innervate the posterior scalp bilaterally. The lesser occipital nerves are branches of the ventral rami of C2 and C3. Like the greater occipital nerves, the lesser occipital nerves ascend cranially from the neck in the fascial plane between the inferior oblique muscles and the splenius capitis muscles. The lesser occipital nerves provide innervation to the scalp just posterior to each ear (Figure 11.1).

General Technique

For a *supraorbital nerve block* (SONB), we generally position the patient supine with the head of the bed up. The supraorbital notch can then be palpated over the medial third of the supraorbital ridge, roughly directly superior to the midpoint of the pupil. The injection is given by advancing a needle just above the notch until contacting the orbit. The needle is then withdrawn slightly, the syringe is aspirated to confirm negative aspiration, and injection mixture is then administered.

For an *auriculotemporal nerve block* (ATNB), positioning can be accomplished either as described previously or with the patient sitting up, depending on both provider

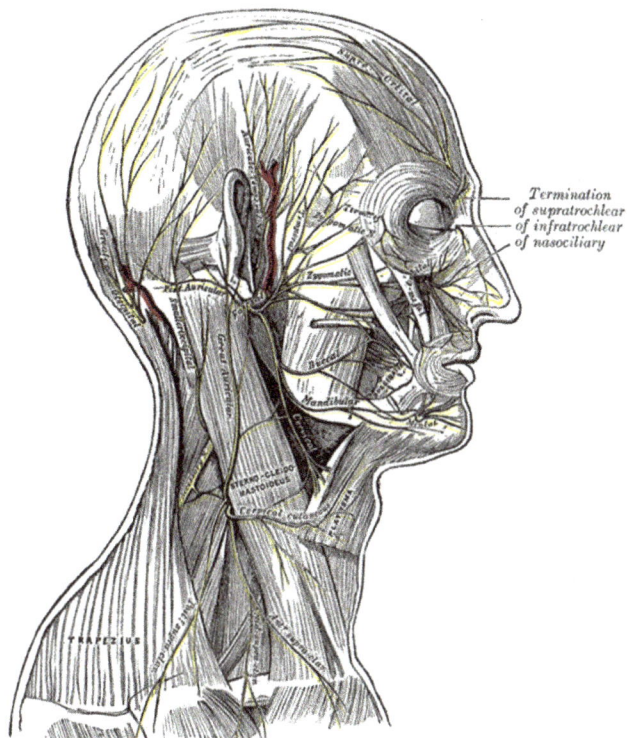

FIGURE 11.1 Nerves of the scalp, face, and side of neck. (From Rathmell JP. Atlas of Image-Guided Intervention in Regional Anesthesia and Pain Medicine (2nd ed.). Philadelphia: Wolters Kluwer/Lippincott Williams & Wilkins Health; 2012.)

and patient preference. The region of the scalp immediately superior to the ear in a line directly above the tragus of the ear is then cleansed with alcohol, after which a 27-gauge 1.25-inch needle is advanced perpendicular to the skin just until contact with bone is made. At that point, the needle is slightly withdrawn, and following negative aspiration, 1 to 2 mL of injectate is then administered.

For *greater and lesser occipital nerve block* (GONB/LONB), the region of the greater occipital nerve along the occipital ridge midway between the occipital protuberance and the mastoid process is palpated. After the occipital artery is palpated, a 25- to 27-gauge 1.25-inch needle is then inserted in a perpendicular fashion just medial to the artery until bone is contacted. The needle is then withdrawn slightly and, following negative gentle aspiration, 2 to 3 mL of injectate is administered. To achieve blockade of the lesser occipital nerve, another injection may be completed 2.5 cm lateral to the location of the greater occipital nerve along the occipital ridge.

Nerve Block	Needle Gauge	Needle Length	Injection Mixture and Volume
SONB	25–30 gauge	0.5–1.25 inches	2–4 mL of 1% lidocaine or 0.25–0.5% bupivacaine with or without 1 ML of dexamethasone 10 mg or methylprednisolone
ATNB			
GONB			
LONB			

Botulinum Toxin (Botox) for Migraine Headache Prophylaxis

Indications

Botulinum toxins are produced by the gram-negative anaerobic bacterium *Clostridium botulinum*. They produce paralysis of muscle by preventing the presynaptic release of acetylcholine (Ach) at the neuromuscular junction. In 2010, the US Food and Drug Administration (FDA) approved the use of botulinum toxin for the treatment of chronic migraine. To qualify for Botox for migraine treatment, patients generally have to meet the criteria of migraine attacks occurring 15 days or more monthly for at least 3 months, with the attacks lasting for 4 hours or more. A decrease in migraine frequency may be observed for 3 months or greater versus placebo.

General Technique

Each vial of nonbotulinum toxin A contains 100 units of vacuum-dried toxin without preservative. The toxin is reconstituted in 2 mL of sterile saline before injection. Using 1-mL syringes, the reconstituted toxin is drawn up so that the concentration is 5 units/0.1 mL. We then utilize 30-gauge needles for injection of each site. There are 31 sites in total, and each site is injected with 5 units of toxin (155 units total are injected).

Risks

Risks with botulinum toxin injections for migraine mainly include neck pain (9%) and eyelid droop (4%), both of which will resolve over 1 to 3 months. Very rarely, botulinum toxin injections can lead to difficulty breathing, swallowing, or allergic reaction.[8]

Blocks of the Trigeminal Nerve and Trigeminal Nerve Branches

Indications

Diagnostic blocks confirm presence of trigeminal neuralgia. Therapeutic blocks for intractable trigeminal neuralgia after failure of medication management may include steroid and are often performed before neuroablative or surgical procedures on the trigeminal nerve to predict efficacy of such procedures.

General Technique

Generally performed under fluoroscopic guidance, the C-arm is rotated to obtain a submental view with a slight oblique tilt toward the affected side until the foramen ovale is visualized—generally medial to the mandibular process. A needle (generally a 22- to 25-gauge 3.5-inch blunt-tipped stimulating needle is advanced toward the foramen ovale under intermittent fluoroscopy. A finger in the mouth will aid in preventing oral mucosa penetration by the needle. When the needle tip is within the foramen ovale, motor stimulation will elicit jaw muscle twitches, and 0.5 to 1 mL of contrast dye is then injected under live fluoroscopy to rule out vascular spread and to confirm proper positioning. One to 2 mL of 0.5% bupivacaine with or without steroid is then administered with close monitoring of the patient's hemodynamics.

Risks

Because of the close approximation of the needle to the dura mater when inside the foramen ovale, the potential for high spinal or brainstem anesthesia does exist. Additionally, intravascular injection of bupivacaine in this area could lead to seizure activity, and close attention must be paid to avoid such an event.

NECK PROCEDURES
Stellate Ganglion Block

Indications

The stellate ganglion is formed by the fusion of inferior cervical and the first thoracic sympathetic chain ganglia and is usually located between the seventh cervical and first thoracic vertebrae anterolateral to the vertebral bodies. This paired structure, one on the left and one on the right, transmits efferent sympathetic signals to the ipsilateral head, face, and arm. Infiltrating the ganglion with local anesthetic medication can aid diagnosis and also treatment of sympathetically mediated pain conditions, which include some forms of complex regional pain syndrome (CRPS). A stellate ganglion block can reduce pain severity in conditions that are sympathetically mediated, including some forms of CRPS. Although the pharmacologic effect of local anesthetics lasts only hours, blocking the ganglion can provide prolonged relief and increased functional activity that last weeks to months. This ganglion has also been blocked to manage hyperhidrosis, and case reports have identified other applications such as treating ventricular storm (episodic ventricular tachycardia and/or fibrillation).

General Technique

Classically, landmark and fluoroscopic approaches (Figure 11.2) have targeted the prominent anterior transverse process of the sixth cervical vertebrae (C6) known

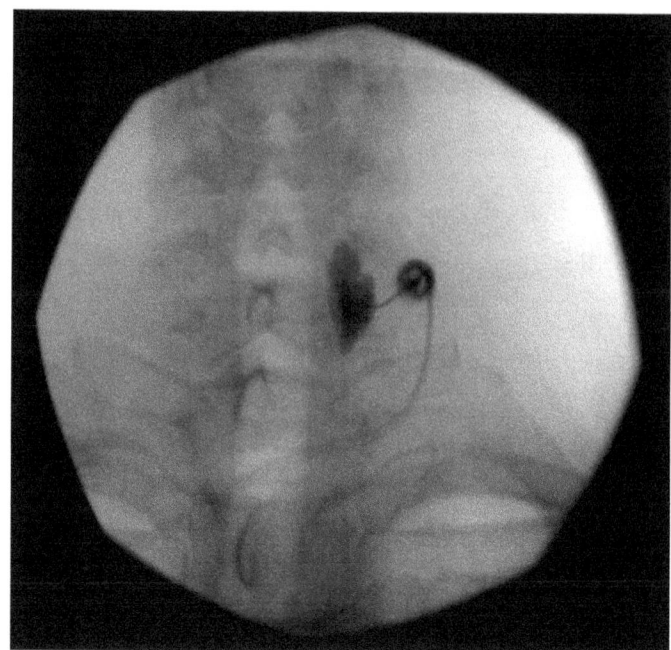

FIGURE 11.2 Stellate ganglion block with fluoroscopy (contrast dye highlights dye spread lateral to C7 facet along the sympathetic chain).

as Chassaignac tubercle. The needle is advanced, often from an anterior approach, until contacting this bony landmark. More recently, ultrasound-guided techniques have been described with infiltration of local anesthetic at soft tissue targets over the C6 or C7 vertebral body. Specifically, this target has been described as the plane between the lateral part of the longus colli muscle posteriorly and the prevertebral fascia covering the posterior aspect of the carotid sheath anteriorly. This technique may enable closer proximity to the ganglion and, therefore, a more complete block. With either approach, caudal spread of local anesthesia aids in blocking the stellate ganglion.

With both landmark and ultrasound techniques, when the block needle reaches the target position, negative syringe aspiration and nonvascular contrast dye spread (when using fluoroscopy) ensure that the needle tip is not in a blood vessel. With ultrasonography, hydrodissection within the appropriate soft tissue plane further indicates appropriate needle tip positioning. Often, about 10 mL of 1% lidocaine is injected in 2-mL aliquots, pausing to rule out side effects such as mental status changes and to ensure that negative aspiration has been maintained. Endpoints of a successful block include cutaneous temperature change in the distal ipsilateral extremity and ipsilateral Horner syndrome.

Risks

The risks of the procedure are related to the vital structures adjacent to the target site. The thyroid lobe, esophagus, and cervical nerve roots can be injured in this procedure. Vascular structures in close proximity include the carotid artery, internal jugular vein, and vertebral artery. Injection to the vertebral artery can lead to neurotoxicity, and damage to the vessel can result in stroke.

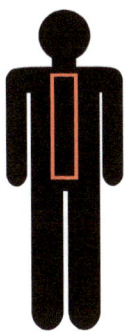

NEURAXIAL PROCEDURES
Epidural Steroid Injection (Cervical, Lumbar, and Thoracic)

Indications

Epidural steroid injections (ESIs) are among the most common interventions performed in chronic pain management clinics. They are utilized to treat spine-related ailments such as radicular pain and radiculopathy. When intervertebral disks herniate posterolaterally, the displaced disk material can press on and mechanically injure adjacent neural elements. At this interface, inflammatory changes can add further insult. This condition may manifest as pain, numbness, and tingling in a dermatomal distribution along the extent of the involved nerve root. Introducing steroid into the area can antagonize the inflammatory process. Additionally, local anesthetic can dull pain sensations, and normal saline can dilute the existing inflammatory milieu. Evidence generally supports the use of ESIs in alleviating lumbosacral radicular pain in the acute to subacute phase of symptomatic disk herniation. The utility of ESIs in treating chronic lumbosacral radicular pain and radiculopathy, as well as other spinal diseases such as spinal stenosis, is controversial.

General Technique

The epidural space lies within the bony canal formed by the posterior vertebral bodies and laminae, and it surrounds the dura matter, which contains the spinal cord and cerebral spinal fluid (Figure 11.3). The epidural space extends from the foramen magnum to the sacrum, so ESIs can be performed at the cervical, thoracic, lumbar, and sacral spinal levels. This space can be reached from interlaminar or transforaminal approaches.

In either approach and with fluoroscopic guidance, the patient is usually positioned prone, and the needle is advanced in a general posterior to anterior direction. In the interlaminar approach, an epidural needle is advanced either in the midline or paramedian to the ipsilateral side of pain and also at or near the level of symptomatic pathology. Serial fluoroscopic images identify an appropriate target site and also ensure that the desired needle path is maintained along the intended trajectory as it is advanced. The needle is then advanced between two laminae, and a loss-of-resistance

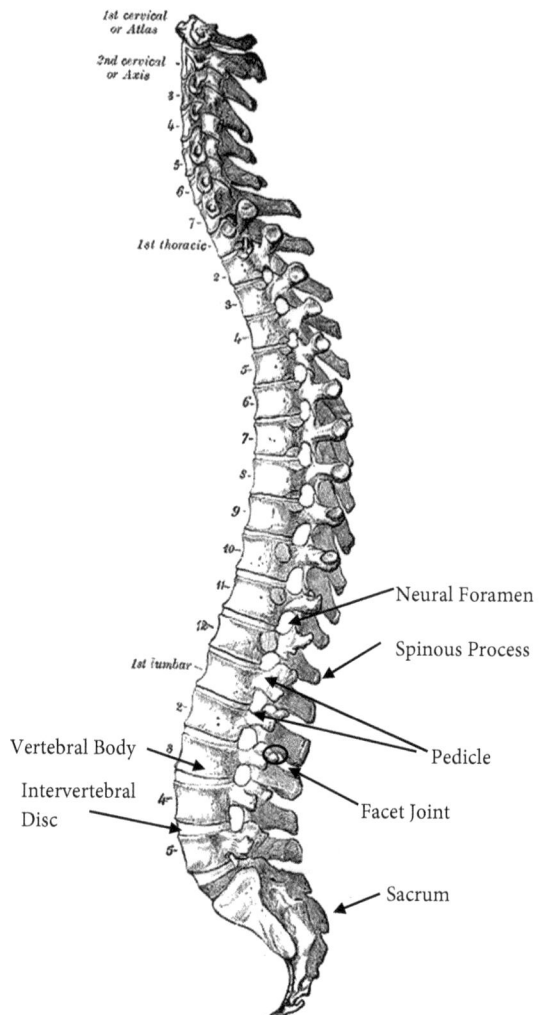

FIGURE 11.3 The spinal column. (From Rathmell JP. Atlas of Image-Guided Intervention in Regional Anesthesia and Pain Medicine (2nd ed.). Philadelphia: Wolters Kluwer/Lippincott Williams & Wilkins Health; 2012.)

syringe preloaded with saline or air is attached to the hub. An inability to depress the syringe sharply gives way to an ability to do as the epidural needle advances through posterior spinal ligaments and into the epidural space. Multiplanar fluoroscopy then demonstrates appropriate needle depth. Contrast dye spread verifies position by appropriate spread within the epidural space while simultaneously ruling out both vascular uptake and intrathecal administration (Figure 11.4). After these checks, the mediation mixture, often 1 to 2 mL of steroid mixed with 1 to 2 mL of normal saline and/or 1 to 2 mL of local anesthetic, is delivered to the epidural space.

In the transforaminal approach, a spinal needle is directed toward the foramen on the ipsilateral side of pain at or near the level of symptomatic pathology. Because foramina are oriented laterally, the skin insertion site for the spinal needle is more lateral compared with the interlaminar approach, and the needle takes a more oblique path toward its target as it is advanced. Because thick ligaments do not shield the neural

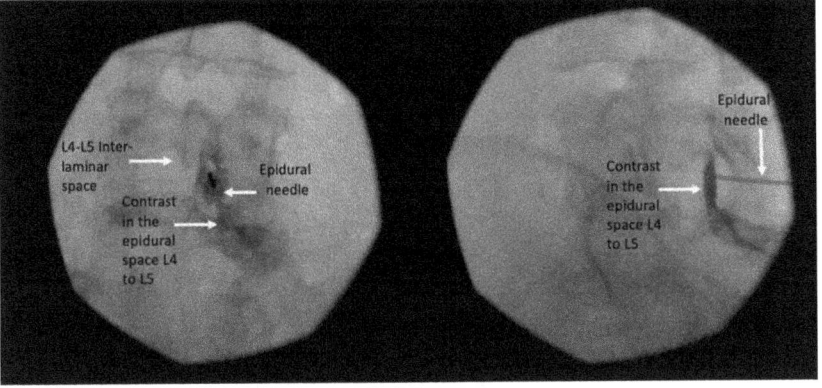

FIGURE 11.4 Interlaminar lumbar epidural steroid injection at L4–5, right of midline.

foramen, a loss-of-resistance syringe is not used in the transforaminal ESI approach. Multiplanar fluoroscopy demonstrates appropriate needle depth, and contrast dye verifies the position with appropriate spread before 1 to 2 mL of steroid mixed with 1 to 2 mL of normal saline and/or 1 to 2 mL of local anesthetic is administered.

Risks

Advancing the epidural needle past the dura and into the thecal sac can result in a dural puncture, which can lead to headache and spinal cord or nerve root (depending on the spinal level) trauma. With transforaminal ESIs, the spinal needle can pierce the nerve root, leading to radiculopathy, although this usually resolves when the needle is slightly withdrawn. Additionally, the spinal needle can pierce the intervertebral disk, which may lead to discitis. Although rare, ESIs can also result in devastating neurovascular injury. Inadvertently injecting particulate steroid into spinal radicular arteries can result in spinal cord infarction and paraplegia. Inadvertently injecting particulate steroid into the vertebral artery can result in cerebellar or brainstem stroke.

Intra-Articular Facet Joint Injection (Cervical, Lumbar, and Thoracic)
Indications

Degenerative arthritic changes of the spine, or spondylosis, accumulate with age and may contribute to chronic axial pain. Joint degeneration can occur at the posterior articulations between vertebral levels. Therapeutic injections into these zygapophyseal (or facet) joints may provide short-term or prolonged relief.

General Technique

First, clinical and radiographic data are analyzed to determine which facet joint or joints are to be targeted for injection. Patients lie prone on the procedure table, and the fluoroscope is angulated to optimize visualization of the targeted facet joints. A spinal needle is then advanced under tunnel view toward the lucent area between adjacent articular processes (Figure 11.5). The interventionalist may appreciate the sensation

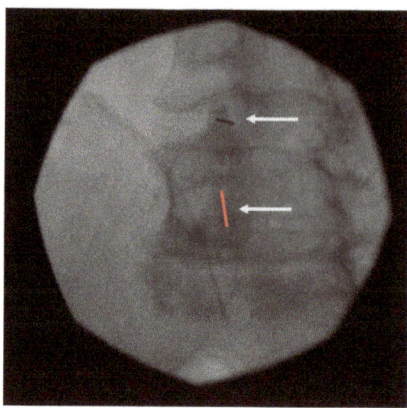

FIGURE 11.5 Intra-articular facet injection, needle inserted at L4–5 facet joint on the left (*superior white arrow*); L5–S1 facet joint (*red line, inferior arrow*).

of the needle tip slipping past the joint capsule and into the joint space. Multiplanar fluoroscopy demonstrates appropriate needle position, and a small amount of contrast dye shows joint space spread. Typically, a 1- to 2-mL mixture of local anesthetic and steroid is then delivered to each joint targeted. Because it may be difficult to confidently know that only a single facet joint level is symptomatic a priori, often two or more adjacent spinal levels (e.g., L4–5 and L5–S1) are treated in a single procedure visit. In a related technique, facet joint cysts, which often communicate with the facet joint and may cause pain by impinging on adjacent neural structures, can be ruptured by overpressurizing the joint until the cyst wall gives way.

Risks

The proceduralist must use caution to ensure that proper depth is achieved. Inadvertent epidural or intrathecal access can occur if the needle passes through the facet joint and into the neuraxis.

Medial Branch Block and Radiofrequency Ablation (Cervical, Lumbar, and Thoracic)

Indications

As with intra-articular facet joint injections, medial branch blocks (MBBs) are performed in the setting of spondylosis and chronic axial pain. However, unlike joint injections, MBBs are generally performed with diagnostic, rather than therapeutic, intent. The medial branch of a given spinal nerve divides from the main nerve root and provides partial sensory innervation to the facet joint both above and below it. It follows that each facet joint is dually innervated from the medial branch above and below. Infiltrating adjacent branches with local anesthetic numbs entire facet joints temporarily for 3 to 5 hours. If patients experience significantly decreased pain during this anesthetic phase, RFA of the medial branches can be performed. In this procedure, medial branches are lesioned with a heating probe that reaches 80° C in order to interrupt pain signaling to the brain. Peripheral nerves can regenerate over time, and if pain returns because of regeneration, then RFA can be repeated. This procedure essentially converts the effect of a brief diagnostic MBB into a therapeutic procedure with prolonged effect for an average of 6 months or longer.

General Technique

In the cervical spine, MBBs can be performed with the patient in a lateral or prone position. The needle enters at the level of the vertebral body waist or indentation, and the proper depth is at the center of the lateral body on lateral view. In the lumbar spine, the needle is directed to the junction of the superior articulating process and the transverse process. On lateral view, the needle remains posterior to the intervertebral foramen. Often, needles placed at three adjacent levels are used to treat two adjacent facet joints, respectively. With MBBs, local anesthetic is injected to numb the targeted nerves for a short-lived diagnostic period of time in which the patient assesses any improvement in pain relief and activity tolerance.

Patients who respond favorably to two diagnostic MBBs may proceed to medial branch RFA. In this procedure, insulated probes are directed to the same targets treated in the MBB procedures. Only the distal tip of the probe is exposed and in proximity with the targeted medial nerve root branches. Then, sensory and motor testing are carried out. Sensory stimulation elicits pain or pressure and predicts medial branch sensitivity (or efficacy). Motor stimulation demonstrating lack of distal radicular muscle contraction predicts specificity (or safety). After these tests, ablation is carried out at 80° C for 90 seconds.

Risks

Specific risks of MBBs include nerve root irritation and anesthetic blockade. Specific risks of medial branch RFAs include nerve root irritation and denervation.

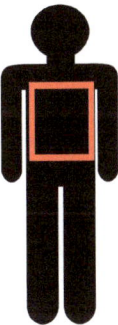

TRUNK PROCEDURES
Intercostal Nerve Block

Indications

Intercostal nerves branch off from their thoracic nerve roots and continue laterally along the inferior aspect of the respective rib along the costal groove. Along this course, they give off further divisions that innervate the lateral and anterior chest and abdominal wall. Painful conditions related to this area can be diagnosed and treated by blocking respective intercostal nerves that correspond to the affected dermatome. Because they do not innervate deeper structures such as lung and abdominal organs, response (and lack thereof) can distinguish superficial, somatic pain from deeper, visceral pain. Patients can have chronic pain within the distribution of intercostal nerves due to trauma such as rib fracture, neuroma after surgery such as thoracotomy, and idiopathic causes such as slipping rib syndrome. Intercostal injections can help to diagnose and treat pain mediated by intercostal nerves.

General Technique

To target pain in the distribution of an intercostal nerve, imaging helps determine the dermatome of the thoracic level in which a painful area predominately lies. Often, the level above and the level below are also treated because of potential adjacent level crossover. Within the costal groove, the nerve lies caudal to the vessels, while the pleura lies deep. With the patient lying prone and using fluoroscopy, a needle is advanced to the targeted rib several centimeters lateral from midline. After making contact with bone, the needle is minimally pulled back, directed caudally, and readvanced so that it "walks off" the surface of the rib. The needle is then minimally advanced deeper so that it reaches the area of the nerve. However, care is taken to avoid penetrating the pleura. Contrast dye injection demonstrates spread along the costal margin laterally and also lack of vascular uptake. Diagnostic blocks with local anesthetic only can establish whether or not pain is mediated by the intercostal nerves. Therapeutic injections with steroid and radiofrequency treatments have also been described.

Risks

Interventions in this area also carry unique risks. Performing the procedure too medially can lead to epidural or subarachnoid block. Lung puncture can lead to pneumothorax and, potentially, life-threatening tension pneumothorax. Also, significant reabsorption from the intercostal blood vessels may increase the risk for local anesthetic toxicity and decrease the duration of analgesia after a local anesthetic infiltration.

Ilioinguinal and Genitofemoral Nerve Block

Indications

The ilioinguinal and iliohypogastric nerves are formed from the anterior rami of the L1 nerve root. The nerves course from the neuraxis and around the abdomen inferomedially in a plane between the internal oblique and transversus abdominis muscles. They travel together above the ilium and pass near the anterior-superior iliac spine (ASIS). The iliohypogastric nerve lies medial and the ilioinguinal nerve lies lateral in this region. The iliohypogastric nerve innervates the abdominal wall in the hypogastric or suprapubic region, which is below the level of the umbilicus and above the inguinal ligament. The ilioinguinal nerve innervates the abdominal wall along the inguinal ligament in the groin.

The genitofemoral nerve is formed from anterior rami of the L1 and L2 nerve roots. It courses from the neuraxis and through the psoas muscle before reaching the anterior abdomen. Just above the inguinal ligament, it divides into genital and femoral

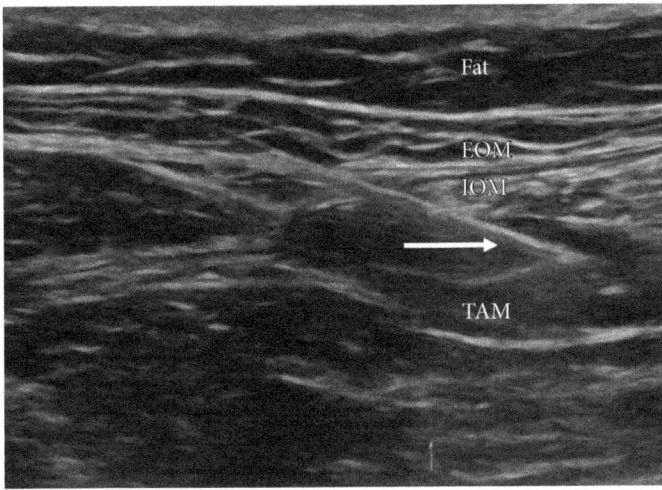

FIGURE 11.6 Ultrasound-guided ilioinguinal nerve block with local anesthetic spread around the needle tip placed in the inguinal nerve plane over the transversus abdominus muscle (TAM). EOM = external oblique muscle; IOM = internal oblique muscle.

branches. The genital branch enters the inguinal canal and innervates the scrotum in men and labia majora in women. The femoral branch enters the femoral sheath and supplies sensory innervation to the proximal medial thigh.

General Technique

The ilioinguinal and iliohypogastric nerves are often blocked together in an area medial to the ASIS. Although landmark techniques exist, ultrasound-guided blocks have the advantage of visualizing the needle tip reaching the desired tissue plane and then injection medication collecting in that space. A linear ultrasound probe is placed oblique to the transverse plane with one end visualizing the ASIS and the other pointing toward the umbilicus. The needle is then advanced in a plane superomedial to inferolateral until reaching the plane between the internal oblique and transversus abdominis muscle (Figure 11.6).

Techniques to block the genitofemoral nerve have been described, but typically, the genital branch of the genitofemoral nerve is blocked. Here, landmark technique is still common, but ultrasound-guided blocks are also becoming more commonplace.

Risks

With proper technique, risks for intravascular injection, intraperitoneal injection, or nerve injury are low.

Celiac Plexus Block
Indications

Celiac plexus blocks are often performed for visceral pain from upper abdominal cancers, including pancreatic cancer. They can be performed percutaneously, often from a posterolateral approach utilizing fluoroscopy or CT. Alternative approaches include performing the block during an endoscopic ultrasound. Current evidence suggests demonstrable but limited benefit compared with oral analgesics in appropriate patient populations, so an emphasis on patient selection is warranted in order to maximize the benefit-to-risk ratio.[9]

General Technique

In the percutaneous technique, the patient lies prone on an imaging table. The needle is advanced 5 to 7 cm lateral from the spinous process of the first lumbar vertebrae and advanced toward the vertebral body until reaching the desired depth. In the classic retrocrural variant, the needle is advanced until the tip is just anterior to the superior third of the vertebrae in lateral view. In the anterocrural approach, the needle advances further until it is on the anterior side of the aorta. With either approach, a diagnostic block using local anesthetic such as lidocaine 1% can establish the extent to which a patient's pain is mediated from the celiac plexus. A therapeutic block using neurolytic medication such as ethanol can then be given for long-lasting pain relief. A successful sympathetic block can manifest with hypotension and diarrhea.

Risks

There are several risks with this technique related to the structures surrounding the target area. Piercing vascular structures such as the aorta can lead to retroperitoneal hematoma and systemic toxicity from intravascular injection. Delivering local anesthetic to the intrathecal or epidural space can lead to temporary weakness, whereas delivering neurolytic agents can lead to paraplegia. Perforation of nearby organs such as lung and kidney risk pneumothorax and renal hematoma, respectively.

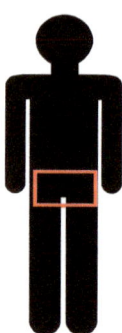

PELVIC PROCEDURES
Sacroiliac Joint Injection, Nerve Block, and Radiofrequency Ablation

Indications

The sacroiliac joint is formed by the articulation of the sacrum medially and ilium laterally. The joint is curved, with the posterior aspect medial and the anterior aspect lateral. It is also undulated, and the contours of the two bones interlock to form a stable position. Movement within the joint is further limited by strong stabilizing ligaments. Nevertheless, it is a true synovial joint, and joint degeneration and inflammation within and around it can contribute to pain in the lower back, buttocks, and upper thighs. It is innervated from anterior and posterior rami of L5 and S1–3 providing sensation to the anterior and posterior aspects of the joint, respectively. Because the anterior aspect is in proximity to pelvic organs, only the posterior joint and contributing nerve branches are typically targeted in pain management practice.

General Technique

Because of the arcing and irregular shape of the sacroiliac joint, intra-articular joint injection can be difficult to achieve. Many techniques have been described to optimize the injection, including oblique angulation of the fluoroscope. Diagnostic injections with local anesthetic into the joint space can help clarify the cause of a patient's lower back pain. Steroid may be added to augment possible longer term relief. If duration of relief is brief, four nerve blocks (Dreyfuss technique) with local anesthetic at the ipsilateral L5–S1 facet joint and lateral to the S1, S2, and S3 foramina may provide diagnostic relief in preparation for thermal ablation of these same nerve roots.

Risks

Risks include bleeding, infection, and nerve root irritation.

Pudendal Nerve Block

Indications

The pudendal nerve supplies sensory innervation to the rectum, perineum, and genitalia. It also provides motor function involved in urination and intercourse. The nerve passes near the ischial spine and enters Alcock canal, and irritation in these areas due to nerve entrapment may present with pain in the distribution of the pudendal nerve, worsened with sitting and relieved with lying down (e.g., pudendal neuralgia).

General Technique

Traditional pudendal nerve blocks are performed by gynecologists transvaginally. The nerve may be accessed transgluteally in males and females by fluoroscopic approach. The patient lies prone, and the lower pelvis is visualized on fluoroscopy. The ischial spine is visualized and optimized with slight oblique tilting. A 22-gauge spinal needle is advanced to the tip of the ischial spine. The needle can then be walked off the spine slightly deeper to penetrate the sacrospinous ligament. A diagnostic block with local anesthetic only, such as 5 mL bupivacaine 0.25%, can help establish the presence of pudendal neuralgia. A therapeutic mixture of local anesthetic such as 4 mL bupivacaine 0.25% with or without 1 mL methylprednisolone 40 mg may be injected to prolong relief.

Risks

The unique risks of pudendal nerve blocks relate to structures surrounding the pudendal nerve and the structures that the nerve innervates.

Piriformis Injection
Indications

The piriformis muscle is a lateral hip rotator that lies in the region of the gluteal muscles. It originates from the anterolateral sacrum and inserts on the ipsilateral greater trochanter. The sciatic nerve, which is derived from L4–S3 spinal nerves and supplies sensation and motor function to the lower leg, typically passes deep to the piriformis muscle. However, in some patients the sciatic nerve partially or entirely pierces the piriformis muscle. It is theorized that irritation to the muscle leads to inflammatory mediators that can secondarily affect the nerve. Patients with piriformis syndrome present with buttock pain in the area of the piriformis muscle and also referred pain down the leg (i.e., sciatica).

General Technique

A piriformis injection is performed with the patient lying in the prone position. A fluoroscope shows the lateral sacrum and greater trochanter on the affected side. A 22-gauge spinal needle is inserted between the two landmarks in an area that is 1 to 2 cm inferior and 1 to 2 cm lateral to the inferior aspect of the ipsilateral sacroiliac joint. This site is in close proximity with the sciatic nerve. On the lateral view, the needle is advanced until it is just anterior to the anterior sacral margin. Appropriate contrast dye spread will reveal muscular striations that are parallel to the piriformis muscle insertions. A mixture of local anesthetic such as 4 mL bupivacaine 0.25% with 1 mL methylprednisolone 40 mg is then delivered to the muscle.

Risks

The sciatic nerve is the largest of the human body, and inadvertent trauma to the nerve risks both temporary paresthesia and permanent neuropathy. Even with a successful injection, local anesthetic near the nerve can lead to blockade.

LARGE JOINT PROCEDURES
Shoulder Injections: Subacromial Subdeltoid Bursa and Glenohumeral Joint Injections
Indications

The subacromial subdeltoid bursa lies underneath the acromion medially and the deltoid muscle laterally as well as above the supraspinatus tendon. It is an extra-articular

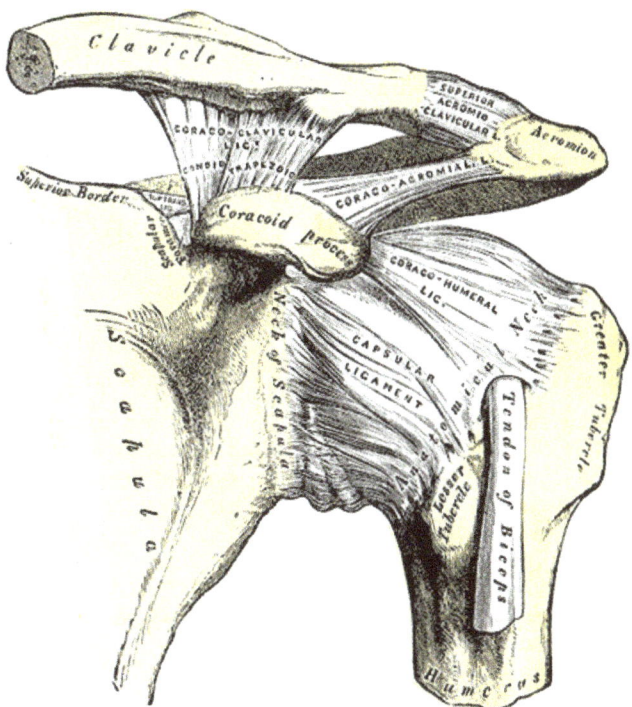

FIGURE 11.7 The left shoulder and acromioclavicular joints, and ligaments of the scapula. (From Rathmell JP. Atlas of Image-Guided Intervention in Regional Anesthesia and Pain Medicine (2nd ed.). Philadelphia: Wolters Kluwer/Lippincott Williams & Wilkins Health; 2012.)

synovial sac that decreases friction between the deltoid muscle and supraspinatus tendon as they move relative to one another during shoulder movements. When this bursa becomes inflamed because of acute trauma or insidious overuse injury, it can lead to pain and impingement. The goal of a subacromial subdeltoid bursa is to relieve pain and improve mobility due to bursitis.

At the glenohumeral joint, the humeral head articulates with the glenoid fossa of the scapula. Pain conditions related to this joint include arthritis, both rheumatologic and osteoarthritic, and also frozen shoulder (also known as adhesive capsulitis). Glenohumeral joint injections can be performed for shoulder pain related to these three diagnoses. See Figure 11.7 for review of shoulder anatomy.

General Technique

The subacromial subdeltoid bursa injection can be performed using a number of different techniques. The needle can approach the joint from an anterior, posterior, or lateral position. Additionally, landmark technique or ultrasonography may be employed. Ultrasonography may have advantages, including optimizing needle approach and confirming that the injection mixture spreads within the joint. A common approach for this bursa injection is the lateral approach with ultrasound guidance. A linear transducer is oriented in the coronal plane on the affected side, with the linear transducer directed toward the contralateral hip. The optimal view has the bony shadow of the acromion over the edge of the screen, and the rest of the image shows the deltoid muscle overlying the supraspinatus tendon, which overlies the humeral head. A 3.5-inch, 22-gauge spinal needle is advanced in plane and in real time with the ultrasound transducer until reaching the plane between the deltoid muscle and supraspinatus tendon just lateral to the shadow of the acromion. After negative aspiration, a mixture of local anesthetic such as 4 mL bupivacaine 0.25% with 1 mL methylprednisolone 40 mg is delivered.

The glenohumeral joint injection can be performed using a number of different techniques. The needle can approach the joint from an anterior, posterior, or lateral position. Additionally, landmark technique, fluoroscopy, or ultrasonography may be employed. Image-guided techniques may have advantages, including optimizing needle approach and confirming that the injection mixture spreads within the joint. The most common approach for this joint injection utilized at our clinic is the posterior approach with ultrasound guidance. A linear transducer is oriented in the transverse plane just caudal to the posterolateral aspect of the acromion on the affected side until the concave glenoid, triangular-shaped labrum, convex humeral head, and both infraspinatus and deltoid muscles are in view. A 3.5-inch, 22-gauge spinal needle is advanced in plane and in real time with the ultrasound transducer until reaching the joint space. After negative aspiration, a mixture of local anesthetic such as 4 mL bupivacaine 0.25% with 1 mL methylprednisolone 40 mg is delivered.

Risks

For the subacromial subdeltoid bursa injection, risks for inadvertent involvement of neurovascular structures is minimal with the lateral approach. For the glenohumeral joint injection, risks include neurovascular trauma and intravascular injection. The posterior approach may pose less risk to inadvertent involvement of neurovascular structures than the anterior approach. Additionally, the trauma to the labrum can be incurred by the needle but perhaps avoided with ultrasound visualization.

Knee Intra-Articular Joint Injection

Indications

Indications for knee intra-articular joint injections may include inflammatory arthritis and osteoarthritis. Intra-articular knee injections may aid in the treatment of arthritic pain that is refractory to physical therapy and medication management.

General Technique

Injections may be performed by landmark technique, ultrasound, or fluoroscopy. Utilizing fluoroscopy, the joint space is visualized between the articulation of the femoral and tibial condyles. A 3.5-inch, 22-gauge spinal needle is then inserted into the joint space, on either the medial or lateral side, and 0.5 to 1 mL of contrast dye is then injected to confirm proper joint spread and lack of intravascular uptake. Subsequently, a mixture of local anesthetic 1 to 5 mL and steroid (e.g., methylprednisolone 40 mg) is injected into the joint, and the needle is then removed.

Risks

Risks may include infection or bleeding, especially in patients who have ongoing infections and who are on anticoagulant therapy.

SURGICAL PAIN PROCEDURES
Neuromodulation (Spinal Cord Stimulation)
Indications

Spinal cord stimulator (SCS) systems are electronic devices implanted for many chronic pain conditions, including failed back surgery syndrome (FBSS), CRPS/causalgia, and peripheral neuropathy.[10] An SCS system consists of a battery connected to one or more leads with several metal contacts that emit electric output. The leads are placed in the posterior epidural space, and the output from the metal contacts occurs posterior to the spinal cord near the sensory dorsal columns, or transforaminally in the case of a dorsal root ganglion (DRG) stimulator with output adjacent to the DRG (Figure 11.8). This output leads to neuromodulation, whereby afferent and efferent pain signaling processes in the spinal cord are altered, leading to a reduction in chronic pain signaling. The location of the contacts, which contacts are activated, and electric output characteristics, including pulse frequency, duration, and amplitude, may all contribute to SCS efficacy. Major device manufacturers have developed proprietary SCS programs to maximize patient benefit. The stimulation from conventional programs elicits paresthesias, but other programs stimulate in a way that is imperceptible so that paresthesias are not felt.

General Technique

Before proceeding with a procedure, a thorough psychological evaluation is obtained to assess a patient's social support, psychological well-being, expectations with spinal stimulation, and any concerns for implantation of a foreign body. After a successful

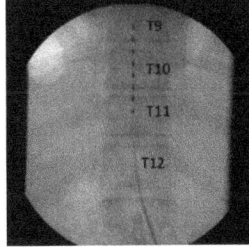
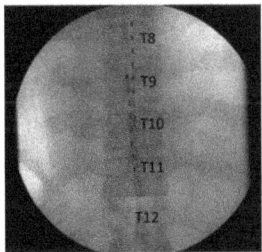
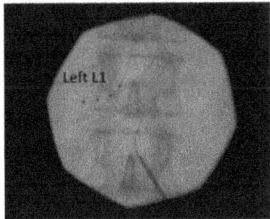

FIGURE 11.8 Spinal cord stimulator trial lead placements (indications and techniques). *Left image:* chronic left femoral neuropathy after femur fracture repair and history of spine surgery, traditional spinal cord stimulation to T9; *middle image:* chronic low back and lumbar radiculopathy after spinal surgery and not a repeat surgical candidate, high-frequency spinal cord stimulator;

right image: left ilioinguinal neuralgia/causalgia after inguinal hernia repair, dorsal root ganglion stimulator placed transforaminally on the left at L1 with lead loops to prevent lead migration. (From Gray H, Lewis WH, Gray H. Anatomy of the Human Body (20th ed.). Philadelphia: Lea & Febiger; 1918.)

screening, SCS implantation occurs in two phases. First, a removable system is placed for a trial period, which generally lasts 1 week. Stimulator leads are introduced percutaneously through an epidural needle so that the distal metal contact end lies in the epidural space or over the DRG, while the proximal end emerges from the skin. The epidural space is accessed in a manner similar to the technique used for an epidural steroid injection (discussed previously). The proximal ends of one or more leads are then attached to an external battery, which is secured to an elastic belt worn under the clothes for the trial period. Several output programs and other settings are adjusted throughout the trial in order to obtain maximal benefit before the leads are removed percutaneously.

Patients who respond to the SCS trial with significant benefit (e.g., >50% reduction in their chronic pain) may proceed to the second phase, permanent surgical implantation. Here, percutaneous leads are inserted, similar to the trial, or contacts on a paddle array are inserted by laminotomy. These leads are then either sutured to ligamentum flavum or secured to lamina, respectively. Next, a subcutaneous battery pocket is created, often below the waist. The proximal ends of the leads are tunneled subcutaneously to the pocket and attached to the battery.

Risks

Risks of spinal stimulation include but are not limited to infection, bleeding, nerve injury, postdural puncture headache, lead migration, and diminishing relief.

Intrathecal Drug Delivery System

Indications

Intrathecal drug delivery is used in the treatment of severe refractory pain in cancer pain and noncancer pain, in patients who have failed conservative treatments. In patients whose life expectancy is less than 2 to 3 months, a percutaneous catheter and pump are generally used. When life expectancy is more than 3 months, an implantable system with an implanted spinal catheter connected to a medication reservoir pump implanted under the skin may be utilized.

Many diagnoses may benefit from intrathecal drug delivery techniques, including metastatic cancer, spinal cord injury, severe spasticity, diabetic neuropathy, CRPS, postherpetic neuralgia, and phantom limb pain. Additionally, mixed nociceptive and neuropathic conditions such as postlaminectomy pain syndrome or chronic pancreatitis, as well as nociceptive pain conditions such as chronic vertebral compression fractures and severe spinal degeneration, may also be appropriate in some circumstances.

A key benefit to intrathecal drug delivery for pain management is a lower overall dose of medication required for adequate pain control. Also, less systemic and cognitive side effects allow for a more comfortable, interactive, and lucid patient, especially at the end of life.

General Technique

A trial is typically performed before permanent system placement. Trial options include a single-bolus intrathecal injection, multiple-bolus injections, or a continuous infusion through a percutaneous intrathecal or epidural catheter.

Implantation is carried out under local anesthesia, spinal anesthesia, or general anesthesia. First, a location for the pump itself must be determined before anesthetizing the patient. A location away from bony prominences and away from the belt line is determined. Also, if the patient is a side sleeper, locating the pump on the opposite side is generally preferred.

During the procedure itself, the intrathecal space is located with a Tuohy needle. The intrathecal catheter is then threaded into place, and if the patient is awake, the patient can confirm that there are no paresthesias or pain with placement. When the catheter is confirmed to be in the intrathecal space radiographically and by free flow of cerebrospinal fluid, injection of 20 to 30 mg of lidocaine will provide adequate spinal anesthesia for both the posterior midline incision and abdominal pump pocket incision.

Risks

Risks include bleeding, infection, wound dehiscence, and neurologic injury. There is also risk for cerebrospinal fluid leakage, migration of the intrathecal catheter, and pump site complications such as seroma formation. Granuloma formation (0.49% incidence) has also been described, wherein aseptic inflammatory masses with granulation tissue develop within the dural sac. This may cause loss of analgesic effect, progression of neurologic symptoms from mass effect on the spinal cord, and permanent neurologic injury. Risk factors for granuloma formation include high dose and high concentration infusion of all opioids except for fentanyl, and it most commonly occurs with morphine.

SUMMARY

Interventional and surgical pain management techniques using image or landmark guidance may provide diagnostic and therapeutic relief for patients suffering from pain. Performed by formally trained and experienced proceduralists, interventions, in conjunction with other multimodal strategies such as medications, physical therapy, and behavioral therapies, can be useful techniques for helping patients achieve improved function and pain relief. Benefits may be short or longer term, depending on the interventional strategy utilized. Indications, evidence, and risks must be considered when choosing the most appropriate interventional options for a patient.

REVIEW QUESTIONS

1. A 43-year-old woman has had more than 2 months of low back pain radiating into her right leg and foot. She has been unable to be physically active like she used to be and enjoys biking and running. She denies any bowel or bladder symptoms and is able to go to work. She completed 6 weeks of physical therapy and continues to have pain. An MRI demonstrates a right-paracentral L4–5 disk herniation with nerve impingement. What is the best interventional treatment to help her with acute pain relief?
    a. Lumbar facet injection
    b. RFA of the lumbar nerve root
    c. Lumbar sympathetic nerve block
    d. Interlaminar lumbar epidural steroid injection

2. A 64-year-old man underwent lumbar fusion and laminectomy surgery 2 years ago and presents with chronic back pain radiating into his right knee with persistent numbness and tingling in the right thigh and knee since his surgery. He has tried various injections with temporary relief. Medications have caused side effects, and he has not made any progress in physical therapy. He has difficulty walking, working, and sleeping because of pain. Repeat imaging does not demonstrate any surgical issues. What best interventional option might be pursued next?
   a. Spinal cord stimulation trial
   b. Lumbar sympathetic neurolytic injection
   c. Intrathecal pump trial
   d. Sacroiliac joint radiofrequency ablation

REFERENCES

1. Rathmell JP. Atlas of Image-Guided Intervention in Regional Anesthesia and Pain Medicine (2nd ed.). Philadelphia: Wolters Kluwer/Lippincott Williams & Wilkins Health; 2012.
2. Benzon HT. Practical Management of Pain (5th ed.). Philadelphia: Elsevier/Mosby; 2014.
3. Krames E, Peckham PH, Rezai AR. Neuromodulation: Comprehensive Textbook of Principles, Technologies, and Therapies (2nd ed.). London: Academic; 2018.
4. Narang S, Weisheipl A, Ross EL. Surgical Pain Management: A Complete Guide to Implantable and Interventional Pain Therapies. Oxford; New York: Oxford University Press; 2016.
5. Fishman S, Ballantyne J, Rathmell JP, Bonica JJ. Bonica's Management of Pain (4th ed.). Baltimore, MD: Lippincott, Williams & Wilkins; 2010.
6. Karmakar MK, Soh E, Chee V, Sheah K. Atlas of Sonoanatomy for Regional Anaesthesia and Pain Medicine. New York: McGraw-Hill Education; 2018.
7. Narouze SN. Interventional management of head and face pain: nerve blocks and beyond. New York: Springer; 2014.
8. Key facts about Botox. Accessed at: https://www.botoxchronicmigraine.com/botox-chronic-migraine-benefits-safety-and-side-effects.
9. Arcidiacono PG, Calori G, Carrara S, et al. Celiac plexus block for pancreatic cancer pain in adults. Cochrane Database Syst Rev. 2011(3):CD007519.
10. Verrills P, Sinclair C, Barnard A. A review of spinal cord stimulation systems for chronic pain. J Pain Res. 2016;9:481–492.

12 Rehabilitation Approaches to Pain and Applications in Outpatient Practice

Marlis Gonzalez-Fernandez,
Katherine S. Wright, Bernard Abrams,
Ada L. Yao, Amira Noles,
and Beth B. Hogans

You never know how strong you are until being strong is your only choice.
—Bob Marley

LEARNING OBJECTIVES

At the completion of this chapter, the learner should be able to discuss:

- The principle modalities of treatment used in the rehabilitative treatment of pain
- Appropriate conservative treatments that can be recommended to patients
- The prevalence of complementary and alternative medicine (CAM) use and some basic information about the major types of CAM, including modalities such as acupuncture, meditation, dietary supplements, and manipulative methods
- The definitions of impairment, disability, and handicap and the multiple scales for assessing impairment and disability
- The role of the physician in the disability determination process
- The multiple effects of litigation on recovery and response to pain treatments
- The application of rehabilitative principles and coordinated care patient-centered approaches to pain care in outpatient settings
- Placebo, nocebo, and expectancy effects related to pain treatment

CASE SCENARIO

A 64-year-old woman is referred for treatment of severe, persistent, treatment-resistant headaches. The headaches began when she was undergoing a cardiac stress test. While on the treadmill at a high intensity of effort, she developed a severe posterior headache, 9/10. The treadmill was stopped, and the patient was observed for 30 minutes, during which time the headache abated partially but did not resolve. She was instructed to go home and rest. When the headache persisted and even worsened 3 days later, she presented to the emergency department, where tests were run and medication was given. She had some relief from the headache and was told tests were normal; she was discharged home. The headache returned the next day and continued to plague her for ensuing weeks and months as she was repeatedly evaluated and told that all tests results were normal. The patient is seen by you 2 years after the treadmill incident, at which point she describes the headache as follows: pressure-like pain, over the top of her head, never less than 4/10, peaking at 8/10 with occasional 10/10 spikes, and continuous despite waxing and waning. The pain is exacerbated by movement, especially bending over forward at the waist, and exercise. The pain is relieved slighted by over-the-counter analgesia and refraining from activity. She does not have associated symptoms except for some mild nausea when the pain is most severe. She was a lifelong competitive amateur tennis player. She cannot play matches now because every time she bends over to pick up a tennis ball, her head pain spikes. She has a stable supportive family, and her husband recently retired. They are considering legal action against the cardiologist supervising the treadmill test because of all the pain and suffering associated with the headache. Nonetheless, the patient notes that her primary goal is to make sure that nothing's wrong and to gain control over the headaches. The patient's pain-focused exam shows no neurologic deficits; she has some scattered trigger points in the cervical muscles and some allodynia (tenderness to mild pressure) over the temporal region bilaterally.

1. What are your first steps with this patient?
2. How will you organize your treatment plan?
3. How will you explain the rehabilitative approach to pain care to this patient?

INTRODUCTION: THE REHABILITATION APPROACH

Pain is a significant threat to a person's overall functional abilities and quality of life. It is not only a negative or distressing sensory experience but also affects a person's mobility, ability to perform daily activities, and participation in society. Given the complexity of pain, management must be mechanism based, multimodal, tailored to patient's goals and needs, and aimed at optimizing overall daily function while providing pain relief and minimizing adverse effects.[1,2] With its challenges, pain management should be an open collaboration among a number of clinical specialties, including nonsurgical, interventional, surgical, and psychological or therapy-based practitioners. Rehabilitation interventions are geared toward ameliorating pain-related dysfunction and disability even when the source of the pain cannot be eliminated. In those cases, facilitating participation in daily activity and fulfilling life roles, despite the pain, is the main goal. In general, a patient-focused multimodal approach to improve function and quality of life is the cornerstone of rehabilitation and physiatry.

This approach is well suited and complementary to other modalities to manage pain, and these same principles are useful in primary care settings.

PAIN MANAGEMENT AND REHABILITATION

Rehabilitation of people with pain includes a range of interventions targeting somatic, behavioral/psychological, and neurochemical pathways. The focus of this chapter is on nonpharmacologic interventions.

Physical interventions aim to enhance a patient's physical capacity and functional ability through mobility, progressive exercise, and manual therapy because these interventions reduce negative pain outcomes.[3] Physical, occupational, ergonomic, and psychological interventions can be used as appropriate to address factors that contribute to how a particular person experiences pain. Current evidence suggests that combining multiple approaches addressing preventive strategies, strengthening, and education can be successfully used to manage pain.[4]

It is critical to consider psychological factors as a component of pain management.[4,5] For example, cancer patients might be reluctant to raise concerns about pain or discomfort limiting function. These can be address with psychobehavioral interventions. Communication barriers include fear of pain indicating any form of disease progression or recurrence, not wishing to have treatment reduced or to look weak, not wanting to disappoint or to distract the care providers, disbelief that something can be done for pain, or not desiring to appear to be seeking drugs.

PHYSICAL THERAPY FOR PAIN MANAGEMENT IN THE REHABILITATION SETTING

As previously mentioned, physical therapy (PT) can contribute to effective pain control, starting with early mobilization, which helps curb the development and worsening of pain through physical and psychological inputs.[3,4] Because of underlying pathology or comorbidities, exercise tolerance may be limited. Traditional aquatic therapy or gravity-reducing treadmills (using air or water) can be an initial therapeutic intervention.[6] Exercise can then progress to land therapy, including range of motion and strengthening exercises.[7] Therapeutic modalities such as kinesiology taping, electrical stimulation, laser, dry-needling, and manual therapy can also be employed to reduce pain and foster progress toward achieving functional goals.[8–10] Exercise, when combined with nutrition interventions, can also result in weight loss, which is known to improve lower limb joint pain (most commonly knee pain).[11] There is evidence to suggest that physical interventions are useful for pain reduction. Examples include using kinesiology taping for patellofemoral pain and knee arthritis; aquatic therapy for neck and shoulder pain in breast cancer survivors; and transcutaneous electrical nerve stimulation, enhanced mobility, and activity for knee arthritis.[10]

Psychologically Informed Physical Therapy

Rehabilitation through a combined approach is reasonable considering the intricacies of pain. There is increasing evidence that patients can benefit from therapy team–led cognitive behavioral self-management approaches. Psychologically informed physical therapy (PIPT) treatments aim to use psychological techniques to hasten and to enhance the impact of PT and to entrench patient's long-term maintenance of exercise recommendations. Part of this is addressing catastrophizing and acceptance; it focuses on helping patients live well in the face of chronic difficulty and, like cognitive behavioral therapy (CBT), has specific techniques for targeting problematic thinking. Acceptance and commitment therapy (ACT) is another cognitive therapy that emphasizes a state of mindful acceptance accompanied by a refocusing of the attention on engaging in meaningful activities that can be accomplished despite pain.[5,12]

PIPT encompasses the whole body, not just specific problem areas. There is recognition that patients' experiences are beyond the physical. This highlights the importance of inner experiences: being more aware of thoughts and feelings and being conscious and mindful of the process of making choices. Patients feel safe and supported, further nurturing open communication lines and motivation to explore barriers to their daily function and quality of life.[5,12]

NEUROCOGNITIVE MODULATION OF PAIN IN THE REHABILITATION SETTING
Behavioral or Psychologically Informed Therapeutic Interventions

Given the limitations of traditional biomedical pain interventions, psychological principles began to be used in the 1960s to help treat pain conditions.[13,14] There is now a large body of empirical research supporting the conceptualization of pain as multidimensional in nature and having biopsychosocial causes and effects.[15,16] Acute and chronic pain is common among many patient populations traditionally treated in rehabilitation settings, including patients with spinal cord injury, traumatic brain injury, stroke, orthopedic and musculoskeletal conditions, and cancer.[17] Before intervention, multimodal assessment of chronic pain is typically conducted through patient interviews and self-report measures and includes evaluation using pain ratings with visual analog or numeric rating scales, cognitive appraisals, negative affect, verbal and nonverbal pain behaviors, pain-related physical and psychological functional status, and coping strategies.[17-19] Reviews of the literature support the use of psychological interventions for pain, with small to moderate effects in improving disability, mood, and catastrophic thinking and, in some cases, reduction in pain, compared with controls.[18] Psychological treatments for chronic pain largely fall under the following four psychological models: (1) operant model, (2) peripheral physiologic models, (3) cognitive and coping models, and (4) central neurophysiologic models.[13,18]

Operant Model

The theory of operant conditioning hypothesizes that behavior is sensitive to changes in the environment, such that the frequency of behavior may increase with reinforcement or decrease if ignored or punished.[14] Contingency management seeks to identify both "pain behaviors" and "well behaviors" and then to eliminate or extinguish the former while reinforcing the latter.[13,15]

Peripheral Physiologic Models

Relaxation, biofeedback-assisted relaxation, and autogenic training are all interventions based in training patients to control autonomic peripheral nervous system activity. Relaxation training was originally developed in the 1930s and later adopted by psychologists in the 1950s for treatment of anxiety and in the 1970s for treatment of chronic pain. Although relaxation can produce short-term improvement in pain through reduction in muscle tension, research has demonstrated that the positive outcomes are associated with a central, rather than peripheral, mechanism of action as patients' self-efficacy increases and stress reduces.[20]

Cognitive and Coping Models

Interventions based on cognitive models hypothesize that behavior can be understood, predicted, and modified by accounting for and working with a patient's beliefs, attributions, motivation, and intentions. Cognitive therapy involves helping a patient monitor and identify patterns of thoughts and ultimately challenging irrational or unhelpful thinking with more adaptive thoughts.[21-23] The dominant psychological treatment for chronic pain is CBT, and there is strong empirical support for the use of both cognitive and behavioral strategies to address pain-related dysfunction through learning to control one's thoughts, behaviors, emotions, and aspects of physiologic processes.[22-24] Psychological interventions based in CBT focus on self-management and include coping skills training, problem-solving training, stress management, communication skills training, graded exposure in vivo, mindfulness-based stress reduction, and ACT. Another intervention technique in this category is motivational interviewing, which is not a stand-alone therapy but rather a style and strategy to help patients explore their own motivations with the goal of increasing their readiness to adopt adaptive coping strategies.[25] CBT can vary in number of sessions and specific techniques but often includes relaxation training, behavioral activation, setting and tracking behavioral goals, activity pacing guidance, problem-solving training, and cognitive restructuring.[24]

Central Neurophysiologic Models

Melzack and Wall's gate control theory hypothesizes that nociceptive pain information interpreted by the brain is modulated at the dorsal horn of the spinal cord, which can "open" or "close" the hypothetical pain gate and change the way pain is experienced.[13] The cortical brain regions that integrate pain information include the prefrontal cortex, which interprets the meaning of pain; the anterior cingulate cortex, which processes affective responses to pain; and the insula, which integrates information about motivation related to one's physical condition. Psychological interventions based on central neurophysiologic models include neurofeedback (biofeedback with electroencephalography or functional magnetic resonance imaging), hypnosis, graded motor imagery, mirror visual feedback, and sensory discrimination training. Aspects of these models are often included as part of education in CBT interventions, particularly using the gate control theory as part of the rationale for practicing self-management strategies that can modulate pain information.[16]

Cognitive Behavioral Therapy

Another approach is CBT. CBT programs have been shown to be beneficial for pain. Strategies aim to reduce pain and disability through addressing fear of movement and increasing self-efficacy. Empirically supported behavioral self-management, problem-solving, cognitive restructuring, and relaxation training compose CBT. Quite similar to PIPT, there are initiatives to have therapy teams integrate CBT into a chronic pain patient's therapy program. Such efforts focus in on the relationship between the body, the mind, one's activity level, designing a graded activity plan, weekly activity, and walking goals. Therapists introduce different cognitive or behavioral strategies to facilitate identifying enjoyable activities (distraction), replacing negative thinking with positive thoughts, finding a balance between rest and activity (pacing), and managing setbacks by recognizing high-risk situations and negative thoughts.[5,12,21-23] This program has been shown to translate to better pain control and functional outcomes in low back surgery patients when started before surgery and when continued at least 6 months afterward.[11,12]

Although psychological interventions have clinically meaningful impact on a patient's functional status and disability, there are still gaps in knowledge regarding which strategies are most effective for which kind of pain and which phase of care.[11]

PREHABILITATION TO SUPPORT PAIN CONTROL
Prehabilitation

Often, medical interventions are debilitating, and the circumstances of a hospital admission can lead to further deconditioning. The rehabilitation physician's approach to patients who are about to undergo a stressful intervention is best initiated, if possible, before the intervention and early in the course of their disease state in order to prevent deconditioning. Prehabilitation is the process of enhancing one's functional and mental capacity to better withstand a significant health-related stressor or treatment (e.g., joint or spine surgery, cancer treatment, solid organ transplantation).[26] Common interventions include exercise, nutritional support, and psychological assistance. A rehabilitation physician's goal is to identify baseline impairments, ameliorate those impairments before the health-related event (if possible), and anticipate future impairments that may occur as a result of medical interventions. Prehabilitation also allows patients to participate in their preintervention care and to be in control of some aspects of their health.

This relatively new approach has not been extensively studied for pain reduction. Nevertheless, pain management interventions included as part of prehabilitation programs have been beneficial for people undergoing elective orthopedic procedures. Pain from postoperative complications has been extensively studied in those undergoing orthopedic procedures. Several studies have shown that dependence on opiates for pain management preoperatively results in increased use of opiates postoperatively compared with their opiate-naïve counterparts and is associated with poor surgical outcomes, including infection, acute kidney injury, prolonged delirium, acute hypotension, ileus, respiratory complications, impaired wound healing, and overall increased morbidity and mortality.[27] Titrating individuals off opiates before elective orthopedic surgery improves outcomes, such that they become similar to opiate-naïve groups.[28] The approach to pain management in the prehabilitation setting should be geared toward titrating patients off opiates, decreasing pain catastrophizing, and decreasing learned helplessness, while providing patients with coping skills, increasing their self-esteem and resilience.[21-23]

Implementation of a Prehabilitation Program

As a relatively new approach, prehabilitation programs are variable and not standardized. However, there is evidence that implementing prehabilitation programs is beneficial for some clinical situations.[29] Prehabilitation programs have been implemented in diverse settings, including home-based therapies, supervised group therapies, and hospital-based therapies; all of which have generated successful results. However, some level of supervision has been shown to improve compliance and can range from intensive supervised inpatient exercises to weekly phone calls.[30]

The individualized trimodal approach to prehabilitation, including exercise, nutrition, and psychological support, has promising results. Most researchers agree that implementing this treatment triad will prove to have superior results.[30] A trimodal comprehensive approach to prehabilitation might entail establishing the patient's baseline functional status, medical comorbidities, and psychosocial obstacles in order to optimize each patient's opportunity for a satisfactory outcome. A highly individualized approach to prehabilitation tailored to address each patient's needs can include exercise programs made up of aerobic and resistance exercises, including walking, biking, weight training, and respiratory exercises to improve total lung capacity and respiratory muscle endurance. Nutritional interventions should include protein supplementation, treatment of anemia, and body mass index optimization. Psychological interventions may include smoking and alcohol cessation programs, anxiety- and pain-reducing programs, and management of depression. Prehabilitation is a promising treatment approach combining well-understood strategies described earlier. Evaluation of specific protocols in formal trials to optimize this intervention is necessary.

COMPLEMENTARY AND ALTERNATIVE MODALITIES FOR PAIN
Active Complementary and Alternative Modalities

Therapeutic exercise, outside of formal PT, can be beneficial for patients with pain. One well-studied exercise regimen is tai chi, which is a low-impact exercise regimen that focuses on breathing and whole-body motion. A related modality, qi gong, is characterized by flowing movements that emphasize dynamic balance. A systematic review by Kong et al. concluded that a regimen of at least 6 weeks of tai chi reduced pain related to chronic low back pain, rheumatoid and osteoarthritis, fibromyalgia, and osteoporosis.[31] Tai chi could also be used as a low-impact strategy to minimize subsequent pain as a result of activation of nociceptive pain receptors during intensive physical and occupation therapy.

Yoga, from the old Sanskrit word *yuj* meaning "to integrate," is a mind–body discipline aimed at synchronizing psychosomatic responses through various postures, poses, and breathing integrations. There is evidence to suggest that yoga has positive outcomes in pain reduction and functional status in people with chronic back pain.[7] Park et al. reported clinically significant improvement in arthritic pain, fatigue, and walking speed after 90 minutes of yoga per week for 8 weeks compared with traditional therapy programs in a pilot randomized controlled trial.[32] Yoga has not been associated with serious adverse events. The addition of yoga to a rehabilitation program for patients with preexisting back pain or join pain is reasonable given the potential benefit and low risk for harm.

Passive Complementary and Alternative Modalities

Acupuncture, both traditional and auricular, uses a meridian-based therapy of fine needles into the body. The principle is to stimulate realignment of the body's energy to promote wellness and anesthesia. A systematic review by MacPherson et al. reported that acupuncture is effective for chronic pain (except neck pain) and can have persistent effects for up to 12 months after last treatment.[33] Cumulative data point to positive therapeutic effect for migraines, osteoarthritic pain, headaches, lumbago, and shoulder pain.[10,33] Auricular acupuncture is also known as "battlefield acupuncture" for its use in the military population for various conditions, including anxiety, pain, and post-traumatic stress disorder.[34] The evidence to support the use of auricular acupuncture for pain management is sparse. However, small pilot studies and randomized controlled trials have reported some clinically significant improvement in pain. Dry-needling is another passive rehabilitative modality that may be especially useful for patients with demonstrable muscle trigger points and pain that limits more successful mobilization and participation in exercise.[7]

REHABILITATION INTERVENTIONS FOR CANCER-RELATED PAIN

Cancer pain is one of the most feared complications for cancer patients.[1] Thus, it should be addressed at diagnosis, as a consequence of therapies, in cancer survivors, or toward the end of life. This type of pain shares the same neuropathophysiologic pathway as noncancer pain. Multiple mechanisms are involved: inflammatory, neuropathic, ischemic, or compressive—and perhaps several mechanisms occurring simultaneously. Pain can be present in different and multiple anatomic sites. A full understanding of its neurophysiology will lead to best practice in pain management.[2] Thus, treatment of cancer pain should also use a multimodal approach. Assessing pain and risk factors for pain is critical early in the disease around the time of diagnosis. Prehabilitation programs may be implemented for general physical conditioning, to improve nutrition, and to provide patients with the psychological tools necessary to handle pain after curative or palliative interventions. Surgery, radiation therapy, chemotherapy, hormones, opioids, nonsteroidal anti-inflammatory drugs, and bisphosphonates are all used to treat cancer-related pain. Some cancer treatments, including surgery, radiation, and chemotherapy, can also cause persistent pain in cancer survivors. Chronic pain after surgery may occur in up to 50% of patients. For breast cancer surgery, risk factors for developing chronic pain include young age, chemotherapy and radiation therapy, poor postoperative pain control, and certain surgical factors. Cranial electrotherapy stimulation–alpha stimulation is a low-level electrical stimulation used for treatment of depression, anxiety, and insomnia. Few studies have evaluated this therapy for the treatment of pain. Pain reduction benefit has been reported in patients with advanced cancer, but less robust effects were seen in other conditions.[35] Combining cancer treatments, pharmacologic interventions, rehabilitation interventions, and complementary and alternative methods is a reasonable approach at all stages of the disease to maintain function and quality of life. Careful attention to personal goals is critical; understanding the specific needs of cancer survivors and the roles they want to fulfill in society is foundational for treatment of cancer survivors and for those in palliative care alike.

DISABILITY, IMPAIRMENT, LEGAL ACTION, AND THE CLINICIAN–PATIENT RELATIONSHIP

The definition of disability may vary depending on the context. In 1980, the World Health Organization provided the following definitions in their International Classification of Impairment, Disability, and Handicap[36]:

Impairment—In the context of health experience, an impairment is any loss or abnormality of psychological, physiological or anatomical structure or function. (Note: "Impairment" is more inclusive than "disorder" in that it covers losses—e.g., the loss of a leg is an impairment, but not a disorder).

Disability—In the context of health experience, a disability is any restriction or lack (resulting from an impairment) of ability to perform an activity in the manner or within the range considered normal for a human being.

Handicap—In the context of health experience, a handicap is a disadvantage for a given individual resulting from an impairment or a disability, that limits or prevents the fulfilment of a role that is normal (depending on age, sex, and social and cultural factors) for that individual.

Disability is defined by CMS as "inability to engage in any substantial gainful activity by reason of any medically determinable physical or mental impairment which can be expected to result in death or which has lasted or can be expected to last for a continuous period of not less than 12 months."[37] Regarding disability, the Social Security Administration follows a multistage process; regarding pain as a cause or contributor to disability, there is an additional two-stage process.[38] In the first stage, the determination team reviews the records for objective evidence of a medical impairment that is expected to be associated with pain. The second stage of assessment involves multiple factors, which are listed in the next box. Impairment is determined clinically as a loss or abnormality in some aspect of health (e.g., impaired vision, impaired cognition). Many times, clinicians can mitigate the impact of impairment through appropriate clinical support, this can include several clinical tasks and may seem time-consuming (see the box that follows). Nonetheless, responding to challenges that interfere with more successful integration into work and school life has a huge impact on patients, caregivers, and families.

Second-Stage Factors Included in Determination of Disability Related to Pain

Objective medical evidence
Medical history
Daily activities
Region, severity, and timing of pain
Worsening and relieving factors
Treatments used and side effects
Measures used for pain
Functional limitations and restrictions

Tasks That Support Patients With Impairment in Remaining Active

Writing work/school notes for time off to address medical concerns
Communicating needs for accommodation to school or employers as requested
Providing referrals for durable medical equipment
Referring patients for prosthetics and following up to ensure safe and effective utilization
Encouraging patients to communicate concerns
Addressing needs to appropriate access to accessible mass transit

---

Disability is the result of an organizational process of being determined unable to work and relies on the rules and requirements of the organization making that determination. Social Security determinations follow specified processes as noted previously. Many times, impairment and disability claims are related to accident, mishap, or injury; in these situations litigation or pending legal action may be at work. It is established based on observational studies that patients presenting with pain who additionally have pending legal action are more likely to have persistent and treatment-resistant pain.[39] There are a variety of factors that may contribute to this: In addition to potential secondary gain, there is stress and uncertainty that result from unresolved legal aspects. The primary obligation of the clinician, in most settings, is to the patient, and it may be helpful to be open with patients about their goals and objectives (Figure 12.1A and B). Some patients, determined to recover, will resolve or dispense with legal action when they are aware of the putative association of pending legal action and nonresolution of pain. Patients need to consider their life objectives carefully. Although a real randomized clinical trial evaluating the effects of litigation on pain resolution cannot be done for ethical reasons, patients may be interested to know that evidence is suggestive of litigation interfering with pain resolution.

APPLICATIONS IN OUTPATIENT CLINICAL PRACTICE

Access to structured pain rehabilitation programs may be limited, and these programs are not appropriate or necessary for all patients. One of the principles of this book is that the tenets of pain care can be applied effectively in primary care settings, given sufficient knowledge, motivation, and opportunity.[40] This chapter has introduced the concepts of pain rehabilitation, but the question of how to apply these in general

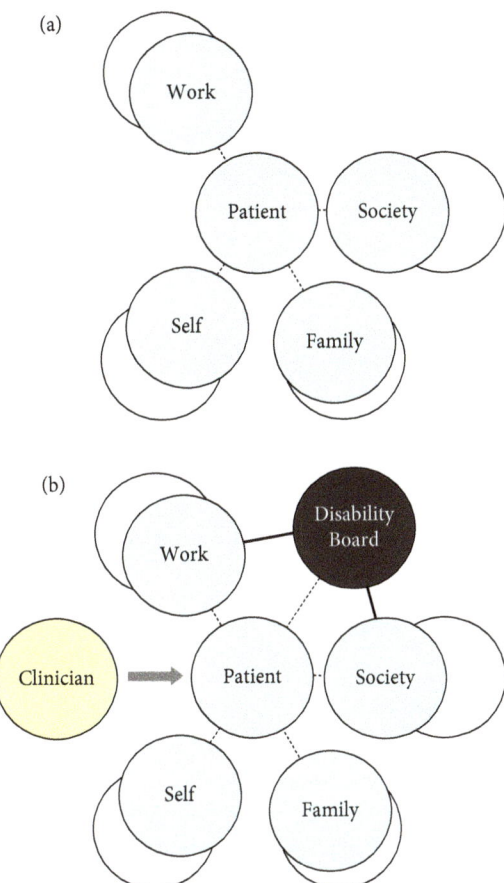

FIGURE 12.1 Relationships of patient to domains of function, healthcare provider, and disability system. **A,** Patient has diminished function in various domains of function during pain-associated illness. Function in domains may be diminished to differing degrees, depending on circumstances, the patient, and the condition. **B,** Clinician's primary responsibility is toward patient with a goal of recovery and resolution or control of pain. The disability board reports to the employer or the government. The patient's sense of well-being is often strongly influenced by the challenges and demands of the disability process.

settings remains. Based on the idea that a comprehensive pain self-management approach is highly empowering and effective for patients with chronic pain, it is possible to assemble such a plan in a primary care context if sufficient support and resources are present.[40,41] It is necessary to have patient education materials and a network of skilled providers, ideally including physiatrists, physical therapists, pharmacists, nursing educators, clinical psychologists, nutritionists, and potentially others. In the absence of a true interprofessional practice, providers can counsel patients about the process of incorporating comprehensive approaches and can work with the patient to develop these inputs simultaneously or in a sequential manner, or, depending on the patient's physical and cognitive capacity, can approach the problem on multiple fronts at once.[42] Some patients are eager for a coordinated solution because the potential benefits of coordinated evidence-based therapies are immediately apparent to them and they may be very interested in minimizing medications. Other patients will be less able to take

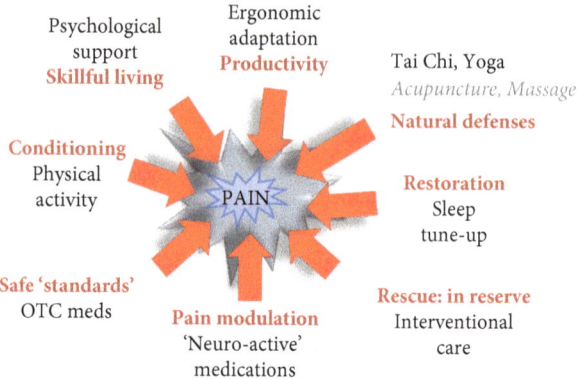

FIGURE 12.2 Coordinated nonopioid, evidence-based pain self-management planning implementable in outpatient primary practice (details in text). Based on the clinician's professional findings of likely nociceptive, inflammatory, or neuropathic pain mechanisms, it is possible to utilize rationally based pharmacologic selection process. In conditions with multiple potential mechanisms, medications may need to be combined for optimal outcomes.

on multiple new therapies at once, but even for these patients, it is very useful for the provider to have a mental roadmap of how such a plan could be assembled. It is then possible to propose therapies in the roadmap to the patient sequentially, depending on the patient's healthcare-related values, preferences, openness to new therapies, or commitment to self-management. Many patients with mild cognitive impairment still relish moderate daily exercise; if this can be incorporated safely, it is important to encourage exercise. Figure 12.2 illustrates the general format on one such roadmap for addressing complex or persistent pain states.

Coordinated Outpatient Pain Self-Management Plans

The basic elements of coordinated outpatient pain self-management are evidence-based and are listed in the following box and described more fully here.

Modalities Included in Coordinated Outpatient Pain Self-Management

Physical activity
Cognitive strategies
Mind–body therapies
Sleep optimization
Medication safety
Healthy surroundings

Physical Activity

Physical activity takes many forms, and there is evidence that moderate daily exercise (i.e., aerobic activity, stretching, and resistance exercise) is beneficial for several types of chronic pain; evidence is especially strong for chronic musculoskeletal pain. Physical activity can take other forms as well, including exercises oriented toward improving balance, a tailored home exercise program, and group activities. Evidence for these forms of physical activity vary by condition and intervention, but evidence is accruing in support of multiple forms of routine exercise. Recent evidence suggests that giving patients a specific exercise prescription may be highly effective for motivating positive behavior change.

Mental Preparation

Mental preparation is an umbrella term to cover the wide range of cognitive and psychological strategies that demonstrate effectiveness against chronic pain. These can be introduced to patients in the context of a primary care appointment if the provider is experienced with specific modalities. Some patients are interested in learning about therapies and will respond positively to suggestions for reading or strategically placed waiting room materials. Selected psychological pain approaches are described in this chapter and in Chapter 5.

Mind–Body Therapies

Mind–body therapies are demonstrating substantive efficacy against certain forms of chronic pain. Yoga is particularly effective in patients with chronic low back pain, and qi gong (slower, more fluid tai chi) is beneficial in patients with fibromyalgia. Other mind–body therapies, including forms of meditation such as mindfulness (mindfulness based stress reduction and mindfulness-oriented recovery enhancement), have demonstrated and continue to be studied for efficacy against pain.

Sleep Optimization

Sleep plays a critical role in pain modulation, and sleep and pain have a fundamental bidirectional relationship. Worse pain interferes with sleep, and poor sleep worsens pain. Steps to improve sleep such as enhancing sleep hygiene through removal of televisions and computers from bedrooms, elimination of blue light (screen) exposure well before bedtime, reduction of noise, increased comfort through padding for those with neck, back, and hip pain, and other measures are important to enhance sleep quality and optimize sleep duration. Sleep studies can be helpful in patients with chronic reports of poor sleep quality and daytime fatigue because this may indicate undiagnosed sleep apnea.

Medication Safety

Medication safety is a fundamental element of any comprehensive pain self-management plan. Patients must know which medications are to be taken on a time-contingent basis (standing dose) and which medications should be used for rescue therapy (as needed). Safe medication storage and refill practices, as well as medication risks, must be clearly explained. Universal precautions, originally developed for opioids, may be appropriate in many settings where pain is managed and pain-active medications are prescribed.

Environmental Factors

Management of the patient's environment and surroundings can have a profound effect on the success of any pain self-management plan. Some patients require additional support from their healthcare providers in order to successfully navigate recuperation from a pain-associated medical event. Whether from a sprain, strain, arthritis, headache, or a spinal issue, patients will vary in terms of their pace of rehabilitation. Some patients need additional ergonomic support, and it is possible for some working patients to have an ergonomic assessment in the workplace; this can make a huge difference for the patient who needs modified seating arrangements or perhaps a standing desk. Environmental factors extend to safety in the home: both from the surroundings (e.g., are there secure handrails on the stairs?) and from the persons who enter or share the patient's living space (e.g., does the patient feel safe at home?).

Taken together, these factors work holistically to build a positive, health-forward plan for pain self-management. Each of these elements must be considered and addressed in order for patients with chronic pain to have the best chance of effective recovery from a chronic pain event. Several examples of applying this approach to chronic pain conditions are provided in Chapter 16.

See Appendix VII for an evidence-based daily pain prevention plan that includes these elements (also see the following box, Text box 12.4).

Weekly Pain Prevention Plan

- *Hamstring stretches.* Find a spot with clear floor and wall space. Lying with your back on the floor, position buttocks close to wall. Stretch your legs up the wall; your body should be perpendicular to the wall and fully supported by the floor. Fold a towel under your head for comfort. Hold this position for several minutes. You will feel your hamstrings stretching. Contracting quads and abdominal muscles intermittently may help the hamstrings relax through reflex action.
- *Crunches twice weekly.* Do not do full sit-ups because these can strain back structures. Start with 3 crunches and build up to 25 twice a week.
- *Bridges twice weekly.* Lying on your back with the arms on the floor at your side, place your feet flat on floor near the buttocks. Using pelvic tilt to stabilize the abdomen and core, press up into half bridge and hold for a few seconds, then relax back down in a controlled manner. Repeat three times, twice a week.
- *Modified push-ups twice weekly.* Lying on your stomach, place the palms on floor on either side as if starting a push-up. Leaving hips and legs in contact with the floor, press through your hands to raise up a little and hold. This will give the spine a good extension stretch and help strengthen your arm muscles. You can use your back muscles to take some of the weight off the arms; this will help strengthen the back.

Table 12.1 Placebo and Related Effects

Effect	Definition
Placebo effect	An effect that results when no treatment or a placebo treatment is given
Nocebo effect	Negative effect resulting from patients' expectations of harm or side effects when no treatment effect exists
Expectancy effect	An effect that occurs as a result of patients' expectations; may be shaped by provider or other factors

EXPECTANCY AND PLACEBO EFFECTS

One factor that is present in every clinical encounter and yet remains very poorly understood is the effect of expectancy (expectation) and placebo. Often thought of in the context of medication effects, placebo and expectancy affect all treatments and health-related interactions (Table 12.1). Patients do respond to the positive effects of relating to healthcare providers. Clinicians hold a position of trust for many patients, and with the establishment of a therapeutic alliance in the course of single or repeated clinical encounters, the clinician can appropriately anticipate that the patient may expect improvements from certain therapies.[42] It is critically important for providers to be familiar with the evidence base associated with the greatest number of relevant therapies in their scope of practice so that they can aid patients in realizing the benefits of various therapies. Placebo effects are very prevalent in pain treatment; for this reason, it often takes a series of visits over several months' time to determine whether specific therapies are going to be needed in the long run. For example, a patient may initially perceive that there is a benefit associated with a certain medication. As the patient engages in a routine exercise program and learns skills associated with appropriate psychological strategies and optimizes sleep and environmental factors, the patient may come to appreciate that the medication is no longer providing added benefit and be able to taper the medication. In practice, it is not always essential to understand whether a specific medication was genuinely altering the pain neurochemistry according to the putative drug mechanism. What matters is the patient's perceived response and ability, in the context of that response, to incorporate positive lifestyle changes that ultimately lead them to be able to overcome pain or live well despite their pain.

IMPACT OF DEMENTIA AND COGNITIVE IMPAIRMENT

As noted previously, dementia and cognitive impairment have a major impact on the organization of a comprehensive treatment plan. It is important that the clinician understand the potential for coordinated care to benefit the patient and then, as Hippocrates noted, to be prepared to make the patient and the peripherals (i.e., caregivers) respond to the plan in a way that would benefit the patient. Some plans can be implemented all at once, and other plans need to be rolled out in a gradual manner. Some psychological strategies will not be accessible to patients with dementia.

Working With Caregivers

Caregivers are often overwhelmed by small changes to a routine when caring for patients with chronic pain. They experience the pain of their charge's suffering, but communication is limited by the dementia, and the caregiver feels helpless in the face of these difficulties. The clinician can work with caregivers to implement a coordinated care plan. Sometimes, written instructions are especially helpful because caregivers are often especially stressed during clinic visits. Make a short list of treatments or rescue strategies for the caregiver to "keep on the refrigerator"—the impact that this simple support can have is enormous.

SUMMARY

Many patients with chronic pain receive the majority of their care in an outpatient setting. In this context, it important to understand the evidence base supporting the most effective approaches to chronic pain management and to recognize the importance of coordinated care incorporating multiple forms of nonpharmacologic therapy as well as appropriate pharmacologic treatments that, taken together, address the patient's needs comprehensively and ultimately more effectively.

REVIEW QUESTIONS

1. Rehabilitation approaches to pain care include the following, *except*:
    a. Dry-needling
    b. PIPT
    c. ACT
    d. Arthroscopic knee surgery
    e. Mobilization

2. Pertaining to CBT, the following are correct, *except*:
    a. CBT can be integrated into a comprehensive rehabilitation program.
    b. CBT arose in the context of earlier behavioral approaches.
    c. CBT involves multiple mental strategies including cognitive reframing.
    d. CBT is not part of PIPT.
    e. CBT and ACT must be used together to be effective.

3. Regarding disability, impairment, and litigation, the following are correct, *except*:
    a. Disability is determined by the healthcare provider.
    b. Impairment refers to the loss of function or health in physical or mental functioning.
    c. Impairments may prompt healthcare providers to provide support for adaptive technology.
    d. Despite impairments, some patients may be able to function with workplace protections.
    e. Litigation is associated with poorer pain outcomes in patients after injury.

4. Treatment modalities included in coordinated pain self-management include:
    a. Physical activity
    b. Mental preparation
    c. Mind–body therapies
    d. Surgical referral
    e. Sleep optimization

REFERENCES

1. Perez J, Olivier S, Rampakakis E, et al. The McGill University Health Centre cancer pain clinic: a retrospective analysis of an interdisciplinary approach to cancer pain management. Pain Res Manage. 2016;2016:2157950.
2. Richeimer S. Palliative care section. Pain Med. 2006;7(4):319.
3. Wilson S, Chaloner N, Osborn M, Gauntlett-Gilbert J. Psychologically informed physiotherapy for chronic pain: patient experiences of treatment and therapeutic process. Physiotherapy. 2017;103(1):98–105.
4. Dadabayev AR, Coy B, Bailey T, et al. Addressing the needs of patients with chronic pain. Fed Pract. 2018;35(2):43–49.
5. Syrjala KL, Jensen MP, Mendoza ME, et al. Psychological and behavioral approaches to cancer pain management. J Clin Oncol. 2014;32(16):1703–1711.
6. Cantarero-Villaneuva I, Fernández-Lao C, Fernández-de-Las-Peñas C, et al. Effectiveness of water physical therapy on pain, pressure pain sensitivity, and myofascial trigger points in breast cancer survivors: a randomized, controlled clinical trial. Pain Med. 2012;11(1):1509–1519.
7. Rayegani S, Bayat M, Bahrami MH, et al. Comparison of dry needling and physiotherapy in treatment of myofascial pain syndrome. Clin Rheumatol. 2014;33(6):859–864.
8. Kalisch BJ, Lee S, Dabney BW. Outcomes of inpatient mobilization: a literature review. J Clin Nurs. 2014;23(11–12):1486–1501.
9. Cho HY, Kim EH, Kim J, Yoon YW. Kinesio taping improves pain, range of motion, and proprioception in older patients with knee osteoarthritis: a randomized controlled trial. Am J Phy Med Rehabil. 2015;94(3):192–200.
10. Skelly AC, Chou R, Dettori JR, et al. Noninvasive Nonpharmacological Treatment for Chronic Pain: A Systematic Review. Rockville, MD: Agency for Healthcare Research and Quality; 2018.
11. Messier SP, Resnik AE, Beavers DP, et al. Intentional weight loss for overweight and obese knee osteoarthritis patients: is more better? Arthritis Care Res. 2018;70(11):1569–1575.
12. Hayes SC, Strosahl KD, Wilson K. Acceptance and Commitment Therapy: The Process and Practice of Mindful Change (2nd ed.). New York: Guilford Press; 2016.
13. Melzack R, Wall P. Pain mechanisms: a new theory. Science. 1964;150(3699):971–979.
14. Fordyce W, Fowler R, Delateur B. An application of behavior modification technique to a problem of chronic pain. Behav Res Ther. 1968;6(1):105–107.
15. Flor H, Turk D. Chronic Pain: An Integrated Biobehavioral Approach [e-book]. Seattle: IASP Press; 2011.
16. Jensen M, Turk D. Contributions of psychology to the understanding and treatment of people with chronic pain: why it matters to ALL psychologists. Am Psychol. 2014;69(2):105–118.
17. Robinson M, O'Brien E. Chronic pain. In Handbook of Rehabilitation Psychology [e-book] (pp. 119–132). Washington, DC: American Psychological Association; 2010.

18. Williams ACDC, Eccleston C, Morley S. Psychological therapies for the management of chronic pain (excluding headache) in adults. Cochrane Database Sys Rev. 2012;(11):CD007407. doi:10.1002/14651858.CD007407.pub3.
19. Fordyce W. Behavioral Methods for Chronic Pain and Illness. St. Louis: Mosby; 1976.
20. Blanchard E, Andrasik F, Appelbaum K, et al. Three studies of the psychologic changes in chronic headache patients associated with biofeedback and relaxation therapies. Psychosom Med. 1986;48(1–2):73–83.
21. Beck A. Cognitive Therapy of Depression. New York: Guilford Press; 1979.
22. Thorn B. Cognitive Therapy for Chronic Pain: A Step-by-Step Guide. New York: Guilford Press; 2004.
23. Burns J, Nielson W, Jensen M, et al. Specific and general therapeutic mechanisms in cognitive behavioral treatment of chronic pain. J Consult Clin Psychol. 2015;83(1):1–11.
24. Ehde D, Dillworth T, Turner J. Cognitive-behavioral therapy for individuals with chronic pain: efficacy, innovations, and directions for research. Am Psychol. 2014;69(2):153–166.
25. Miller W, Rollnick S. Motivational Interviewing: Helping People Change (3rd ed.). New York: Guilford Press; 2013.
26. Santa Mina D, Matthew AG, Hilton WJ, et al. Prehabilitation for men undergoing radical prostatectomy: a multi-centre, pilot randomized controlled trial. BMC Surg. 2014;14(1):89. Accessed at: http://www.ncbi.nlm.nih.gov/pubmed/25394949. doi:10.1186/1471-2482-14-89.
27. McAnally H. Rationale for and approach to preoperative opioid weaning: a preoperative optimization protocol. Periop Med. 2017;6(1):19. doi:10.1186/s13741-017-0079-y.
28. Rozell JC, Courtney PM, Dattilo JR, Wu CH, Lee G-C. Preoperative opiate use independently predicts narcotic consumption and complications after total joint arthroplasty. J Arthroplast. 2017;32(9):2658–2662. doi:10.1016/j.arth.2017.04.002.
29. Silver JK, Baima J. Cancer prehabilitation. Am J Phys Med Rehabil. 2013;92(8):715–727.
30. Hijazi Y, Gondal U, Aziz O. A systematic review of prehabilitation programs in abdominal cancer surgery. Int J Surg. 2017;39:156–162. doi:10.1016/j.ijsu.2017.01.111.
31. Kong LJ, Lauche R, Klose P, et al. Tai chi for chronic pain conditions: a systematic review and meta-analysis of randomized controlled trials. Sci Rep. 2016;6(25325):1–9.
32. Park J, McCaffrey R, Newman D, et al. A pilot randomized controlled trial of the effects of chair yoga on pain and physical function among community-dwelling older adults with lower extremity osteoarthritis. J Am Geriatr Soc. 2016;65(3):592–597.
33. MacPherson H, Vertosick EA, Foster NE, et al. The persistence of the effects of acupuncture after a course of treatment: a meta-analysis of patients with chronic pain. Pain. 2017;158(5):784–793.
34. Yeh CH, Chiang YC, Hoffman SL, et al. Efficacy of auricular therapy for pain management: a systematic review and meta-analysis. Evid Based Complement Altern Med. 2014;2014:934670.
35. Yennurajalingam S, Kang DH, Hwu WJ, et al. Cranial electrotherapy stimulation for the management of depression, anxiety, sleep disturbance, and pain in patients with advanced cancer: a preliminary study. J Pain Symptom Manage. 2018;55(2):198–202.
36. World Health Organization. International classification of impairments, disabilities, and handicaps: a manual of classification relating to the consequences of disease, published in accordance with resolution WHA29. 35 of the Twenty-ninth World Health Assembly, May 1976. (1980).
37. 42 U.S.C. 423(d)(1)(A) and 1382c(a)(3)(A); see also 20 CFR 404.1505(a) and 416.905(a).
38. Consideration of Pain in the Disability Determination Process. Federal Register, Vol. 83, No. 241 / Monday, December 17, 2018 / Proposed Rules 64493.

39. Jacobs MS. Psychological factors influencing chronic pain and the impact of litigation. Curr Phys Med Rehabil Rep. 2013;1:135–141.
40. Dobscha SK1, Corson K, Perrin NA, et al. Collaborative care for chronic pain in primary care: a cluster randomized trial. JAMA. 2009;301(12):1242–1252.
41. Kroenke K, Krebs EE, Wu J, et al. Telecare collaborative management of chronic pain in primary care: a randomized clinical trial. JAMA. 2014;312(3):240–248.
42. Dadabayev A, Coy B, Bailey T, et al. Addressing the needs of patients with chronic pain. Fed Pract. 2018;35(2):43–49.
43. Colloca L. The placebo effect in pain therapies. Annu Rev Pharmacol Toxicol. 2019;59:191–211.

PART IV
PAIN CARE IN CLINICAL CONTEXT

13 Pain Emergencies and Complications of Pain Treatments

Isaac Tong, R. Jason Yong, and Beth B. Hogans

It never occurred to me to call 911 or my physician.... As foolish as it may appear, you are, in a sense, a prisoner of the pain, which was intolerable. You're thinking, "What could I do to relieve myself of it." If it becomes intense enough, you're perfectly willing to accept cardiac arrest as a possible way of getting rid of the pain.
—Michael DeBakey, pioneering cardiac surgeon describing his aortic rupture at age 97, *The New York Times*, December 25, 2006

LEARNING OBJECTIVES

At the completion of this chapter, the learner should be able to discuss:

- The clinical evaluation of acute chest pain and the application of the principles of this assessment to other pain conditions
- Major pain emergencies for the following areas: chest pain, abdominal pain, back/spine pain, head pain, pelvic pain, and limb pain
- Pertinent complications of pain treatments, such as overdose, withdrawal, and pump failure

CASE SCENARIO

A 62-year-old woman is admitted to the emergency department (ED) for evaluation following a single seizure. She has a fever of 38.6° C, pulse is 100 beats/minute, and other vital signs are normal. She is not able to provide a coherent history but nods when asked if she has pain and rubs her hand across her forehead, wincing briefly. She appears sensitive to light. Her husband provides the history that she has had recent dental work and takes one medication for mild hypertension that is well controlled. She drinks one to two drinks daily before dinner and was well until she had single seizure lasting about 2 minutes about 2 hours after dinner this evening, while watching TV. On examination she is mildly confused and slightly sleepy. She is not oriented to date or location. She is able to state her name and name objects. Her speech is mildly slurred. Cranial nerves are intact, and the remainder of the neurologic and general examination is intact.

1. What, specifically would you like to know about her exam (e.g., a pertinent negative)?
2. What is your differential diagnosis?
3. Head computed tomography (CT) and basic labs are normal except for a mild leukocytosis. What is your next diagnostic step?
4. What treatment will you start?

INTRODUCTION

Pain is often an indicator of serious illness and may indicate threats to life. In this chapter, we address both common medical emergencies associated with pain and emergencies arising from complications of pain treatments. Although general examples of emergent pain-associated conditions, such as chest pain, abdominal pain, limb pain, headache, and spine pain, are included here, each area of practice will evince specialist knowledge of pain-associated conditions, and the content here is intended as a general introduction to applying the principles of pain care to understanding and taking first steps in an emergent care setting, with competence and compassion. Local practice patterns vary, and this content is not a substitute for clinical advice, care paths, and practice parameters.

Pain management is practiced in a myriad of locations. Pain emergencies in the pain clinic are quite rare, but when they do occur they can be catastrophic and even deadly. The pain specialist should be familiar with the most common complications. This chapter aims at reviewing the most common pain complications and emergencies so that providers can recognize and provide prompt treatment.

Pain in the Emergency Department

The prevalence of pain among patients seen in the ED has been cited to be as high as 78%.[1] A national telephone survey performed by Todd et al. suggests that 24 million adults with chronic pain visit the ED annually and that 12 million visits are due to exacerbations of chronic pain syndromes.[2] Pain is inherently subjective and complex, and the ED physician is often tasked with the difficult job of assessing pain. Several practical pain assessment tools are available for clinical use. Pain intensity should be assessed for all patients presenting to the ED with either an 11-point numeric rating scale (NRS) or a graphic rating scale (GRS). The NRS is sensitive to short-term changes in pain intensity associated in ED, while the GRS or picture scales are useful for patients with limited literacy and children.[3] Additionally, pain levels should be assessed after therapeutic interventions and at the time of ED discharge.

Effective pain management should include multiple modalities. Simply asking about pain and validating the pain reports have significant effect on patients' satisfaction with ED pain management.[4] In general, it is inappropriate to delay pain therapies until a diagnosis has been established. Therapies and medications should be given as soon as clinically possible. If tolerated, therapeutics by mouth are most commonly used because they are convenient and inexpensive. When pain is severe, analgesics must be given immediately and titrated to effect. The intravenous (IV) rather than intramuscular route is preferred in this context.[5]

Chest Pain

One common example of pain as an indicator of serious illness is chest pain. By the completion of prelicensure preparation for primary practice, the health professions trainee will be familiar with the assessment of acute chest pain. The characteristics of acute coronary syndrome, in particular, will be familiar and rapid assessment well-rehearsed. The principles of pain care are at work here. As the provider quickly assesses the patient. the provider will want to know whether the pain is pressure-like or crushing (quality), if it is felt just under the left of the sternum with possible radiation to the arm or jaw (region), whether it is intense (severity), when it started, if it has been getting worse (timing), and what are the usually associated symptoms (shortness of breath), alleviating factors (rest, nitroglycerin), and worsening factors (activity).[6] These skills can be applied to various forms of pain presentations, emergent and nonemergent, and utilized to develop a differential diagnosis that will guide treatment and evaluation. A brief differential diagnosis of acute chest pain is provided in Table 13.1; by extracting key characteristics from the pain narrative, it is possible to obtain useful clues to diagnosis.

From a pain standpoint, large-scale cardiac outcomes research in recent years has changed the role of morphine from a standard part of acute coronary syndrome protocols to a secondary role to the overarching importance of restoring vascular integrity.[7] Although one recent retrospective study purported to show that morphine was no different from nonmorphine treatment outcomes, the group receiving morphine fared worse by multiple measures, with consistently lower Kaplan-Meier survival outcomes. However, according to a priori analysis, this difference did not reach statistical significance, suggesting the study was not sufficiently powered to reveal a difference, which was estimated as 4%.[8] At this point, based on the available retrospective data, it is not possible to exclude the possibility that patients treated with morphine have worse outcomes, and it is likely that this issue will require large-scale randomized studies to resolve because of the complex interactions of pain, revascularization, and ischemia.

Abdominal Pain

Abdominal pain is common in emergency care settings. The causes of abdominal pain range from life-threatening to benign. With the advent of spiral CT scans, a dramatic change came over the management of acute abdominal pain. In previous decades, it was common to refrain from providing analgesia to patients with acute abdominal pain in order to observe the course of pain and thereby discern diagnostic clues. This

Table 13.1 Chest Pain Emergencies, Differential Diagnosis Based on Classical Presentations, Selected Conditions

Condition	Quality	Region	Severity	Timing	Usually Associated With
Acute coronary syndrome	Crushing, pressure-like	Substernal, just left of midline, radiating to left arm or left jawline	Severe, crescendo	Begins acutely over minutes, mid to late morning predominance	Shortness of breath, diaphoresis
Aortic aneurysm rupture	Tearing, profound	Radiating to mid-back	Severe	Abrupt	Unstable vital signs, rapidly impending death
Pneumonia	Deep, aching to sharp	Based on chest well	Moderate to severe	Acute with insidious or sudden onset	Decreased oxygenation, abnormal chest radiograph
Pulmonary embolus	Variable		Moderate to severe	Abrupt or step-wise	Decreased oxygenation, recent immobility
Gastroesophageal reflux disease	Deep aching to sharp	Substernal	Moderate to severe	Acute to insidious, hours after last meal (nighttime)	Relief with Histamine-2 receptor antagonist
Costochondritis	Aching to sharp	Parasternal	Moderate to severe	Acute to chronic	Reproduced or worsened with local palpation

meant that patients who presented to the hospital with abdominal pain, expecting relief, would often wait for hours, writhing in agony until the clinical condition was "clear." This changed with the availability and relatively low radiation risk of spiral CT as well as the widespread availability of diagnostic ultrasound. With spinal CT and diagnostic ultrasound, the use of stat imaging in evaluation of acute abdominal pain has made it possible to quickly evaluate for acute processes such as appendicitis and to plan treatment, including analgesia, accordingly. The exception to this rule is in women of childbearing age, in whom pregnancy status must be established before CT or radiographic imaging. In the event of pregnancy or undetermined status, it is possible to plan a diagnostic strategy based on ultrasound. Nonetheless, it is useful to recognize the classical presentations of various abdominal pain–associated emergencies, summarized in Table 13.2.

Limb Pain

Acute limb pain may herald serious infection or vascular-ischemic events and should be addressed promptly. Physical examination, in particular inspection of the affected limb, is critically important for distinguishing various causes, but assessment begins with elicitation of the patient's pain narrative. Trauma is usually evident from the patient's history, but in patients with altered mental status, cognitive impairment, or polytrauma, history may not be sufficient. Patients may experience an insect bite without being aware. Soft tissue abscess can be caused by injection or penetrating trauma, so it is important to understand potentially relevant circumstances and whether the patient has had recent vaccination for tetanus. On examination, it is important to inspect the limb for evidence of focal or diffuse swelling (tumor), discoloration (rubor or purpura), thermal changes that may manifest as increased temperature (calor) or cooling of the limb, presence or absence of a pulse, vascular perfusion, chronic changes such as nail thickening or hair loss, and pain at rest, with movement, and with palpation or compression.[9] If discrete focal infection (e.g., abscess) is suspected, a soft tissue ultrasound is potentially helpful. In cellulitis, more common in patients with diabetes, chronic immobility, and immunosuppression, Doppler ultrasound may be less helpful, and diagnosis should incorporate clinical observations.[10] If vascular processes, either arterial or venous, are suspected, a vascular ultrasound, either portable Doppler, arterial flow with Doppler studies, or ankle-brachial index (ABI) study, is appropriate. Chronic vascular impairment may precede gangrene, which may rapidly progress to life-threatening sepsis and require amputation, depending on circumstances and responses to limb-sparing therapies.

Pelvic Pain

Acute pelvic pain can signal impending life-threatening illness, much in the way that chest or abdominal pain may herald critical illness. In women of childbearing-age, pregnancy is always a concern, and the hazards of pregnancy, including ectopic pregnancy and damage to the placenta, uterus, or fetus, and other aspects of obstetric care should be addressed. The details are beyond the scope of this text. One benign cause of sharp abrupt pain in the anterior pelvis during or after pregnancy is laxity of the anterior symphysis pubis, which can present as severe pain provoked by stepping or even

Table 13.2 Selected Abdominal Pain Emergencies, Differential Diagnosis Based on Classical Presentations

Condition	Quality	Region	Severity	Timing	Usually Associated With
Cholecystitis	Colicky, cramping	Right upper quadrant	Severe in waves	Worsens over days to weeks	Worse after fatty meal (fertile, female, in 40s)
Pancreatitis	Deep, boring to sharp	Upper abdomen	Moderate to severe	Acute with insidious or sudden onset	Elevated amylase, worse with eating/drinking
Appendicitis	Variable	Initially diffuse focuses to right lower quarter	Moderate to severe	Abrupt or progressive	With or without fever
Renal stone	Aching to sharp	Flank	Unbearably severe in waves	Acute onset	Personal or family history of stones
Ruptured ectopic pregnancy	Aching to profound	Lower abdomen	Moderate to severe	Insidious with abrupt worsening	Anemia, signs of pregnancy

any movement.[11] This may be responsive to strengthening of the adductor muscles of the thigh or other physical therapy. An analogous syndrome in the posterior pelvis (i.e., dysfunction of the sacroiliac) occurs in both males and females and may present with acute onset as sharp pain in the lateral low back or posterior pelvis. This condition may respond well to manual therapy, as performed by chiropractors, physical therapists, and some osteopathic practitioners. Repeated or persistent dislocation may not respond as well to manual repositioning as the first episodes, so core strengthening is important in order to prevent recurrence. Infections such as urinary tract infection, pelvic inflammatory disease, or epididymitis may present with pain in the pelvic area, and appropriate diagnostic testing should be considered. The distal gastrointestinal tract passes through the pelvis, and pathologies here may present with pelvic pain. Neuropathic syndromes such as pudendal neuropathy exist, but these typically present with a more chronic timeframe; however, in some situations, the pain is noted to abruptly become intolerable, prompting the patient to seek immediate care.

Headache

Acute severe headache with fever or neurologic impairment represents a pain emergency. Major causes of emergent headache include stroke, neoplasm, and infection. Stroke and infection are typically characterized by abrupt and rapidly evolving neurologic deficits, whereas neoplasm may present more indolently.

Stroke may begin with headache; most commonly, intracranial hemorrhage (ICH) is associated with headache, although headache may accompany ischemic stroke as well. In addition, subarachnoid hemorrhage (SAH) classically presents with "thunderclap headache," a severe, dramatically abrupt headache often described as the worst in the patient's life, occasionally with a transient alteration of consciousness. SAH results typically from a release of blood from a vascular aneurysm. These events are very important to recognize because the mortality associated with unrecognized SAH is high. The presence of blood in both the subarachnoid space and ICH (parenchyma) is visualized by head CT. The sensitivity of head CT for SAH and ICH, although high, is not 100%, and local practice patterns dominate decision-making regarding the requirements for additional testing. CT combined with lumbar puncture (LP) for evaluation of cerebrospinal fluid (CSF) for blood and blood products is considered definitive to exclude SAH, but LP would not be appropriate for patients with ICH. Interpretation of spinal fluid results is summarized in Table 13.3. Most patients with SAH will require additional imaging to assess for the potential presence of intracranial vascular aneurysms, which may require interventional or surgical management. In many cases, neurosurgery or interventional radiology will be consulted. In patients with hemorrhagic stroke (ICH), acute neurologic deficits or stroke signs are evidence. For ICH, tissue plasminogen activator (tPA) is not appropriate, but acute care management is required. These patients may need aggressive blood pressure control. If the patient does well in the early stroke period and no further bleeding occurs, these patients often have dramatic functional recovery as blood is resorbed; by contrast, if revascularization is not attained, ischemic stroke will result in permanent loss of brain centers, and recovery may be protracted or quite limited. The establishment of acute stroke centers has contributed to reducing the burden of stroke impairment, but rapid, competent assessment is essential for good outcomes.

Table 13.3 Cerebrospinal Fluid Analysis of Headache and Back Pain Emergencies, Differential Diagnosis Based on Classical Presentations

Condition	Red Blood Cells	White Blood Cells	Protein	Glucose
Meningitis*	Variable	Markedly elevated, neutrophils early, lymphocytes later	Elevated	Decreased
Viral encephalitis*	Variable, elevated in herpes simplex encephalitis	Elevated, lymphocytic predominance	Elevated	Normal
Fungal*	Variable	Variably elevated, lymphocytic	Elevated	Variably decreased
Tuberculous*	Variable	Variably elevated, lymphocytic	Elevated	Variably decreased
Abscess*	Variable	Variably elevated, lymphocytic	Elevated	Normal
Guillain-Barré syndrome	None	Normal	Elevated, 100 mg/dL	Normal

*Additional testing may include cultures, polymerase chain reaction, or staining procedures as appropriate.

Headache associated with neoplasm was traditionally described as headache that was worse upon awakening; however, support for this in the evidence-based literature has been limited. Neoplasms may be associated with progressively worsening neurologic deficits, but when the nondominant hemisphere (in most people the right hemisphere) is involved, symptoms may be subtle and detection delayed. Tumors that involve speech centers (the dominant hemisphere) may present with slurring of speech, agrammatical speech, speech arrest, or word-finding difficulties. Neoplasms based in the cortex (outer, cellular layer of the brain) may lead to seizures as the first incontrovertible symptom; these patients will require anticonvulsant therapy in addition to the therapy necessary to manage the neoplastic process. Glioblastoma multiforme is the most common primary brain tumor in adults; pediatric primary brain tumors vary by age and location in the brain. Brain metastases are not uncommon in other cancer syndromes such as lung, breast, and melanoma, in approximately 33, 22, and 11%, respectively. Other, less common primary cancers include renal, uterine, and colon adenocarcinoma.

Infections leading to emergent headache syndromes include meningitis and encephalitis. Meningitis involves a bacterial infection based in the meninges and characterized by severe acute headache, photophobia, and neck stiffness. Neck stiffness can be assessed by passive range of motion testing, moving the head in flexion and extension as the patient is told to relax and allow the motion to occur. Fever is commonly present but may be variable; thus, the classic triad of headache, fever, and neck stiffness may not always be present, and an index of suspicion should pertain according to clinical context. Additional symptoms of photophobia, nausea, and vomiting are common; whereas rash and neurologic deficits are observed often but less frequently. Encephalitis is often a viral infection of the brain, and as such, evidence of brain dysfunction, such as seizures, neurologic deficits, and depressed alertness, may be seen. Neck stiffness is less common but does not preclude encephalitis. Therefore, the classical presentation of encephalitis is headache, fever, and new neurologic deficit. This triad may also be present in other syndromes, such as brain abscess. The analysis of stat brain imaging and CSF is useful in establishing the diagnosis. Common causative agents of viral encephalitis include herpes simplex, but West Nile virus is increasing in prevalence.[12] Bacterial meningitis is a true emergency, and treatment should not be delayed because death may ensue rapidly if treatment is not given. For this reason, it may be necessary to start empiric antibiotics before obtaining CSF for analysis. This may eliminate the possibility of identifying the causative organism by culture but may be life-saving. Common causative agents, such as *Streptococcus pneumoniae, Neisseria meningitidis,* and group B *Streptococcus,* should be considered likely; *Listeria* species infection may be more common in older adults, and consideration of Lyme disease and syphilis depends on clinical context prevalence of syphilis, which is rising dramatically in some regions.[12]

Spine Pain

Acute spine pain may arise from a variety of processes: Infection, neoplasm, spontaneous fracture, and vascular compromise are all potential causes, depending on the clinical context (e.g., patient factors and setting). The first step, after airway, breathing, and circulation are secured, is to ensure the stability of the spine. In most patients admitted for trauma evaluation, the patient is already immobilized on arrival to the ED. Spinal column integrity and stability are critically important to preventing permanent paralysis, and the column should be "cleared," that is, evaluated for stability, according to local protocols before mobilization of the patient.

Infection as a cause of spine pain is uncommon but potentially catastrophic. Epidural abscess can arise most commonly in patients with immunocompromise, such as those who have previously undergone transplantation or those with alcoholism. New focal pain at or slightly above the level of involvement, tied to neurologic deficits, such as upper motor neuron deficits (weakness with hyperreflexia), and occurring in the context of signs of or risks for infection warrants urgent investigation. Treatments include prolonged antibiotics and possible needs for stabilization or surgical débridement. Transverse myelitis can occur either as an isolate infectious/autoimmune process, and it is associated with more diffuse pain and distal (caudal) neurologic deficits.

Metastatic involvement of the spine is common in patients with advanced neoplastic disease. Spinal metastatic disease can be very painful, and advanced cancer care is appropriate. Depending of the extent and site of involvement, therapies can include radiation, systemic medications, focal instillation, or nerve-directed blocks or ablation procedures.

Spontaneous and trauma-evoked vertebral fractures are typically very painful and require several weeks to resolve. There is substantive controversy over the use of glue-based fillers to stabilize fractured vertebrae. Although some have advocated for this as an effective pain-reducing intervention, there are recent reports that find modest support for this intervention.[13]

Shingles is a common cause of acute back pain that may respond to immediate treatment. This is discussed in Chapter 14.

Guillain-Barré syndrome is an emergent postinfectious ascending paralysis that can present with new onset of diffuse low back pain. It is important to recognize this condition quickly, and weakness progressing to failure of respiratory effort can lead to death. The clinical hallmarks are new onset of diffuse low back pain, with ascending weakness that is rapidly progressive (hours to days). On examination, reflexes may be absent in the lower extremities. Emergent referral for CSF assessment and admission for acute management including IV immunoglobulin and respiratory support as needed are appropriate.

Spinal cord stroke is uncommon but can occur either in the context of surgical manipulation of the aorta or otherwise. Vascular supply to the cord consists of one anterior spinal artery, which is partially anastomotic at levels between the rostral anterior spinal artery forming at about C2 and the artery of Adamkiewicz at about T10, and two dorsal spinal arteries. Anterior spinal artery occlusion can result in paralysis, most typically paraplegia, with some sensory loss; pain may or may not be present.

Cauda Equina Syndrome Cauda equina syndrome is caused by compression or injury to the nerve roots distal to the level of spinal cord compression. It usually involves the lumbar and sacral nerve roots. Cauda equina syndrome, while rare, may stem from many etiologies: intervertebral disk herniation, spinal metastases, spinal hematoma, epidural abscess, traumatic compression, acute transverse myelitis, or abdominal aortic dissection.[14] Symptoms result from compression of multiple lumbosacral nerve roots below the level of the conus medullaris. The patient may initially present with radicular pain in the lower extremities in a sciatic distribution, weakness, gait disturbances, abdominal discomfort from urinary retention, and overflow incontinence. The physical exam demonstrates saddle anesthesia, which is diminished sensation in the buttocks and perineum, diminished anal sphincter tone, and evidence of urinary retention. The severity of the symptoms depends on the degree of compression and the precise nerve roots that are being compressed. Tumors affecting the cauda equina, unlike conus tumors, produce slowly and irregularly progressive signs and symptoms of compression. The diagnosis should be made with the aid of magnetic resonance imaging (MRI), which should include imaging of the entire spine because of the possibility of spinal cord compression at higher levels.[14] Cauda equina syndrome can be classified as a rare neurosurgical emergency that requires urgent decompressive surgery to reduce the possibility of permanent neurologic sequalae (Figure 13.1).

Sickle Cell Disease

A sickle cell crisis is one of the most common reasons for ED visits by patients with sickle cell disease. Vaso-occlusive pain crises, caused by vessel occlusion by sickled red blood cells leading to decreased tissue oxygenation or ischemia, exemplify the syndrome of pseudoaddiction—a condition resembling drug addiction but caused by underprescription of drugs to treat pain, causing the patient to seek more. Patients with sickle cell disease may face substantive stigma; in one survey study, 53% of

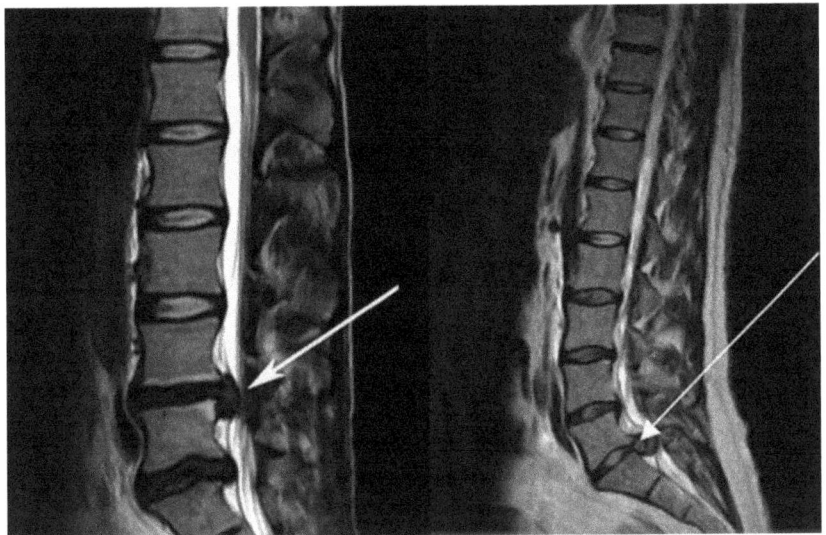

FIGURE 13.1 Cauda equina syndrome.

emergency physicians believed that more than 20% of sickle cell patients were addicted to opioids.[15] A protocolized approach to opioid administration in the setting of a vaso-occlusive pain crisis has been shown to decrease hospital admission for sickle cell pain, total inpatient days, and hospital stay lengths. An emphasis on continuous opioid infusion and sustained courses of controlled-release opioids may be needed to treat sickle cell crisis. It is important to incorporate treatments that address the pathophysiology of the disorder, such as oxygen supplementation and hydration. For long-term management, dedicated programs that support patient self-management strategies may be valuable.

COMPLICATIONS OF PAIN TREATMENTS

Medication Complications

See Table 13.4 for a summary of pain emergencies and their consequences.

Table 13.4 Pain Emergencies: Differential Diagnosis Based on Classical Presentations, Side Effects, and Consequences of Systemic Opioids

Common	*Undesirable Consequences*
• Mild respiratory depression	• Respiratory arrest
• Sedation	• Generalized muscle rigidity
• Nausea	• Myoclonus
• Vomiting	• Hyperalgesia
• Pruritus	• Neurotoxicity
• Constipation	• Nystagmus
• Dependency and tolerance	• Abuse and addiction

Opioid Overdose

Opioids are used for the treatment of moderate to severe pain and may cause numerous side effects, such as constipation, nausea, vomiting, sedation, and respiratory depression as well as lead to the risk for misuse and abuse. Over the past several decades, opioid use for nonmalignant pain has increased dramatically.

The most common side effect of opioid overdose is sedation. Sedation most frequently occurs at initiation of an opioid regimen or when a dose increase occurs. Symptoms frequently resolve within a few days. Sedation for extended periods may occur when comorbidities, such as dementia or impaired metabolism, or other sedating medications are used. Many medications, including antihistamines, antidepressants, and anxiolytics (e.g., benzodiazepines), can contribute to sedation.

The most feared complication of an opioid overdose is respiratory depression and respiratory arrest. The US Food and Drug Administration (FDA) advises that opioids pose a high risk for harm because of their risk for causing respiratory depression. Opioids act on respiratory centers in the brainstem to produce respiratory depression to the point of apnea.[16] Tolerance to respiratory depression develops with prolonged use, as with many other opioid side effects, so that respiratory depression is less common in patients on stable, chronic opioid regimens. When hypoxia occurs in a patient with long-term opioid use, other causes should be explored, such as pneumonia, pulmonary embolism, or the overdose of another sedating medication such as a benzodiazepine. The treatment of opioid overdose is the use of an opioid antagonist such as naloxone. Naloxone may need to be readministered, given its short half-life versus the longer half-life of most opioids.

Opioid overdose in the context of addiction to prescription medications or IV opioids such as heroin presents a particularly critical encounter to address a patient's substance abuse. Often, additional psychiatric, social, and infectious comorbidities also need to be treated. Addiction services and counseling are not always available in the emergency setting, but patients and families need to be engaged in conversation and motivated to seek long-term treatment.[17] Intramuscular or intranasal naloxone (Narcan) should be prescribed at hospital discharge to the patient who has survived an opioid overdose (regardless of the clinical scenario). Naloxone has not been shown to increase the risk for further misuse or abuse but has been demonstrated to save lives.

Serotonin Syndrome

Serotonin syndrome is a life-threatening condition that occurs as a result of excess serotonin in the serotonin neural system. The condition is classically associated with the concomitant use of a monoamine oxidase inhibitor (MAOI) with another antidepressant such as a selective serotonin reuptake inhibitor (SSRI), selective serotonin/norepinephrine reuptake inhibitor (SNRI), or tricyclic antidepressant (TCA), but it can occur with any drug that increases serotonin in the body. This syndrome is a clinical diagnosis and usually consists of a triad of symptoms: cognitive changes, neuromuscular excitability, and autonomic instability (see the following box). There is a broad range in the severity of presentation. Although life-threatening complications are rare, they can include disseminated intravascular coagulation, leukopenia, thrombocytopenia, tonic-clonic seizures, multiorgan failure, rhabdomyolysis, and respiratory failure. The most current diagnostic criteria require three of the following: agitation, mental status changes, myoclonus, shivering, tremor, hyperreflexia, ataxia, diarrhea, or fever.[18] The differential diagnosis includes neuromuscular malignant syndrome, delirium tremens, anticholinergic toxicity, and sympathomimetic overdose.

The treatment of serotonin syndrome is primarily supportive. Usually, the syndrome resolves with discontinuation of the serotonergic medications alone, with 70% of patients recovering within 24 hours, 40% requiring intensive care unit admission, and 25% requiring intubation.[18] Benzodiazepines are first-line treatments to decrease myoclonus and the muscle rigidity that can lead to respiratory compromise and rhabdomyolysis. Second-line treatments for muscular rigidity include nondepolarizing neuromuscular blocking agents or paralytics. ß-Blockers may be used to blunt autonomic instability.

Common Signs of Serotonin Syndrome

- Agitation
- Mental status changes (confusion, hypomania)
- Myoclonus
- Shivering
- Hyperreflexia
- Ataxia
- Diarrhea
- Fever

Neuraxial Complications

Complications From Epidural Steroid Injections

Epidural steroid injections (ESIs) are one of the most commonly used interventional techniques for the management of radicular pain. The overall incidence of complications from ESI is low; however, catastrophic complications may occur.[19] Complications and side effects can be generalized into two categories: injectate side effects and complications associated with needle placement.

ESIs may lead to adverse events such as hyperglycemia, Cushing syndrome, hypertension, venous thrombosis, secondary infections, psychological disorders, epidural lipomatosis, osteoporosis, and numerous other endocrine and dermatologic manifestations. ESIs have been shown to affect native cortisol concentrations for up to 30 days after a single injection. This effect is likely due to the suppression of the hypothalamic-pituitary-adrenal axis.[20] The total dose of steroids given during a specific time is highly associated with steroid complications. There is also growing evidence that particulate steroids have an increased incidence of vascular events.

It is general practice to limit the total annual dose of steroids to the smallest efficacious dose possible. There is no evidence that large doses of steroids are superior to low doses. Some have recommended limiting the amount of annual steroid dose to 3 mg/kg of triamcinolone or equivalent.[21]

Cervical spine transforaminal ESIs have been reported to result in catastrophic complications such as stroke, paralysis, and death. While the mechanism is unclear, it is thought to be from trauma to a radicular artery supplying the anterior or posterior spinal arteries or from embolism and vasospasm resulting from particular steroids. Some interventional pain specialists use nonparticulate steroid solutions such as dexamethasone when performing transforaminal epidural injections in the cervical, thoracic, or lumbar spine.[22]

Complications associated with epidural needle placement have been noted. Complications such as pneumocephalus, pneumothorax, intravascular injection, epidural hematoma, subdural injection, epidural abscess formation, nerve damage, spinal cord trauma, cerebrovascular infarction, vasovagal episodes, and increased pain have all been reported during and after epidural injections. Epidural hematoma formation is a significant but uncommon complication in patients receiving anticoagulation therapies. Epidural hematoma formation has been estimated to occur in 1 in 150,000 to 220,000 patients undergoing neuraxial procedures.[23]

Complications From Intrathecal Delivery of Drugs

During the past decades, implantable drug delivery devices (designed for long-term continuous infusions of medications administered by a subcutaneous pump reservoir connected to an intrathecally implanted catheter) have been adopted as a tool in the management of chronic pain syndromes (Figure 13.2). Intrathecal drug delivery systems were initially indicated for cancer pain, but their use has expanded to include treatment of patients with noncancerous chronic pain conditions as well as those with neurologic disorders such as spinal and cerebral origin spasticity (e.g., secondary to spinal cord or cerebral origin spasticity, Parkinson disease, and others).[24] While intrathecal delivery of drugs has changed the lives of thousands of patients, and most systems are managed by a specialist such as a pain management interventionalist or neurosurgeon, the potential for complications must be recognized by anyone in contact with patients with this spinal drug delivery system.[25]

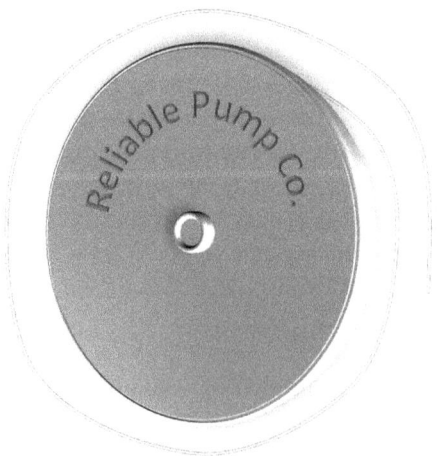

FIGURE 13.2 Intrathecal pump, mock-up.

Postimplantation Surgical and Bleeding Complications

Bleeding is a risk with any surgical procedure. Severe bleeding is a rare postoperative complication seen with implantation of intrathecal drug delivery systems. All patients should be screened for risk factors that could cause intraoperative and postoperative bleeding. As always, a careful review of the medical history should be done. Laboratory studies such as platelet count, prothrombin, and partial thromboplastin time should be evaluated if the patient has any risk factors for abnormal bleeding.[26]

Wound hematoma or seroma develops more commonly than clinically significant epidural bleeding. A wound hematoma is usually due to inadequate hemostasis. A wound hematoma usually manifests by local pain, pressure, and swelling over the surgical wound. Most wound hematomas or seromas can be managed conservatively and will resolve spontaneously. A large collection can be surgically evacuated or percutaneously aspirated. In the event of a wound hematoma or seroma, early pump refills should be limited because puncture of the skin increases the risk for infection. A large hematoma overlying the pump will make accessing the refill port difficult and increase the chance of accidental subcutaneous injection of the medication.

An epidural hematoma is a rare but potentially catastrophic complication that occurs when accessing the epidural or intrathecal space. The incidence of epidural hematomas is significantly increased when patients are anticoagulated. The incidence of epidural hematoma has historically been cited at 1:150,000 for epidural anesthesia and 1:220,000 for spinal anesthesia, but a recent study estimates the incidence to be as high as 1:3,600 in certain patient populations. Incidence is increased at least 10- to 100-fold in the setting of anticoagulation. If left untreated, an epidural hematoma can progress and result in numbness, weakness, increased pain, and ultimately paralysis. If the development of an epidural hematoma is suspected, immediate MRI and surgical evaluation should be done. Prompt hematoma evacuation should be performed within 8 hours of the onset of symptoms because evacuation within this time frame has been associated with better neurologic outcomes.[26]

Infectious Complications

The incidence of infection following intrathecal drug delivery system implantation is low. Most wound infections present early as pain, swelling, erythema, and tenderness over the surgical incision, with or without purulent drainage. If an infection of the pump pocket occurs, the device and the catheter should be removed. If there is no extension of the infection toward the lumbar catheter insertion site, it is possible to leave the intrathecal catheter in situ and occlude it just above the fascial insertion site. When the infection has resolved, the catheter can be revised and a new pump implanted to a site remote from the previous infection. The safest and most conservative approach is to reimplant the entire system after the infection has resolved. Meanwhile, the provider must have a strategy to prevent any withdrawal syndromes, such as reinstitution of systemic analgesics.

Meningitis After Pump Implantation

Meningitis is a rare but lethal complication following a pump implantation. There are sparse data regarding the incidence of meningitis after an intrathecal pump implantation. Ghosh et al. report a 6% incidence of meningitis in 119 children undergoing intrathecal pump implantation for administration of baclofen.[27] Epidural abscess is a rarely reported complication of epidural corticosteroid injection for treatment of radicular back pain, and the incidence remains undetermined.[28]

The clinical presentation of bacterial meningitis includes fever, chills, intractable, headache, nausea, vomiting, and nuchal rigidity. If meningitis is suspected, LP should be performed to obtain a culture, and broad-spectrum antibiotics should be started. The most conservative approach is to remove the hardware. If there is no evidence of pump infection, some clinicians may elect to remove only the spinal catheter and leave the pump intact. In this case, the pump should be emptied, filled with preservative-free saline, and set to run at a minimum flow rate.[29]

Cerebrospinal Fluid Leak and Postdural Puncture Headache

CSF leak and postdural puncture headache are known and expected consequences of intrathecal pump implantation. Headaches are more commonly associated with multiple attempts and dural puncture sites. CSF can also leak around the catheter where it enters the dura. Some implanters try to minimize the leak by placing a pursestring suture around the catheter below the fascial insertion site.

Postdural puncture headache is classically described as a positional headache that is worsened in the upright position. Initial management includes bed rest, fluid administration, and use of an abdominal binder. Medications such as IV caffeine and IV hydration have been shown to be effective. In some cases, patients may present with a CSF hygroma beneath the lumbar incision. Outpatient management involves similar strategies with bed rest, hydration with caffeinated beverages, and medication. Initially, short courses of Fioricet (butalbital, caffeine, and acetaminophen) can be given. In refractory cases, a Medrol dose pack may attenuate symptoms. The majority of these cases will resolve spontaneously. Normally, cases of postdural puncture headache can be managed with an epidural blood patch to prevent continued CSF leak; however, with hardware in place, most providers will only perform an epidural blood patch as a last resort.

Intrathecal Opioid Effects

True anaphylaxis is extremely rare with the use of intrathecal opioids. The most common side effects experienced by patients receiving intrathecal opioids mirror those from oral opioids: respiratory depression, gastrointestinal symptoms, urinary dysfunction, hormonal alterations, and itching. Respiratory depression results from the supraspinal interaction of the opioids with μ_2-receptors in the brainstem. It can also occur with systemic absorption into the blood and redistribution to the CNS. This is most likely to occur in patients who have opioid tolerance. Respiratory depression can occur as soon as 4 hours after initial intrathecal dosing and as late as 24 hours after dosing. Treatment of respiratory depression consists of respiratory support and the use of a μ-opioid receptor antagonist such as naloxone.

Urinary retention has been reported in up to 20 to 40% of patients receiving intrathecal opioids.[30] This is due to a reduction in detrusor muscle tone and detrusor urethral sphincter dyssynergia. The urinary effects are usually self-limited and resolve within 24 to 48 hours. Treatment entails intermittent bladder catheterization until the issue resolves.

In the case of a malfunctioning intrathecal pump or abrupt discontinuation of opioids leading to opioid withdrawal, withdrawal symptom management may include measures to minimize a patient's discomfort—though there is no direct emergency related to opioid withdrawal. Symptoms such as tachycardia, gastrointestinal distress, and sweating may be attenuated with the use of other agents (e.g., tizanidine, clonidine).

Intrathecal Baclofen Withdrawal

Intrathecal baclofen may be administered for severe spasticity symptoms. If abruptly discontinued, intrathecal baclofen withdrawal is a life-threatening complication. Baclofen withdrawal usually presents with spasticity and progresses to rigidity, pruritus, hyperthermia, and drowsiness. Life-threatening complications such as respiratory depression, rhabdomyolysis, acute renal failure, acute multiorgan failure, and even death can ensue.[31] The differential diagnosis of baclofen withdrawal includes autonomic dysreflexia, sepsis, narcoleptic malignant syndrome, and malignant hyperthermia. Making an accurate diagnosis before initiation of treatment is essential because management differs between acute baclofen withdrawal and other conditions. Early recognition is essential. The pillars of treating baclofen withdrawal are aimed at diminishing exacerbations in muscle spasticity, treating blood pressure lability, and treating seizures and delirium. Currently, there is not a definitive approach to treating acute baclofen withdrawal. Numerous agents have been shown to have success in the prevention and treatment of baclofen withdrawal symptoms, including oral and intrathecal baclofen, benzodiazepines, cyproheptadine, and dantrolene.

Treatment includes the restoration of the intrathecal baclofen infusion. In patients with severe baclofen withdrawal, oral baclofen alone is inadequate for replacing large intrathecal doses. Oral baclofen is often not effective in the early stages of acute baclofen withdrawal because of its slow onset of action (3–4 days) and time to peak effect (5–10 days). In such cases, a lumbar spinal catheter and infusion should be started. A commonly used intrathecal bolus dose is 50 µg, with maintenance infusion doses ranging from 12 to 2,000 µg/day. In cases in which resumption of an intrathecal infusion is not possible, acute treatment of baclofen withdrawal may necessitate medications other than baclofen to prevent the deleterious effects of withdrawal. High doses or a continuous infusion of benzodiazepines or propofol may be necessary for those with severe withdrawal requiring intensive care monitoring and management.[32]

Intrathecal Clonidine Withdrawal

Clonidine may also be included in an intrathecal infusion for management of chronic pain. Clonidine withdrawal has been reported to have significant side effects as well. Abrupt cessation of clonidine has resulted in rebound hypertension in patients with higher doses. It has been suggested that patients receiving intrathecal clonidine be given oral clonidine in case of withdrawal.

Refill Complications

Common complications when refilling an intrathecal pump include subcutaneous administration, accidental intrathecal injection, and pump programming errors. These can be avoided by following a strict protocol. It is essential to interrogate the intrathecal pump and confirm correct refill medication. Refills should only be performed with the appropriate needles that are provided in the refill kit.

Inadvertent injection in the subcutaneous tissue around the pump has been reported. If the pump solution contains high-dose opioids, a pocket refill may lead to significant respiratory depression. If subcutaneous injection occurs, an opioid antagonist may be indicated. If a direct injection into the CSF has occurred, the patient should be admitted to the hospital for observation and frequent monitoring. If the patient develops significant respiratory depression, the patient may require endotracheal intubation and ventilatory support.[33]

SUMMARY

Pain emergencies can have disastrous consequences. Diagnosis and decisive treatment of pain emergencies should be initiated promptly to avoid catastrophic patient outcomes. Patient education about specific signs and symptoms of pain emergencies and complications of pain treatment is essential to ensure early recognition and treatment. Pain specialists should practice with techniques that minimize complications. When evaluating a patient with suspected complication of pain treatment, systemic or focal, a focused history and physical examination should be done to elucidate any acute neurologic change. There should be a low threshold to refer any patient with acute neurologic changes for further imaging and appropriate consultation.

REVIEW QUESTIONS

1. A 57-year-old male presents with left-sided chest pain that is sharp and hurts worse when you press on the left side of the sternum. You suspect the patient may have:
    a. Acute coronary syndrome
    b. Gastroesophageal reflux (GERD)
    c. Costochondritis
    d. Pneumonia

2. A 46-year-old woman presents with a throbbing headache on the left side of her head. She says this is more intense than her usual headaches. As you are examining her, her speech becomes slurred so that you have trouble understanding her, and you notice that the right side of her mouth is drooping, which it was not when you started your exam. You rush her to CT and expect to see:
    a. Nothing, this is a seizure and seizures don't show up on CT
    b. Blood in the subarachnoid space
    c. A tumor in the midline cerebellum
    d. A small to moderate-sized hemorrhage in the left thalamus

3. A 27-year-old who was prescribed a pain-active antidepressant for chronic pain presents to the ED for an overdose of that antidepressant. The working diagnosis is serotonin syndrome. You expect all the following, *except*:
    a. Fever
    b. Agitated confusion
    c. Delayed reflexes
    d. Diarrhea

REFERENCES

1. Cordell WH, Keene KK, Giles BK, et al. The high prevalence of pain in emergency medical care. Am J Emerg Med. 2002;20:165–169.
2. Todd KH, Cowan P, Kelly N, Homel P. Chronic or recurrent pain in the emergency department: a national telephone survey of patient experience. West J Emerg Med. 2010;11:409–416.
3. Paice J, Cohen F. Validity of a verbally administered numeric rating scale to measure cancer pain intensity. Cancer Nurs. 1997;20:88–93.
4. Todd KH, Sloan EP, Chen C, et al. Survey of pain etiology, management, and satisfaction in two urban emergency departments. Can J Emerg Med. 2002;4:252–256.
5. Kelly AM. A process approach to improving pain management in the emergency department: development and evaluation. J Accid Emerg Med. 2000;17:185–187.
6. Chamber JB, Sprigings D. Acute chest pain. In: Sprigings D, Chambers JB, eds. Acute Medicine: A Practical Guide to the Management of Medical Emergencies (5th ed.). New York: John Wiley & Sons; 2018.
7. Anderson JL, Adams CD, Antman EM, et al.,; American College of Cardiology Foundation/American Heart Association Task Force on Practice Guidelines. 2012 ACCF/AHA focused update incorporated into the ACCF/AHA 2007 guidelines for the management of patients with unstable angina/non-ST-elevation myocardial infarction: a report of the American College of Cardiology Foundation/American Heart Association Task Force on Practice Guidelines. Circulation. 2013;127:e663–e828.
8. Bonin M, Mewton N, Roubille F, et al.; CIRCUS Study Investigators. Effect and safety of morphine use in acute anterior ST-segment elevation myocardial infarction. J Am Heart Assoc. 2018;7(4).
9. LeBlond R, Brown D, DeGowin R. DeGowin's Diagnostic Examination (9th ed.). New York: McGraw-Hill Professional; 2008.
10. Belleza M. Cellulitis. September 26, 2017. Accessed March 24, 2019 at: https://nurseslabs.com.
11. Hogans BB, Nugent J, Gonzalez-Fernandez M, et al. Ava: anterior pelvic pain during pregnancy. September 1, 2017. NIH Pain Consortium Center of Excellence in Pain Education module. Accessed April 2, 2019at: http://painmeded.com/jh_ava/.
12. National Institute of Neurological Disorders and Stroke. Meningitis and encephalitis fact sheet. Accessed March 24, 2019 at: https://www.ninds.nih.gov/Disorders/Patient-Caregiver-Education/Fact-Sheets/Meningitis-and-Encephalitis-Fact-Sheet.
13. Yuan WH, Hsu HC, Lai KL. Vertebroplasty and balloon kyphoplasty versus conservative treatment for osteoporotic vertebral compression fractures: a meta-analysis. Medicine (Balt). 2016;95(31): e4491.
14. Chau AM, Xu LL, Pelzer NR, Gragnaniello C. Timing of surgical intervention in cauda equina syndrome: a systematic critical review. World Neurosurg. 2014;81(3–4):640–650. doi: 10.1016/j.wneu.2013.11.007.

15. Shapiro BS, Benjamin LJ, Payne R, Heidrich G. Sickle cell-related pain: perceptions of medical practitioners. J Pain Symptom Manage. 1997;14(3):168–174.
16. Dy SM, Shore AD, Hicks RW, Morlock LL. Medication errors with opioids: results from a national reporting system. J Opioid Manage. 2007;3:189–194.
17. Cherny N, Ripamonti C, Pereira J, et al. Strategies to manage the adverse effects of oral morphine: an evidence based report. J Clin Oncol. 2001;19:2542–2554.
18. Ener RA1, Meglathery SB, Van Decker WA, Gallagher RM., Serotonin syndrome and other serotonergic disorders. Pain Med. 2003;4(1):63–74.
19. Abdi S, Datta S, Lucas LF: Role of epidural steroids in the management of chronic spinal pain: a systematic review of effectiveness and complications. Pain Physician. 2005;8(1):127–143.
20. Knight CL, Burnell JC. Systemic side-effects of extradural steroids. Anaesthesia. 1980;35(6):593–594.
21. Deer T, Ranson M, Kappural L, Diwan SA. Guidelines for the proper use of epidural steroid injections for the chronic pain patient. Tech Reg Anesth Pain Manage. 2009;13(4):288–295.
22. Rathmell JP, Aprill C, Bogduk N. Cervical transforaminal injection of steroids. Anesthesiology. 2004;100(6):1595–1600.
23. Horlocker TT, Wedel DJ, Benzon H, et al. Regional anesthesia in the anticoagulated patient: defining the risks (the second ASRA Consensus Conference on Neuraxial Anesthesia and Anticoagulation). Reg Anesth Pain Med. 2003;28(3):172–197.
24. Smith HS1, Deer TR, Staats PS, et al. Intrathecal drug delivery. Pain Physician. 2008;11(2 Suppl):S89–S104.
25. Bolash R1, Udeh B, Saweris Y, et al. Longevity and cost of implantable intrathecal drug delivery systems for chronic pain management: a retrospective analysis of 365 patients. Neuromodulation. 2015;18(2):150–155.
26. Manchikanti L, Falco FJ, Benyamin RM, et al. Assessment of bleeding risk of interventional techniques: a best evidence synthesis of practice patterns and perioperative management of anticoagulant and antithrombotic therapy. Pain Physician. 2013;16(2 Suppl):SE261–318.
27. Ghosh D, Mainali G, Khera J, Luciano M. Complications of intrathecal baclofen pumps in children: experience from a tertiary care center. Pediatr Neurosurg. 2013;49:138–144. doi: 10.1159/000358307.
28. Hooten WM, Kinney MO, Huntoon MA. Epidural abscess and meningitis after epidural corticosteroid injection. Mayo Clin Proc. 2004;79(5):682–686.
29. Deer TR, Provenzano DA. Recommendations for reducing infection in the practice of implanting spinal cord stimulation and intrathecal drug delivery devices: a physician's playbook. Pain Physician. 2013;16(3):E125–E128.
30. Raffaeli W, Marconi G, Fanelli G, et al. Opioid-related side-effects after intrathecal morphine: a prospective, randomized, double-blind dose-response study. Eur J Anaesthesiol. 2006;23(7):605–610.
31. Heetla HW, Staal MJ, Proost JH, van Laar T. Clinical relevance of pharmacological and physiological data in intrathecal baclofen therapy. Arch Phys Med Rehabil. 2014;95(11):2199–2206.
32. Ross JC, Cook AM, Stewart GL, Fahy BG., Acute intrathecal baclofen withdrawal: a brief review of treatment options. Neurocrit Care. 2011;14(1):103–108. doi: 10.1007/s12028-010-9422-6.
33. Gofeld M, McQueen CK. Ultrasound-guided intrathecal pump access and prevention of the pocket fill. Pain Med. 2011;12(4):607–611. doi: 10.1111/j.1526-4637.2011.01090.x.

14 Acute Pain
Postoperative, Trauma-Related, and Obstetric Pain

Nantthasorn Zinboonyahgoon and Kristin Schreiber

The magnitude of pleasure reaches its limit in the removal of all pain.
—Epicurus

LEARNING OBJECTIVES

At the completion of this chapter, the learner should be able to discuss:

- The prevalence of acute pain
- The neurobiological, endocrine, and metabolic responses to pain and injury, especially segmental and suprasegmental reflexes and increases in cortisol and catechols
- The multiple approaches used for surgical pain, including oral, intravenous (IV), local, and epidural administration of analgesic and anti-inflammatory agents
- Studies showing that premedication and rigorous pain control decrease the incidence of chronic pain and improve functional measures

CASE SCENARIO

A 28-year-old primipara woman at 40 weeks' gestation presents in labor. She declines an epidural when offered, stating that she has prepared for "natural childbirth"; this is documented in the prenatal visits as well. Many of the other laboring mothers present on the ward are managed with epidurals. Your attending assigns you to this patient as a "learning case." A private doula (trained labor coach) and the patient's life partner are present at the bedside throughout. The patient, doula, and life partner communicate throughout the contractions to provide encouragement to the patient to breathe through the contractions, and to apply external pressure support to the pelvis during labor, partially relieving the pain. As labor progresses, the contractions appear very painful for the patient. Each contraction begins to look like barely controlled anarchy as the patient shouts, pants, and calls out for more pressure on her hips. Despite the apparent struggle with contraction pain, the labor progresses normally, and delivery is uneventful. The infant is born with normal assessment scores and appears fully awake.

1. At what stage of labor is it too late for an epidural to be placed?
2. What pain management options are available to this patient if a cesarean delivery is needed?
3. What are the advantages of laboring without an epidural?
4. The night after the delivery patient repeatedly requests perineal ice packs from the maternity ward staff, in excess of the normal amount allowed by nursing protocol. What is your suggestion?

INTRODUCTION

Pain is the most common reason that patients seek medical care. As noted, pain is defined as an unpleasant sensory and emotional experience associated with actual or potential tissue damage or described in terms of such damage.[1] Pain in this sense is an experience, but the impact of pain may reach well beyond an isolated experience. Three common events in which patients experience acute pain are after surgery, after a traumatic accident, or in the course of childbirth, and the healthcare provider needs to be able to use a variety of tools to reduce this pain. Inadequate pain control in these situations not only results in low patient satisfaction but also is detrimental in terms of harmful physiologic changes, poor perioperative outcomes, and long-term negative sequalae, including chronic pain. As such, thoughtful and comprehensive treatment of acute pain after trauma, or in the perioperative and perinatal period, can reduce morbidity and even mortality.

The Joint Commission (TJC) has recognized patients' right to pain management, implementing standards for assessment, monitoring, and treatment of pain. In 2001, pain management became a standard requirement for hospital accreditation,[2] an official recognition of the importance of pain that was long overdue.

PHYSIOLOGIC IMPACT OF POSTOPERATIVE PAIN AND TREATMENT CONSIDERATIONS

Pain not only affects patient satisfaction and emotional state but also has a major impact on nearly all physiologic systems. Much of the evidence for the negative impact of pain comes from comparison studies, where, for example, comparison is made between outcomes in people receiving versus not receiving an epidural or peripheral nerve block (where nerves carrying the painful stimuli are inactivated).

> *Cardiac:* Pain evokes stimulation of the sympathetic nervous system, resulting in tachycardia, hypertension, and increased propensity to cardiac arrhythmias,

all of which increase myocardial oxygen demand, while decreasing myocardial oxygen supply and increasing the risk for myocardial infarction. Adequate pain management, for example, with thoracic epidural analgesia, has been shown to decrease the risk for cardiovascular morbidity (cardiac arrhythmia, myocardial infarction) in patients undergoing various surgical operations.[3,4]

Pulmonary: Pain from upper abdominal and thoracic incision or injury (i.e., rib fracture) prevents patients from deep inspiration and coughing, which may lead to atelectasis, pneumonia, and respiratory failure. As such, adequate pain management with regional block such as thoracic epidural or paravertebral blocks decreases the risk for respiratory complications in patients undergoing high-risk operations such as coronary artery bypass graft or vascular surgery.[3,4] In multiple rib fractures, thoracic epidural analgesia decreased incidence of pneumonia and decreased ventilator days.[5] Thoracic paravertebral blocks, in the same setting, improved oxygenation and respiratory function and had comparable outcomes to thoracic epidural block.[6,7]

Gastrointestinal Tract: Stress hormones, sympathetic neurotransmission, and opioids inhibit gastrointestinal tract motility. The incidence of postoperative ileus is quite prevalent (up to 90%) in the days after abdominal surgery, and ileus is the most common factor delaying hospital discharge. Analgesic treatment with epidural, rather than systemic, opioids, during and after abdominal surgery has been shown to speed the return of bowel function by 24 to 37 hours.[3,4]

Endocrine: Pain increases cortisol levels and results in elevated blood glucose, sodium water retention, and protein catabolism.

Musculoskeletal system: Because pain can prevent a patient from early ambulation after surgery or trauma, adequate pain management can enhance physical therapy and recovery. For example, continuous femoral nerve block for analgesia for knee replacement improved patient's ambulation and physical performance and decreased length of stay.[8–10]

Nervous system: Inadequate pain control is a risk factor for postoperative delirium. Moreover, uncontrolled pain in the postoperative period (acute pain) is also associated with chronic postsurgical pain.[11] Adequate pain control with epidural analgesia for thoracotomy and paravertebral block for mastectomy is associated with decreased risk for persistent postsurgical pain.[12]

Immune system: Pain, stress, inflammation, and opioids all suppress the cell-mediated immune response. Several studies have showed that adequate pain control by regional anesthetic technique may reduce immunosuppression and decrease incidence of postoperative infection,[4] and one study has suggested that it may also reduce cancer recurrence.[13]

PAIN ASSESSMENT

Given the subjective nature of pain, for adults, a self-report tool such as the numeric rating scale is most commonly used. There is little evidence that any given pain assessment system is superior to others. However, for certain patient populations such as pediatric, cognitively impaired, sedated, or intensive care unit patients, where self-report is difficult or impossible, adapted scales or behavioral tools may be used instead.

ACUTE PAIN MANAGEMENT
Pain Pathways and Signaling

Nociceptive input from an injured area transmits along peripheral nerve axons (primarily of the Aδ or C type) to the spinal cord. These peripheral nociceptors synapse on spinal cord neurons, and the signal is then transmitted through the spinothalamic tract to the thalamus and ultimately to the somatosensory cortex and limbic system, as noted in Chapter 1.[14] Understanding the location of the nociceptive transmission pathway for any given injury, surgery, or delivery is an important first step in managing pain during trauma, surgery, or childbirth (Figure 14.1).

Equally important is an understanding of the mode of transmission along this nociceptive pathway, which involves a complex array of ion channels, receptors, enzymes, and second messengers (e.g., sodium channels, N-methyl-D-aspartate, glutamate, substance P, neurokinin, gamma-aminobutyric acid, μ-opioid, cyclooxygenase [COX]); see Chapter 2 for details. By applying what is known about pain anatomy, physiology, and pharmacology, one may interrupt the transmission of the pain signal through interventions (peripheral nerve block, neuraxial block) or modify the signal through pharmacologic or enzymatic blockade by administration of analgesic drugs by mouth

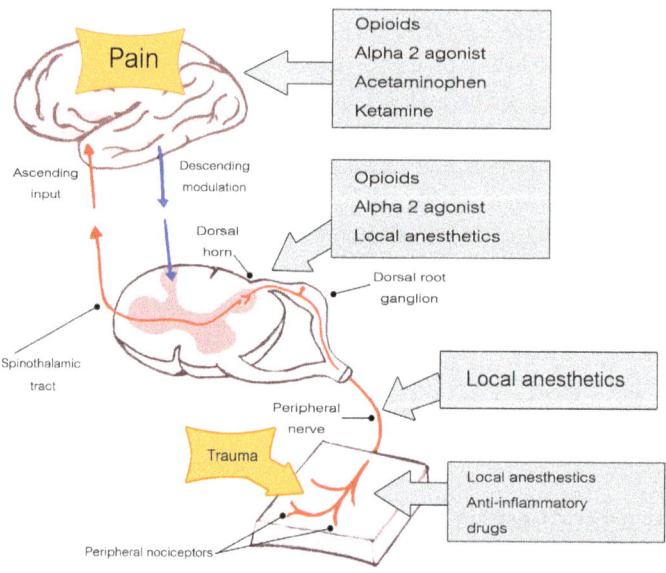

FIGURE 14.1 Overview of the pain processing system illustrating the peripheral transduction of pain generator signals, pain transmission, modulation, and perception in the peripheral and central nervous systems. (From http://www.pharmacology2000.com/Central/Opioids/Advanced_opioids2.htm; retrieved October 2, 2014.)

or intravenously. Interruption of nociceptive transmission may occur at many points along the pain pathway.

The design of acute pain management is ideally multimodal, incorporating elements that engage complementary modes of action to deliver optimal pain control while minimizing side effects. Elements of acute pain management are discussed next.

Nonpharmacologic Therapies

There are many nonpharmacologic approaches and modalities to attenuate pain and pain-related distress, such as application of cold, transcutaneous electrical nerve stimulation (TENS), relaxation therapy, music therapy, meditation, and acupuncture. These modalities may act at peripheral, spinal, or supraspinal sites along the pain pathway. The evidence for analgesic benefit of most of these modalities is variable and context specific. Additional well-designed studies are needed to investigate the efficacy and mechanisms underlying these therapies. Moreover, certain modalities such as acupuncture or hypnosis require specific training and are not widely available or reimbursed in many settings.[15]

Pharmacologic Management

Nonopioids

Nonopioid medications include nonsteroidal anti-inflammatory drugs (NSAIDs), such as ibuprofen and celecoxib, and less commonly known drugs such as ketamine and gabapentin, which alleviate pain at different targets and receptors along the pain pathway. Although they are often viewed as less potent than opioids, their use can reduce opioid use (opioid-sparing effect), importantly decreasing the side effects from opioids. NSAIDs, COX2 inhibitors, and ketamine are associated with reduced incidence of nausea, vomiting, and sedation from opioids.[4]

To yield the best analgesic effect with minimal side effects, many nonopioids can be combined together. This is termed *multimodal analgesia,* an approach involving use of several medications,[16] usually nonopioid, and interventions (nerve block, epidural) for pain management. Common nonopioid analgesics and their side effects are shown in Table 14.1. See Chapters 9 and 10 for additional details.

Opioids

Opioids are potent analgesics, primarily activating μ-opioid receptors in the brain and spinal cord, which inhibits transmission of the nociceptive signal. Opioids can be administered by many routes. The most common are oral and IV, but intramuscular (IM), subcutaneous, buccal, transdermal, or neuraxial (spinal, epidural) routes may also be used. Commonly used opioids for acute pain are shown in Tables 14.2 and 14.3. See Chapter 9 for details on opioids.

Opioids have many side effects, ranging from mild to lethal, most of which are dose dependent. Cautious use and appropriate monitoring should accompany opioid administration for pain. Common side effects include the following:

Table 14.1 Common Nonopioid Analgesics

Agents	Mechanism of Action	Route	Precautions	Side Effects
Acetaminophen	Central COX inhibitor	PO, PR, IV	Liver failure	Minimal, unless overdose (<3–4 g/day)
NSAIDs (ibuprofen, naproxen, ketorolac)	Central and peripheral COX inhibitors	PO, IV	Allergy to NSAIDs. Decrease dose in renal impairment, elderly, or body weight <50 kg	GI bleeding, renal failure, surgical bleeding. Use for no longer than 5 days because of increased risk for complications.
COX2 inhibitors (celecoxib)	COX2 inhibitors	PO	Cross allergy with sulfonamide	Less GI side effects than NSAIDs. Minimal effect on platelet function. Similar renal risk as NSAIDs. Increased cardiovascular death after long-term use.
Ketamine	NMDA receptor antagonist	IV, IM, PO	Patient with psychosis	Hallucination, delirium, hypertension, tachycardia
Gabapentin, pregabalin	Calcium channel blockers	PO	Adjust dose for renal function (CrCl <60 mL/min), elderly	Somnolence, dizziness
Clonidine, dexmedetomidine	α_2-Agonist	PO, patch, IV (dex)	Usually used for <1 week; if used for longer period, monitor for rebound hypertension	Hypotension, sedation, bradycardia

COX = cyclooxygenase; CrCl = creatinine clearance; GI = gastrointestinal; IM = intramuscular; IV = intravenous; PO = per oral (route); PR = per rectum; NSAID = nonsteroidal anti-inflammatory drug.

Table 14.2 Common Opioid Analgesics

Agents	Mechanism	Comment
Codeine	Weak μ-agonist	5–10% of population doesn't respond to codeine because of lack of the CYP2D6 enzyme, which converts codeine to morphine. Use in children is no longer advised[17].
Fentanyl	μ-Agonist	Intravenous delivery in acute pain, more potent and shorter half-life vs. other intravenous agents. Transdermal route (fentanyl patch) results in 12 hr of onset and offset delay, not recommended for acute pain but useful for basal delivery in opioid-tolerant patients
Morphine	μ-Agonist	Contraindicated in end-stage renal disease
Hydromorphone	μ-Agonist	May produce less nausea and vomiting than morphine in some patients
Methadone	μ-Agonist (L), NMDA antagonist (D)	Long half-life; analgesic dose is twice or three times a day and once daily as methadone maintenance therapy for management of opioid addiction; may also have NMDA antagonist effect, thus decreasing opioid tolerance
Oxycodone	μ-Agonist	Often coformulated with acetaminophen (Percocet), requiring caution in patients when there is a potential to take larger than recommended dose; patients should be warned about not also taking acetaminophen (Tylenol) simultaneously when these coformulations are used
Hydrocodone	μ-Agonist	Often co-formulated with acetaminophen (Vicodin), see caution above.
Nalbuphine (Nubian)	μ-Antagonist κ-Agonist	Contraindicated in chronic opioid users (precipitating withdrawal) Used in labor and delivery because of lower risk for neonatal respiratory depression. Low dose (5 mg IV) used for treatment of pruritus (side effect) from other narcotics.
Buprenorphine (Subutex)	Partial μ-agonist κ-Antagonist	Lower risk for respiratory depression, used in patients with previous problems with opioid addiction (combined with naloxone, known as Suboxone). High affinity to μ-receptor, preventing euphoric/analgesic effect from other opioids, should stop 3 to 5 days before major operation secondary to possible antagonistic effects and monitor for withdrawal symptoms

IV = intravenous; NMDA = *N*-methyl-D-aspartate.

Table 14.3 Common Opioids and Equianalgesic Doses*

Agents	Route	Equianalgesic Dose (mg)	Onset (hr)	Duration (hr)
Codeine	PO	200	0.25–1	3–4
Fentanyl†	IV	0.1	0.1–0.2	1–1.5
Morphine	IV	10	0.25	2–3
	PO	30	0.5–1	4
Hydromorphone	IV	1.5	0.25	2–3
	PO	7.5	0.5–1	4
Methadone‡	IV	10	0.2–0.3	4–6
	PO	10–20	0.5–1	4–8
Oxycodone	PO	20	0.5	4–6

*Equianalgesic dosing[20] and onset and duration[21] are discussed in the text.

†Transdermal fentanyl is not recommended for acute pain because of slow onset and offset (12 hr).

‡Conversion for chronic use, from oral morphine to oral methadone, is variable from 4:1 to 20:1 depending on dose of morphine (higher dose needs higher ratio).

IV = intravenous; PO = per oral (route).

Sedation: The sedation from opioids can combine with other sedative agents administered within the same time frame. Sedation usually precedes, and thus can be a warning sign for, impending respiratory depression. Oversedation can also prevent patients from ambulating early in the post-treatment period, which may slow recovery after injury, surgery, or childbirth.

Respiratory depression: Opioids directly stimulate μ receptors in the brainstem and thus cause respiratory depression. Sedation and then hypoventilation (both decreased respiratory rate and depth) usually proceed apnea. Monitoring the sedation score and respiratory rate is therefore standard for opioid administration and is especially important for high-risk patients (i.e., elderly, morbidly obese, those taking sedating medications or coadministered neuraxial opioids, those with comorbid respiratory disease, e.g., chronic obstructive pulmonary disease). Patients should not have more than moderate sedation (still responding to verbal commands), and respiratory rate should be greater than 8 breaths/minute before additional opioids are given. If respiratory depression is present, opioids should be stopped and resuscitation begun, including stimulation, airway and ventilatory support, and naloxone administration (see the following box), if necessary, to counter the effects of opioids.

Naloxone, a μ-receptor antagonist, should be administered by slow titration 40 to 80 μg every 2 to 3 minutes until patient becomes more alert and the respiratory rate is more than 8 breaths/minute. However, naloxone administered in large doses can precipitate severe pain, hypertension, and pulmonary edema. Importantly, naloxone has a 1- to 2-hour half-life, and caution should be used when long-acting opioids are present because patients are at risk for recurrent respiratory depression.[18]

Pruritus (itching): Pruritus is a direct side effect of μ-receptor activity. Administration of a low-dose μ-receptor antagonist (low-dose naloxone 40–80 μg IV) or nalbuphine (5–10 mg IV or IM)) will alleviate symptoms. Antihistamines such as diphenhydramine (Benadryl) will further sedate patients and are typically not helpful.

Urinary retention: Urinary retention is more common with neuraxial opioid administration. This may necessitate a urinary catheter for the first 24 to 48 hours but tends to be self-limited and resolves over time.

Nausea and vomiting: Opioid administration may cause nausea and vomiting from stimulation of opioid receptors in the enteric nervous system (gastrointestinal), leading to decreased bowel movement and constipation. Nausea, vomiting, and the resultant inability to take water and food by mouth are one of the most common reasons to delay home discharge in ambulatory patients after surgery.

Constipation, ileus: Agonism of enteric opioid receptors decreases gastrointestinal motility. This can be countered with laxatives, stool softeners, and, if needed, peripheral μ-receptor antagonist (subcutaneous methylnaltrexone).

Addiction: Iatrogenic addiction from brief use of opioids in the treatment of acute pain after surgery or trauma is uncommon but does occur. It is estimated that the risk for inducing an addictive disorder with short-term opioid therapy is about 3 per 1,000. Development of addiction is multifactorial, a combination of genetic and psychological vulnerability, and also depends on molecular structure, dose, route, and duration of drugs administered.[19]

Immune modulation: Experimental studies have shown that opioid use leads to immunosuppression of both humeral and cell-mediated immune response, which in turn is associated with increased incidence of perioperative infection and cancer recurrence. However, stronger clinical evidence for the relevance of this effect is still needed.[13] Some opioids are associated with mast cell degranulation and histamine release. Morphine, but not fentanyl, is associated with histamine release and other mast cell responses to the extent that higher doses of morphine administered through chronic intrathecal catheters can result in granuloma formation.

Patient-Controlled Analgesia

Patient-controlled analgesia (PCA) is a tool for self-administering opioid analgesics using a secure pump programmed with medication administration limits for safety. By pressing a button, patients may self-administer opioid analgesics usually by the IV route. Compared with conventional care (nurse IV administration), the PCA may provide better pain control and improve patient satisfaction; however PCA, does not decrease the overall amount of opioid administered nor decrease overall opioid-related side effects. Safety features inherent in PCA administration of opioids include patient oversedation, self-limiting the ability to press a button for further administration; an appropriate lock-out period between doses; and maximal doses limits programmed into the PCA machine.[15] It is important to instruct family members not to push the PCA button if the patient is asleep because this can contribute to oversedation.

Regional Anesthesia

Regional anesthesia is an anesthetic technique involving application of local anesthetic agent to nerves supplying a specific area of the body, resulting in a temporary loss or decrease in sensation in that area. Regional anesthesia can be divided into central (neuraxial block: epidural, spinal anesthesia) and peripheral (plexus blocks, nerve blocks) and can be used as the primary technique to cause anesthesia or analgesia during labor, after trauma, or during a surgery or procedure. Regional anesthesia aims to block the incoming pain stimulus at the level of the peripheral sensory nerve, thus preventing the activation of pain sensation in the spinal cord and brain as well as blunting activation of the sympathetic nervous system stress response and its associated negative sequalae.

Epidural Analgesia

Epidural analgesia employs local anesthetics (such as lidocaine or bupivacaine) to block sodium channels in the nerve cell membrane most likely of peripheral nerve roots entering the spinal cord, thus decreasing conduction and providing analgesia in the corresponding vertebral level (Figure 14.2A and B). Blocking nociceptive input at this level blunts the stress response to traumatic, surgical, or childbirth-related injury, decreasing its impact on physiologic systems (as outlined earlier). Importantly, providing excellent pain control, especially limiting pain evoked by movement, can lead to earlier ambulation and improved lung mechanics. Patients require less use of opioids for pain control, leading to less sedation, nausea, vomiting, and ileus.

Side effects of epidural analgesia may include pruritus, respiratory depression (when neuraxial opioids are used along with the local anesthetics), hypotension (from resultant sympathetic block), urinary retention, postdural puncture headache, epidural hematoma, epidural abscess, nerve injury, and local anesthetic toxicity (with inadvertent intravascular injection). Epidural placement is contraindicated if the patient refuses, the patient is coagulopathic, there is infection at the puncture site or along the trajectory of catheter placement, or there is hemodynamic instability. To decrease the risk for complications during epidural block placement, patients should not be overly

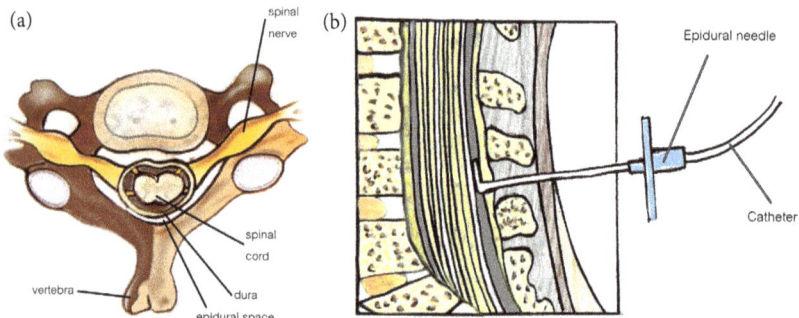

FIGURE 14.2 Anatomy of epidural space and epidural block. **A,** Cross-sectional anatomy of cervical spinal column (note short spinal roots indicative of cervical region) illustrating the relation of the spinal cord to the epidural, intradural, and intrathecal spaces. **B,** Midline sagittal anatomy of the mid-lumbar to lumbosacral spine illustrating the epidural catheter overlying the dural sac, which contains the long spinal nerve roots of the cauda equina. (From http://surgerycenter.ssmedgroup.com/epidural_injection.html.)

sedated in order to be able to report symptoms of local anesthetic systemic toxicity (tinnitus, perioral numbness), lower extremity weakness or numbness (inadvertent spinal local anesthetic administration), or paresthesia (indicating contact of needle with nerve roots, which may increase nerve injury risk). Moreover, standard American Society of Anesthesia (ASA) monitors (noninvasive blood pressure, oxygen saturation, electrocardiogram) are applied to the patient to detect intravascular or intrathecal (spinal) injection of local anesthetics or vasovagal reaction (fainting) to needle puncture. Application of neuraxial block techniques may provide pain control after surgery, after trauma, or during labor and delivery.

EPIDURAL USE IN OBSTETRICS

The anatomic source of pain from labor and delivery varies according to different stages of labor. In stage 1 of labor, visceral nociceptors in the contracting uterus transmit pain signals through the T10–L1 spinal segments (contraction pain). During stage 2, as the baby descends in the birth canal, somatic nociceptors in the cervical and vaginal area transmit though the S2–4 spinal segment. It is important to take into account the anatomic change in pain source as labor progresses, particularly when using regional anesthesia (Figure 14.3), because these segments are somewhat far apart on the neuraxis and an additional bolus of local anesthetic through the epidural catheter, as well as a change in the patient's body position (sitting to encourage lower level of epidural block), will allow local anesthetic to reach the desired level.

Epidural analgesia for labor and delivery not only alleviates pain and stress for the mother but also allows her to be better rested and able to engage in infant care. Use is

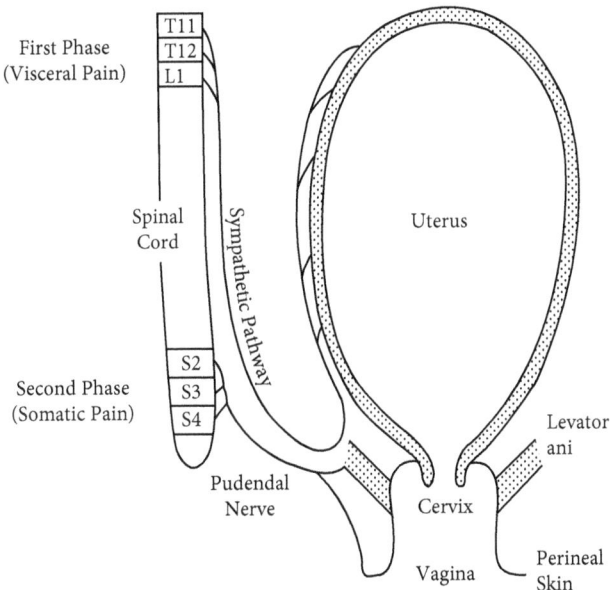

FIGURE 14.3 Anatomic diagram of nerve supply during the labor and delivery process illustrating the spinal levels associated with early and later stages of labor (details in text). (From http://www.indianjpain.org/article.asp?issn=0970-5333;year=2014;volume=28;issue=2;spage=71;epage=81;aulast=Reena, retrieved 10/2/14.)

associated with better postpartum outcome, including lower risk for postpartum depression and higher chance of successful breastfeeding. However, epidural analgesia in larger doses may prolong the duration of the second stage of labor and the rate of instrument-assisted vaginal delivery, but not the rate of cesarean delivery.[22] Women express high rates of preference for natural childbirth, yet rates of epidural analgesia remain high. Alternative models, such as continuous support during labor, demonstrate positive effects, and further study is warranted.[23]

PERIPHERAL NERVE BLOCK

Peripheral nerve block is a technique in which local anesthetics are applied to peripheral nerves to provide analgesia or anesthesia in the corresponding nerve territory. This technique can provide pain control to many regions of the body, including the extremities (brachial plexus block, femoral and sciatic nerve blocks) and truncal area (transversus abdominis plane block, paravertebral block). As with epidural block, this technique not only is used for postoperative pain control but also may significantly decrease pain from traumatic injury such as hip fracture (femoral nerve block)[7] or rib fracture (paravertebral block).[6]

Compared with the use of systemic opioids, peripheral nerve blocks provide superior analgesia without sedation and opioid-related side effects. This technique also avoids the potential side effects of neuraxial blocks such as hypotension, urinary retention, pruritus, epidural hematoma, or abscess. Additional benefits may include enhancement of physical therapy and earlier home discharge (femoral nerve for total knee replacement)[8-10] and prevention of persistent postsurgical pain (paravertebral blocks for breast surgery).[12] Common peripheral nerve blocks and applications are shown in Figure 14.4 and Table 14.4.

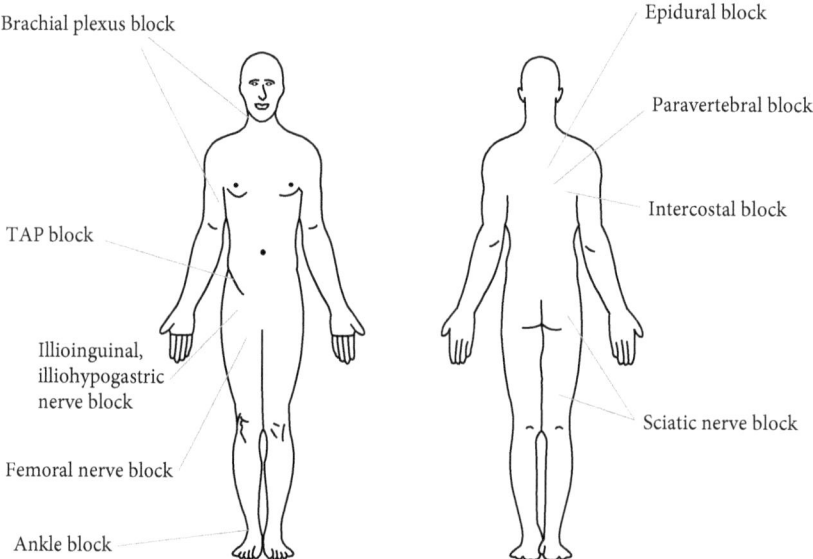

FIGURE 14.4 Common peripheral nerve blocks for acute pain and surgery illustrating the variety of somatic regions where peripheral nerve blocks may provide acute analgesia. TAP = transversus abdominis plane.

Table 14.4 Common Peripheral Nerve Blocks for Acute Pain and Surgery

Nerve Block	Type of Surgery	Specific Complications
Brachial plexus block (interscalene, supraclavicular, infraclavicular, axillary blocks)	Upper extremity and shoulder surgery	Pneumothorax (supraclavicular), diaphragmatic paralysis (interscalene), Horner syndrome
Femoral nerve block Fascia iliaca block	Lower extremity (hip, knee, anterior thigh), hip fracture	Quadriceps weakness, postoperative fall risk[10]
Sciatic nerve block	Lower extremity (leg, except medial part, which is covered by saphenous nerve)	Hematoma (considered deep, noncompressible space)
Transversus abdominis plane block (TAP block)	Abdominal surgery, cesarean delivery	Visceral organ puncture
Paravertebral block	Breast, thoracic, and abdominal surgery, rib fracture	Pneumothorax

Ultrasound Guidance of Peripheral Nerve Blocks

Peripheral nerve blockade requires that a needle is introduced percutaneously and advanced to the target nerve, where local anesthetic is injected around that nerve (Figure 14.5). Previously, this process was guided by anatomic landmarks and nerve stimulation, but in the past decades, the use of ultrasound has become more common to guide these blocks. Ultrasound provides real-time visual guidance of the needle's path to its target, and its use is associated with an improved success rate, quicker block onset, reduced number of needle passes, lower local anesthetic dose requirement, and easier avoidance and detection of intraneural and intravascular injection. In patients with abnormal or challenging anatomy, ultrasound has made the reliable block possible.[24] Ultrasound machines are also portable and do not expose patients to radiation.

Block-specific potential complications, based on the specific anatomy involved, are listed in Table 14.4. Generally, complications from peripheral nerve blocks are quite uncommon, but they may include nerve injury, hematoma, infection, and local

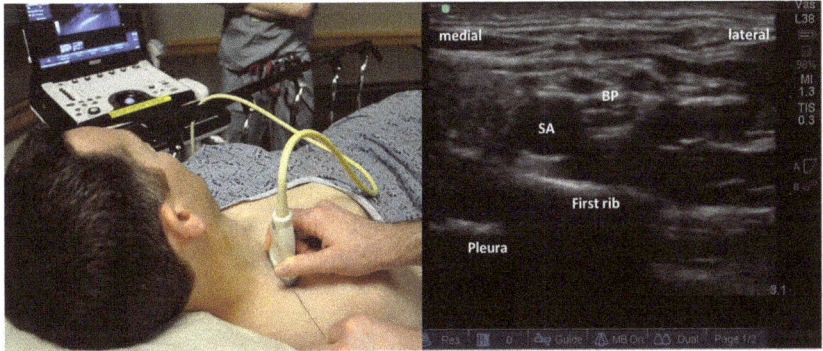

FIGURE 14.5 Ultrasound-guided supraclavicular brachial plexus block, which could be applied for wrist fracture or hand surgery. BP = brachial plexus; SA = subclavian artery.

anesthetic systemic toxicity (LAST). LAST can manifest with neurotoxicity (agitation, auditory changes, metallic taste, seizures, drowsiness, coma, or respiratory arrest) and cardiac toxicity (hypertension, tachycardia, ventricular arrhythmias, bradycardia, conduction block, hypotension, asystole).[25] Prevention, early recognition, and treatment of LAST are important to protect patients from these potentially devastating complications. The lowest effective dose of local anesthetic should be used and the maximum recommended doses (lidocaine 4.5 mg/kg, bupivacaine 2.5 mg/kg)[26] should not be exceeded. A thorough knowledge of anatomy and ultrasound investigation of veins and arteries in the block path and site may allow the practitioner to avoid intravascular injection. Routine safe practice includes incremental injection of local anesthetic, 3 to 5 mL at a time, with aspiration on syringe to assess and reassess for intravascular placement between injections, and epinephrine 10 to 15 µg/mL may be added as a marker for intravascular injection. Patients must also be closely monitored for symptoms of toxicity around the time of block because LAST can present immediately (intravascular injection) or more than 15 minutes (systemic absorption) after block placement. Treatment involves effective airway management and cardiopulmonary support to prevent hypoxia and acidosis, which are known to potentiate LAST. Lipid emulsion (Intralipid), which chelates local anesthetic in the bloodstream, should be administered at the first signs of LAST, after airway management (1.5 mL/kg 20% lipid emulsion bolus, then 0.25 mL/kg/minute of infusion, continued for at least 10 minutes after circulatory stability is attained).

Absolute contraindications to peripheral nerve block include patient refusal. Relative contraindications include coagulopathy if the block will be in a deep or incompressible space, such as paravertebral block, transgluteal sciatic nerve block, or infraclavicular brachial plexus block, or in patients at risk for acute compartment syndrome (ACS) because dense blocks may delay early detection and treatment of ACS. However, use of low-concentration local anesthetics in a block and careful monitoring of signs and symptoms (pain through the block, perfusion, and compartmental pressure) have not been shown to delay the diagnosis of ACS.[27]

NEURAL CHANGE AND PERSISTENT POSTINJURY OR POSTSURGICAL PAIN

Ongoing nerve injury and inflammation from trauma or surgery result in increased nociceptive signaling, thus triggering plasticity in the synaptic efficacy of neurons in the nociceptive pathway. Generally, this afferent barrage of nociceptors triggers enhanced excitability in central nociceptive circuits (central sensitization). This neuronal sensitization manifests as enhanced pain sensitivity, such that painful stimuli become more painful (hyperalgesia) and nonpainful stimuli are perceived as painful (allodynia) for a variable period of time after the initial nociceptive stimulus. In some cases, this pain becomes a chronic condition, lasting longer than 3 to 6 months. Persistent postsurgical pain occurs in 10 to 60% of patients depending on type of surgery (60% postamputation, 20–40% postmastectomy, 40–50% post-thoracotomy, 10% post–cesarean delivery).[28] It is important to recognize that even with identical surgical stimuli, each patient carries a different risk for developing chronic postsurgical pain. This risk appears to depend on a variety of factors, including age, sex, genetics, preexisting pain, and individual psychological factors (depression, anxiety, and catastrophizing) and inherent psychophysical factors (pain sensitivity). Patients who have poor postoperative pain control; higher depression, anxiety, and catastrophizing; and lower pain threshold appear to have a higher incidence of persistent postsurgical pain.[29]

Theoretically, adequate analgesia during a critical period around the injury or surgery induced nociceptive input may prevent this central sensitization (preventive analgesia). Preventive analgesia focuses on blocking the processes that lead to sensitization during and in the days immediately after the initial injury or activation.[30] Preventive analgesia may employ multimodal analgesia, using several drugs or techniques to control pain and attenuate sensitization, while minimizing individual drug side effects. Multimodal analgesia combining regional anesthesia and multiple medications around the time of trauma or surgery may minimize the impact of nociceptive transmission and accomplish the dual goal of acute and chronic pain reduction. Chronic pain, whether the result of surgical, accidental, or childbirth-related trauma, has a huge impact physically, psychologically, and economically on patients. Good prediction models assessing risk for development of persistent pain are needed in order to direct preventive interventions to patients at highest risk.

Acute Pain in Patients Taking Chronic Opioid Medications

One challenge to managing acute pain in patients taking chronic opioid medications is opioid tolerance, whereby higher doses of opioid are required to achieve analgesia. These patients experience the same side effects (e.g., respiratory depression) at these higher doses, effectively narrowing the therapeutic index of opioids. Opioid tolerance is a physiologic phenomenon and should not be confused with addiction. However, many physicians are reluctant to administer larger doses, citing concerns of potential abuse, and legitimate concerns about risk for overdose. On the other hand, inadequate pain control and stress are also associated with relapse of addiction,[31] underlining the need for a balanced approach.

Goals for pain management of opioid tolerant patients in the acute pain setting include the following:

- Establish a comprehensive plan for pain management before or at the outset of the procedure, labor, or surgery and seek input from primary care or consultation with a pain specialist.
- Continue patient's daily opioid dose to maintain baseline analgesic coverage and prevent withdrawal, which can reinforce addiction. If the patient cannot take baseline coverage by mouth, convert to an IV form with equianalgesic dose. The exception is that opioids with partial antagonists such as buprenorphine should be stopped 3 to 5 days before major surgery so that antagonistic effects at the opioid receptor may be diminished. However, for minor procedures with little expected pain, it is recommended that patients continue this medication to prevent withdrawal symptoms.[18]
- Implement nonopioid analgesics such as NSAIDs, neuropathic agents, ketamine, and regional anesthesia.
- Expect higher required doses of opioid, while closely monitoring for sedation and respiratory depression.

- Switch to different opioids for less tolerance (use equianalgesic dose with 25 to 50% reduction because of incomplete cross-tolerance).
- For patients who have a history of addiction, avoid the previous drug of addiction and use long-acting oral opioids to prevent relapse.
- Communicate with primary care about plan for tapering of opioids and consider follow-up with pain specialist or addiction counselor as needed.

SUMMARY

There are many analgesic modalities that may be employed in the management of acute pain during and after trauma, surgery, or childbirth. Patients with the same baseline pain score and procedure but treated with different analgesic technique (regional anesthesia or multimodal nonopioid analgesia vs. opioid only) may have a very different outcome, in terms of relief from both acute and chronic pain and physiologic side effects of pain. The goal of current perioperative pain management is not only to treat the pain in the moment but to also choose wisely among the available techniques and agents to optimize patient outcomes. Pain management is an art, although thoughtful application of sound scientific research may, in the end, greatly enhance the outcomes for patients.

REVIEW QUESTIONS

1. Match the following medications with their typical delivery:
   a. Local anesthetic 1. Oral systemic
   b. NSAID 2. Injected around a nerve
   3. Instilled over the spinal dura (epidural)

2. Which of the following is an absolute contraindication to a peripheral nerve block?
   a. Coagulopathy
   b. Risk for compartment syndrome
   c. Patient refusal
   d. Allergy to morphine

3. Which of the following may be not appropriate adjustments to an acute pain management plan for a patient with substance use disorder?
   a. Modifying opioid regimen preoperatively for buprenorphine maintenance
   b. Reducing the dose of opioids used intraoperatively
   c. Involving addiction medicine supports
   d. Taking a substance use history preoperatively

REFERENCES

1. International Association for the Study of Pain (IASP). Pain definition. Accessed December 1, 2014 at: http://www.iasp-pain.org/Taxonomy?navItemNumber=576#Pain.
2. Accessed November 5, 2014 at: http://www.jointcommission.org/pain_management, retrieved 11/5/14.

3. Pöpping DM, Elia N, Van Aken HK, et al. Impact of epidural analgesia on mortality and morbidity after surgery: systematic review and meta-analysis of randomized controlled trials. Ann Surg. 2014;259(6):1056–1067.
4. Liu SS, Wu CL. Effect of postoperative analgesia on major postoperative complications: a systematic update of the evidence. Anesth Analg. 2007;104(3):689–702.
5. Bulger EM, Edwards T, Klotz P, Jurkovich GJ. Epidural analgesia improves outcome after multiple rib fractures. Surgery. 2004;136(2):426–430.
6. Karmakar MK, Critchley LA, Ho AM, et al. Continuous thoracic paravertebral infusion of bupivacaine for pain management in patients with multiple fractured ribs. Chest. 2003;123(2):424–431.
7. Beaudoin FL, Haran JP, Liebmann O. A comparison of ultrasound-guided three-in-one femoral nerve block versus parenteral opioids alone for analgesia in emergency department patients with hip fractures: a randomized controlled trial. Acad Emerg Med. 2013;20(6):584–591.
8. Richman JM, Liu SS, Courpas G, et al. Does continuous peripheral nerve block provide superior pain control to opioids? A meta-analysis. Anesth Analg. 2006;102:248–257.
9. Chelly JE, Greger J, Gebhard R, et al. Continuous femoral blocks improve recovery and outcome of patients undergoing total knee arthroplasty. J Arthroplasty. 2001;16:436–445.
10. Zinboonyahgoon N, Schreiber K, Zeballos J,et al. Continuous Femoral Nerve Block for Knee Arthroplasty: A Comparison of three evolving regimens. J Med Assoc Thai. 2017;100(9):997–1006.
11. Joshi GP, Ogunnaike BO. Consequences of inadequate postoperative pain relief and chronic persistent postoperative pain. Anesthesiol Clin North Am. 2005;23(1):21–36.
12. Andreae MH, Andreae DA. Local anaesthetics and regional anaesthesia for preventing chronic pain after surgery. Cochrane Database Syst Rev. 2012;(10):CD007105.
13. Heaney A, Buggy DJ. Can anaesthetic and analgesic techniques affect cancer recurrence or metastasis? Br J Anaesth. 2012;109(Suppl 1):17–28.
14. Westlund K. Pain pathways: peripheral, spinal, ascending, and descending pathways. In: Benzon H, Rathmell J, Wu C, et al., editors. Practical Management of Pain (5th ed.). Philadelphia: Elsevier; 2014:87–98.
15. Correll D. Postoperative acute pain management. In: Vacanti C, Sikka P, Urman R, Dershwitz M, Segal B, eds. Essential Clinical Anesthesia. New York: Cambridge University Press; 2011:885–893.
16. Hanna M, Ouanes JP, Tomas VG. Postoperative pain and other acute pain syndrome. In: Benzon H, Rathmell J, Wu C, et al, ed. Practical Management of Pain (5th ed.) Philadelphia: Elsevier; 2014:271–297.
17. Dean L. Codeine therapy and CPY2D6 genotype: medical genetics summaries. Accessed December 7, 2014 at: http://www.ncbi.nlm.nih.gov/books/NBK100662/.
18. Zinboonyahgoon N, Garfield J. Substance abuse and anesthesia. In: Aglio L, Lekowski R, Urman R, eds. Essential Clinical Anesthesia Review: Keywords, Questions and Answers for the Boards. New York: Cambridge University Press; 2015:56–60.
19. Covington E, Bailey J. Pain and addictive disorders: challenge and opportunity. In: Benzon H, Rathmell J, Wu C, et al., eds. Practical Management of Pain (5th ed.). Philadelphia: Elsevier; 2014:669–682.
20. Laughin I, Hickey A. Drug formulary. In: Urman R, Vadivelu N eds. Pocket Pain Medicine. Philadelphia: Lippincott Williams & Wilkins; 2011:chapter 10, 1–23.
21. Hurley R, Adam M. Perioperative pain management. In: Miller R, Pardo M eds. Basics of Anesthesia (6th ed.). Philadelphia: Elsevier; 2011:650–664.

22. Ding T, Wang DX, Qu Y, Chen Q, Zhu SN. Epidural labor analgesia is associated with a decreased risk of postpartum depression: a prospective cohort study. Anesth Analg. 2014;119(2):383–392.
23. Bohren MA, Hofmeyr GJ, Sakala C, Fukuzawa RK, Cuthbert A. Continuous support for women during childbirth. Cochrane Database Syst Rev. 2017;7:CD003766.
24. Chan V, Abbas S, Brull R, Perlas A. Outcome data. In: Chan V, ed. Ultrasound Imaging for Regional Anesthesia: A Practical Guide Booklet (2nd ed.): 43–45.
25. Neal JM, Bernards CM, Butterworth JF 4th, et al. ASRA practice advisory on local anesthetic systemic toxicity. Reg Anesth Pain Med. 2010;35(2):152–161.
26. Freck E, Braveman F. Local anesthetics. In: Urman R, Vadivelu N eds. Pocket Pain Medicine. Philadelphia: Lippincott Williams & Wilkins; 2011:chapter 8, 1–4.
27. Aguirre JA, Gresch D, Popovici A, Bernhard J, Borgeat A. Case scenario: compartment syndrome of the forearm in patient with an infraclavicular catheter, breakthrough pain as indicator. Anesthesiology. 2013;118:1198–1205.
28. Borsook D, Kussman B, George E, Becerra L, Burke D. Surgically induced neuropathic pain, understanding the perioperative process. Ann Surg. 2013; 257:403–412.
29. Schreiber KL, Martel MO, Shnol H, et al. Persistent pain in postmastectomy patients: comparison of psychophysical, medical, surgical, and psychosocial characteristics between patients with and without pain. Pain. 2013;154(5):660–668.
30. Pogatzki-Zahn E, Zahn P. From preemptive to preventive analgesia. Curr Opin Anaesthesiol. 2006;19(5):551–555.
31. May JA, White HC, Leonard-White A, Warltier DC, Pagel PS. The patient recovering from alcohol or drug addiction: special issues for the anesthesiologist. Anesth Analg. 2001;92(6):1601–1608.

15 Urgent Pain Problems

Beth B. Hogans

Of pain you could wish only one thing: that it should stop. Nothing in the world was so bad as physical pain. In the face of pain there are no heroes.
—George Orwell, *1984*

LEARNING OBJECTIVES

At the completion of this chapter, the learner should be able to discuss:

- The principal distinguishing characteristics of urgent headaches, including temporal arteritis, migraine headache, idiopathic intracranial hypertension (pseudotumor cerebri), and selected secondary headache syndromes
- The indications for episodic versus prophylactic treatment of migraine headache
- The indications for evaluation of headache with computed tomography (CT), lumbar puncture (LP), or magnetic resonance imaging (MRI)
- The common serious and neuropathic causes of focal facial and somatic pain
- How multiple structures in the back are innervated (e.g., bones, disks, nerves, muscles) and how these can all contribute to low back pain
- The basic pattern of sensory dermatomes, the rationale for testing reflexes, and the basic mechanics of the straight leg raise exam
- Differences and similarities in the back pain arising from herniated disks
- The properties of some common visceral pain entities
- The primary clinical characteristics of visceral pain and some treatments
- The characteristics of serious muscle pain
- An approach for assessment and management of pain of undetermined origin

CASE SCENARIO

A 23-year-old doctoral nursing student presents to the health clinic with reports of abdominal pain, bloating, and alternating constipation and diarrhea intermittently over the past 6 months. Sleep has been disrupted by increased academic demands in the second year of the doctoral nursing program but even during break, the opportunity to catch up on sleep and exercise did not result in a resolution of symptoms. The patient reports feeling generally fatigued, mildly feverish at times, and unrefreshed by sleep. The abdominal pain comes in bouts lasting as long as 3 days and is diffuse, aching, and relieved only by defecation, which is sometimes delayed by constipation. At other times, bowel movements occur multiple times a day, and there is an increase in painful gas and flatulence. There is no history of foreign travel, jaundice, or change in stool or urine coloration. The review of systems is negative except as noted previously. Weight is stable; academic performance and mood are at baseline.

1. What is your initial diagnostic impression?
2. What other pain syndromes might this patient be at increased risk for?
3. What do you recommend as first treatment steps?
4. The patient is concerned about the cost of the recommended dietary supplement, can you suggest a cost-sensitive alternative?

INTRODUCTION

This chapter covers conditions that require prompt evaluation but are not generally in the group of conditions that are true emergencies.

NEW OR WORSENING HEADACHE

Headache is highly prevalent and often benign in the respect of being painful but not otherwise harmful. Selected exceptions to this rule include the emergent headaches such as meningitis and subarachnoid hemorrhage addressed in the previous chapter. There are causes of headache that require urgent assessment and treatment that are discussed here. The headache causes may include very painful but benign conditions, such as migraine. However, progressive, harmful conditions for which pain is primarily a symptom of disease should also be considered; these could include temporal arteritis, idiopathic intracranial hypertension, glaucoma, tumor, some indolent infectious conditions, autoimmune disease, and others. This chapter discusses benign headaches first, then the serious urgent headaches, and then selected "secondary" headaches.

Benign Headaches

Benign moderate to severe headache is remarkably prevalent. It is reported that most headaches, strictly by population-based prevalence, are likely tension headaches; however, because these headaches are typically moderate in severity and responsive to nonsteroidal anti-inflammatory drugs (NSAIDs) or other over-the-counter (OTC) medications, these headaches are not as prevalent when data are obtained in clinical settings, where migraines are predominant.[1] Migraines are predominant in clinical settings because of the marked pain severity, the disablement associated with them, and the complexities of effective management.

Tension headache is a highly prevalent headache of moderate severity that features band-like or bifrontal pressure that typically worsens during the day. Tension headache patients may demonstrate cervical trigger points (see chronic pain for detailed description) that if treated may reduce the frequency and severity of headaches; this treatment can be performed by a qualified physical therapist, and some patients can learn the techniques of trigger-point self-massage, as noted in Chapter 16. Tension headaches may be associated with increased levels of stress and other lifestyle factors that may be elicited by asking the patient: What do you think is causing your headaches? Motivational interviewing techniques can be used to counsel patients about modifying lifestyle factors such as insufficient sleep, poor diet, substance use, or the need for more daily exercise. If headaches are occurring more often that once a week, additional measures may be needed.

Migraine headaches are the most common form of headache in clinical practice. Widely prevalent, 20 to 25% of middle-aged females and nearly 10% of middle-aged males experience migraine. The patient with a "first or worst migraine" may be an urgent clinic patient because of the severity of migraine pain, associated disability, and the need to exclude dangerous mimics. Migraine usually features severe, throbbing hemicrania with associated intolerance of activity, light, or sound.[2] Nausea and vomiting may be present. Some patients have neurologic symptoms or auras, such as visual distortions (scotomas), that precede pain onset, whereas others do not. Rare patients have associated neurologic deficits such as weakness, slurred speech, or visual loss; these patients require neurologic evaluation. Migraine has strong heritability, running in families. The main key to effective primary care management of migraine is to establish the diagnosis and educate the patient in taking the correct medication as quickly as possible when headache onset is noted. For example, many patients benefit from 400 mg ibuprofen at the first sign of migraine, and if taken within 10 minutes of the first symptom, this may completely abort what would otherwise become a 3-day bout of headache. The challenge of migraine is that after an attack is established, controlling pain may be difficult or impossible, subjecting patients to enduring 2 to 3 days of pain and disability as they seek out a dark, secluded space to endure the intense pounding pain. The mechanisms of migraine remain an area of intensive study and some controversy. There is abundant evidence that both central and peripheral mechanisms contribute, with ion channel mutations contributing to central initiation and calcitonin gene-related peptide (CGRP) release by activated nociceptors (reflexive neuroinflammatory response) contributing to headache perpetuation.[3] Many patients will respond to ibuprofen if taken with consistent promptness; others still require a triptan or other abortive medication. Clinical trials have indicated that prompt delivery of analgesia is essential. Patients should be counseled to take medicine and water with them everywhere (e.g., in the car when commuting, in a bag to movies or sports events) and to avoid known triggers (e.g., wine, bright sunlight without hat or sunglasses). Migraine that is accompanied by neurologic changes should be evaluated by a neurologist; persistent neurologic deficits are not part of common migraine.[2] Newly developed CGRP inhibitors represent additional treatment options for some patients who fail first-line therapy.

Obstructive sleep apnea (OSA) is a potential cause of new or worsening headache, particular in older adults. The prevalence of OSA is 25% in males, and the corresponding estimate is 10% in females. OSA results in decreased oxygen to brain and body during sleep and has numerous deleterious effects on health, so timely evaluation is appropriate. Sleep study referral should be considered for all patients presenting with worsening morning headache, especially after nonbenign causes are excluded as appropriate.

Nonbenign Headache

Nonbenign secondary headaches are common in clinical practice; the differential diagnosis of these headaches depends on features of the headache and the clinical context. Several examples are presented in the following box.

Potential Causes of Headaches With Visual Impairment

Temporal arteritis
Glaucoma
Occipital stroke
Brain tumor
Idiopathic intracranial hypertension
Multiple sclerosis

Temporal arteritis or giant cell arteritis (GCA) is a serious systemic autoimmune condition that can result in permanent visual loss if untreated. GCA often presents with temporal headache and visual loss in the context of weight loss and proximal muscle aches. The classic presentation is an older woman with aches and weight loss with a new unilateral headache and fleeting visual obscuration.[4] It is important to recall that new-onset migraine is uncommon in older adults. Patients with GCA may describe jaw claudication (i.e., fatigue when chewing tough foods) and demonstrate allodynia (i.e., tenderness) to palpation over the temporal region. The erythrocyte sedimentation rate is elevated in most patients and should be tested immediately. Biopsy of the temporal artery to affirm vasculitic changes is essential, and treatment with long-term steroids is necessary. Steroid treatment may precede biopsy, but biopsy should occur promptly when diagnosis is suspected because biopsy findings remit with prolonged steroid treatment.[5] Other autoimmune conditions may also present with headache. Potentially, lupus, rheumatoid, and other forms of vasculitis can all result in headaches. In many cases, the condition will produce associated signs and symptoms, although these may be subtle at initial presentation.

Idiopathic intracranial hypertension (IIH), historically pseudotumor cerebri, is a condition of increased intracranial pressure not associated with a tumor, hence pseudotumor.[6] Diagnosis is suspected in obese female patients of child-bearing age with a steadily worsening headache that may be bifrontal. Females outnumber males by a large margin in this condition. There are a number of factors that increase the occurrence of IIH, including obesity, hypervitaminosis A, and oral contraceptives. There is a risk for visual loss as pressure from the cerebrospinal fluid (CSF) is transmitted to and can compress the optic nerve. It is important to refer those patients suspected of having IIH for neurologic assessment. If this is delayed, CSF pressure assessment may be performed by a qualified interventional radiologist or emergency care center; however, it is important that the patient be recumbent for the measurement of opening pressure, which is the principle diagnostic test for this condition. If the patient is seated upright or at an elevated angle, the measure of opening pressure will not be correct. Some patients with this condition are responsive to pharmacologic management and weight loss; other patients have required shunt placement. Visual loss may result if the condition is not recognized and treated effectively.

Glaucoma is a potential cause of new-onset headache. It is more common in older adults and typically features some change to vision, but may not. It is important to examine the eyes and visual acuity of a patient presenting with new or worsening headache and to counsel patients to have prompt and proper eye exams.

Optic neuritis is a possible cause of new-onset headache; in this condition, visual change may be subtle, involving desaturation of red tones, or more profound. This condition requires prompt assessment and treatment, potentially requiring intravenous steroids as well as magnetic resonance imaging (MRI) of the brain to appraise whether this is a presentation of multiple sclerosis (MS).

MS is also associated with new headache aside from optic neuritis, and this is one of the reasons that it is important to perform a screening neurologic exam of patients with new headache. If the patient demonstrates unexpected findings such as unsteady gait or imbalance, loss of coordination, sensation, or strength, it will be necessary to evaluate the patient with brain MRI and neurologic referral.

Tumors, both benign and malignant, can be a cause of new or worsening headache. As noted for MS, neurologic changes occurring with new or worsened headache require additional evaluation with MRI and neurologic referral. If a tumor is found, local practice patterns will determine whether the patient is referred to a neurologist or directly to a neurosurgeon or oncologist. The classic presentation of worsening headache on awakening may not be discernable.

Some infections are associated with new or worsening headaches: Lyme disease, syphilis, HIV, hepatitis C, common flu, and bacterial infections are all associated with headache. It is important to consider the clinical context carefully when evaluating patients with new or worsening headache (see the following box). Low-grade fever, malaise, and mild elevations or reductions in white blood cell count may all be significant and related.

Screening Neurologic Exam for Headaches

Cranial Nerves

Vision present in each eye
Eyes move well and together
Face sensation symmetric
Smile and eye closure symmetric
Tongue midline

Motor

Arms and legs symmetrically strong

Sensation

Hands and feet all have sensation

Reflexes

Knee and elbow reflexes symmetric

Coordination

Gait steady and able to stand on heels

New or worsening headache in older adults merits prompt evaluation. Stroke and tumor are leading serious causes of headache in this population, making screening neurologic assessment essential; atypical infections may contribute as well. Normal-pressure hydrocephalus is classically described as presenting with a triad of dementia, urinary incontinence, and gait difficulty; headaches are more prevalent in these patients. New diagnosis of migraine in older adulthood is unusual, and caution is urged before proceeding to treatment without thoughtful diagnostic appraisal in the older adult presenting with new headache.

NEW-ONSET FACIAL PAIN: LYME DISEASE, TEMPOROMANDIBULAR JOINT DISORDER, MULTIPLE SCLEROSIS, AND SINUSITIS

Facial pain can result from infectious, inflammatory, or autoimmune conditions, among several potential causes. Trigeminal neuralgia, a major cause of chronic neuropathic facial pain, is described in Chapter 17. In terms of infectious causes facial pain, Lyme disease and syphilis are both capable of producing painful neuropathic injury syndromes. The pain associated with infectious causes of face pain may develop insidiously or come on suddenly; qualitatively, the pain may be deep and difficult to characterize, (i.e., perceived as a mixed burning–cold sensation) or may be lancinating in nature. Sinusitis may present with the patient describing either facial pain or headache. The classical presentation is headache with facial pain that worsens when the patient bends forward so that the face is in a dependent position. Chronic sinusitis can be a complex condition with inflammatory and infectious components; acute sinusitis may result from bacterial infection, which presents with purulent mucus and face pain. Conservative measures and antibiotics may be necessary. Inflammatory syndromes associated with face pain include temporomandibular joint (TMJ) disorder. In this condition, the pain is typically described as an aching pain in the region of the TMJ, anterior to the ear.[7] Classically, the patient will note clicking sensations in the joint and difficulty with chewing. The side area of the face may be tender to palpation. MS may at times present with new onset of facial pain. This condition more commonly presents in early to middle adulthood; for older patients, consideration may be given to atypical small stroke syndromes.

FOCAL AND NEUROPATHIC FACIAL AND SOMATIC PAIN

Atypical focal pain in parts of the body can arise from several conditions, including MS, stroke, tumor, and abscess. As noted previously, MS in younger adults and strokes in older patients can produce syndromes of persistent pain. These neurologic conditions generally require neurologic consultation and MRI to evaluate the patient's needs, risks, and potential for progression. Inflammation of joints, tendons, ligaments, and muscles, including trigger points, may be a cause of atypical focal pain. Tumors and abscesses are also potential causes of atypical focal pain; for this reason, it is recommended to always inspect and gently palpate a part that the patient describes as painful. Palpation may not be appropriate for all patients, and context should be considered. Soft tissue ultrasound may be a useful diagnostic complement for questions of soft tissue abnormalities. Chaperones should be present when appropriate and for certain areas of the body, and specialist referral may be appropriate for definitive examination. Suspected orthopedic conditions may require assessment by a surgeon or physical medicine and rehabilitation physician depending on the situation. Suspected neurologic involvement may require neurologist referral, and pelvic pain may require examination by an obstetrician-gynecologist or pelvic pain specialist. Podiatrists can be instrumental in evaluating painful disorders of the foot or aberrations in stance and weight-bearing; ophthalmologists will need to evaluate most forms of eye pain; and ear, nose, and throat specialists may be needed for ear and sinus pain.

Shingles is a form of focal neuropathic pain that arises from reactivation of dormant varicella-zoster virus that has been resident in the dorsal root ganglion. Typically a condition of patients older than 50 years, its incidence increases with age and is also increased in those with immunocompromise.[8] It is important to recognize this condition quickly because treatment during the early phase is effective in decreasing pain duration and potentially reducing the likelihood of developing postherpetic neuralgia (PHN), a treatment-resistant protracted form of distressing neuropathic pain (see Chapter 17). Treatment should ideally begin with 72 hours of onset, although some support treatment after the 72-hour window, especially for factors of ophthalmic involvement, immunocompromise, or evidence of new lesions. Treatment is primarily with antiviral agents; for details, the prescriber should follow local guidance. Advice on augmentation of treatment with corticosteroids is variable. Cochrane reviews have indicated that there is moderate evidence to indicate no benefit in terms of reducing incidence of PHN; however, others argue that steroids may reduce the pain of the acute episode or reduce swelling in compression-sensitive cranial nerves, if such are involved. Analgesia in the acute phase is important but remains challenging. OTC agents are only effective for mild pain. Some recommend tricyclic antidepressants (TCAs) for acute-phase pain (but side effects may be problematic) and screening electrocardiogram to ensure that no preexisting QTc prolongation is necessary; the onset of TCA efficacy may not be immediate.[9] Nonetheless, the only other option may be opioids, which carry excessive risk, or gabapentinoids, in which case a TCA trial may be reasonable.[10] After the electrocardiogram is cleared and no other contraindications are found, a modest dose of amitriptyline at bedtime (black box warnings) may be a useful adjunct for pain control. Some 20% of shingles patients may experience ophthalmic involvement, in which case proactive management is appropriate because the virus can produce corneal ulcerations that can result over the long term in excruciating pain that is extremely difficult to control.

Diabetic amyotrophy is a neuropathic complication of diabetes, typically in the context of poor diabetic control. Essentially a microvascular infarction of a peripheral nerve, the clinical syndrome is one of profound acute pain and focal weakness. Femoral nerve diabetic amyotrophy, for example, will result in severe anterior-medial thigh pain and quadriceps weakness. This syndrome requires much improved diabetic control and rehabilitation treatment. The medial pain and quadriceps weakness of femoral amyotrophy are in contrast to the neuropathic pain of the lateral thigh, without weakness, that is characteristic of meralgia paresthetica (MP) (Figure 15.1). MP is a nerve compression syndrome of the lateral femoral cutaneous nerve that is seen in those with abdominal obesity or tight belt-wearing, but not necessarily diabetes.

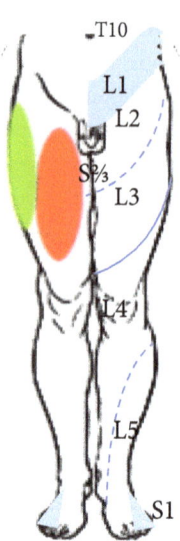

FIGURE 15.1 **Radicular patterns and patterns of femoral amyotrophy pain and meralgia paresthetica pain.** Radicular patterns are shown on the right side of figure, with landmarks including the L1 level pain radiating to lower abdomen and groin, *light blue*; L4 wrapping from lateral thigh across the anterior knee; and S1 radiating down the back of the thigh and calf to the lateral foot, also *light blue*. Pain of femoral amyotrophy radiates to the anterior and medial thigh, *red area*; meralgia paresthetica is associated with pain in the lateral thigh, shown in *green*.

URGENT NECK AND LOW BACK PAIN

Radiculopathy and spinal disk injury are spinal degenerative syndromes that are potentially associated with severe pain. Similar syndromes occur in the cervical and lumbar spine with relative sparing of the thoracic spine because of less mobility and more structural support there. These degenerative spine conditions are remarkably prevalent and are associated with variable presentations across the life span. Activity-associated disk herniation leading to acute radiculopathy is a condition of early to middle adulthood, at which point the disks become more desiccated and less prone to herniation. The classic precipitant is loaded rotation with flexion (i.e., lifting an 80-lb. sack of concrete mix out of a car trunk). Patients experiencing acute disk herniation with nerve root compression typically have high levels of pain and report dermatome-like radiating pain that shoots up with activities of bending, straining, and attempting to arise from a lying position. These patients can be fully disabled from normal activities until the syndrome is recognized and managed. Not all patients require surgery, but urgent assessment and referral for imaging and surgical, chiropractic, interventional, or physical therapy management, along with analgesia, are urgently need for these patients. It is important to balance short-term needs with long-term outcomes. Literature suggests that although interventional management may provide rapid relief that may last for a few weeks, long-term outcomes are unchanged. For this reason, it is important to counsel patients that spine injections are not a stand-alone solution but must be accompanied by physical therapy and home exercise in order to strengthen the spinal musculature, improve posture and ergonomics, and increase the likelihood of durable syndrome resolution.

With advancing age, there are changes in the structures of the spine that lead to multifactorial radicular compression syndromes. Although these changes are "chronic" in nature, some patients will present with a sudden deterioration in mobility that will lead to surprisingly rapid muscle atrophy and loss of functional independence if not addressed promptly. The age-related changes of the spine include loss of disk height, boney spurring and reformation, ligamentous hypertrophy, and fat deposition, all of which may contribute conjointly to cause nerve root compression. This may compress isolated nerve roots, leading to a radicular syndrome, or may ultimately lead to a more extensive set of changes that cause multiple nerve roots to be compressed, a "lateral-recess" variant of spinal stenosis. Some patients have central canal stenosis, which may result from the previously described events. In addition, chronic trauma of vertebral disk may result in protruding calcified disks, which are non-reducible, and as nerves expand naturally during ambulation, this leads to a choking off of blood supply and the condition known as neurogenic claudication. This explains why one of the principal symptoms of spinal stenosis is a progressive decrease in the ability to walk long distances. Reports of pain with spinal stenosis are variable; however, the intense pain associated with simple radiculopathy (isolated nerve root compression) often goes unnoticed: The typical amount of pain associated with a disk herniation-radiculopathy event is 8/10, with a substantive proportion of individuals experiencing pain that is 9/10 or 10/10, and another proportion experiencing pain that is 6/10 or 7/10. Relatively few persons experience only minor pain with radiculopathy.

An aspect of spinal pain that was historically more controversial relates to the lumbar disk. A case series of persons examined by MRI in the 1990s reported that a relatively surprising percentage of people without notable low back pain actually had disk bulges.[11] The population selected for this study was specifically selected on the basis of not having back pain, recruited by responding to a public notice requesting participation of those without low back pain. It is impossible to appraise the degree of selection bias in a study like this, but it may be considerable. In the intervening period, extensive clinical and preclinical work has demonstrated that the chronic stressed and injured disk will be invaded by pain-sensing nerve endings and become sensitized to injury.[12,13] This is because strain on the disk leads to a release of inflammatory signaling molecules, some of which are actually neurotrophins (proteins that support nerve growth) specifically tuned to support in growth of pain-sensing fibers.[14] While it is intriguing to speculate why this might occur on an evolutionary basis, it certainly explains the observation that a 20-year-old linebacker makes a much brisker recovery after a big game than does a 32-year-old football player, and the 42-year-old football player may find that a rough tackle can end his career. The relevance to the ordinary patient is that disks may be very painful after injury. Disk injury can occur through a variety of circumstances, especially trauma, falls, and inappropriate lifting maneuvers. The diagnostic hallmark of disk injury is pain that centralizes to the midline with load-bearing, Valsalva, or change of position. Unlike myelopathic pain, which is diffuse and ill-defined, disk pain is sharp and localized when provoked by movement or loading. It is important to recognize discogenic pain because these patients will typically follow a protracted recovery course. Disks typically require extended periods of time to heal, sometimes taking 2 to 3 months to "simmer down." This is likely due to the presence of activated pain-sensing nerve fibers, inflammatory mediators, limited vascular supply, and constant demands on the spine. Physical therapy and appropriate analgesia are necessary. Most other pain-evoking structures are off the midline, including muscles, facet joints, sacroiliac joints, and nerve pain.

Spinal cord–associated pain conditions are typically of an emergent nature and are addressed in Chapter 14. Emergent causes of low back pain include trauma, epidural abscess, and Guillain-Barré syndrome.

IRRITABLE BOWEL SYNDROME

Irritable bowel syndrome (IBS) is a prevalent condition of abdominal pain and gastrointestinal dysfunction characterized by intermittent diarrhea, constipation, or both. Estimated to affect 20% of the US population, it may be more common in women, but this varies by country globally.[15] People across the life span may experience IBS, and children are not exempt. It has been observed that the majority of those with IBS do not seek medical care and self-manage the condition. Recognition and implementation of conservative management strategies is important to reduce the impact of the condition. Formal criteria for IBS have been established for research purposes and include abdominal pain for 3 or more days each month for at least 12 months and changes in bowel patterns (e.g., stool consistency or frequency). IBS does show heritable features, with increased prevalence in close relatives. Increased stress may contribute to spurring the condition. Stress management, increased fiber and hydration, and probiotics may help patients improve symptoms. If conservative measures are not successful in decreasing syndrome impact, referral for specialist evaluation is appropriate.

MYOSITIS AND MYALGIA

Myositis is inflammation of the muscle. A few specific conditions involve autoimmune muscle inflammation; among these are polymyositis and dermatomyositis. The incidence of these conditions is not especially high. By comparison, an estimated 3 to 5% of persons will develop myalgias while taking statins. Both of these are addressed here. Polymyositis is an autoimmune condition of muscle inflammation that presents with proximal muscle pain and progressive weakness. Diagnosis is made with electromyography and biopsy. Treatment is primarily with immunomodulating agents, including prednisone. Although creatine phosphokinase (CPK) is elevated in the disease, this elevation is not used to guide treatment, which is based on clinical response. Dermatomyositis is a condition of muscle inflammation that is often associated with particular skin changes and increased cancer risk. The classic finding of dermatomyositis is "mechanic's hands," referring to dry, cracked, and reddened skin over the extensor surfaces of the metacarpophalangeal and proximal interphalangeal joints of the hand. Dermatomyositis is associated with increased incidence of cancer. Statin-associated myalgias are a topic of some controversy; nonetheless, a syndrome of muscle destruction and potential rhabdomyolysis is recognized in a minority of patients.[16] Measurement of CPK in patients with reports of muscle pain in response to statins is urgent because left unchecked, substantive muscle damage can occur. One particular statin, Baycol, was associated with high levels of muscle disruption and was removed from the market. Heritable factors play a role because statin-induced myopathy dose occurs at a higher rate in those with SLCO1B1 polymorphisms, but statin myopathy may occur in others as well.[17] Coadministration of medications that inhibit metabolism (CYP3A4 predominantly) may also increase the likelihood of statin-induced muscle destruction (see the following box).[16]

Selected Common Medications Associated With Increased Risk for Statin-Induced Muscle Pain and Damage

Antifungal agents, including fluconazole
Antibiotics, including erythromycin
Selected antidepressants, including fluoxetine and TCAs
Calcium channel blockers, including verapamil

PAIN OF UNDETERMINED PATHOLOGY

Pain can arise at essentially any part of the body because almost all structures in the body are innervated. Exceptions may include the nucleus pulposus and cartilage, although caution in this may be warranted because many structures previously determined to be "un-innervated" have been shown to have phenotypically nociceptive nerve endings in recent years, with various technologic advances improving antigenic characterization and microscopic identification of small structures. A complication arises in that a patient may perceive pain in a place that is not precisely the same as the point of injury that the pain system is signaling: This is because pain is a central nervous system (CNS) representation of neural activation occurring in the peripheral nervous system (PNS), and in some cases the CNS representation does not precisely match the events in the periphery. In other cases, such as trigger points, the pathologic problem acts at a distance through structures such as tendons and fascial layers to cause activation of nerve endings at a site distinct from the causative problem. As noted in the section on neuropathic pain, pain can also arise from abnormalities—macroscopic, microscopic, and molecular—in the nervous system. In neuropathic pain, an aberrant signal arises in a part of the nervous system that is then interpreted by brain systems as being in some part of the body that is not injured but may seem to be in danger. A diligent search for cause, based on the patient's history, relevant clinical examination, and diagnostic testing when appropriate, is essential so that patients are not at risk or consigned to the label "psychogenic." Malingering and factitious disorder are truly rare disorders often reflective of serious psychopathology. Treatment of pain of undetermined pathology is challenging, but initiating treatment can often lead the patient and provider closer to a diagnosis. If a musculoskeletal condition is suspected, these conditions may respond transiently to NSAIDs, but referral to a physical therapist, chiropractor, podiatrist, or orthopedic surgeon may advance the diagnostic and treatment. If a neuropathic condition is suspected, these patients will not respond to NSAIDs, but low-dose gabapentin may provide some symptomatic relief as the workup is proceeding. Referral of patients with suspected neuropathy for electromyelography/nerve conduction studies or neurologic evaluation is appropriate. It is important to ensure that no urgent or emergent conditions are causing the patient's pain, but after safety is assured, preliminary treatment may proceed in parallel with the workup, providing the patient with some pain relief. Figure 15.2 illustrates the process of selecting medications based on suspected pain type. Sometimes, as pain

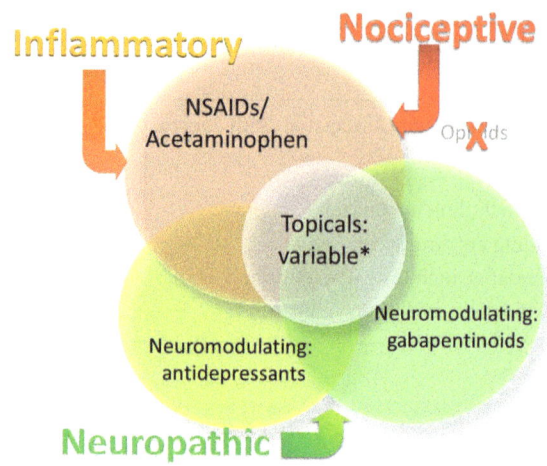

FIGURE 15.2 **Pharmacologic treatment planning based on mechanism-based classification of pain.** For nociceptive pain, acetaminophen and nonsteroidal anti-inflammatory drugs (NSAIDs) are typical first-line choices for mild to moderate acute pain; more severe pain may be selectively managed with NSAIDs, local anesthetics, or a combination of agents. Opioid risks have undergone reappraisal in light of the huge number of opioid-related overdose deaths, and risks may outweigh benefits depending on clinical setting and context (see Chapter 20). Opioids are excluded from the framework presented here and should only be prescribed for clear and compelling indications and with precautions as noted in Chapter 20. Inflammatory pain may respond to NSAIDs, but acetaminophen lacks anti-inflammatory action, and other disease-modifying therapy may be necessary. Neuropathic pain does not typically respond to NSAIDs, so neuromodulating agents such as gabapentinoids and pain-active antidepressants should be considered. Topical agents may prove useful but vary with mechanism. Topical NSAIDs, salicylates, lidocaine, and counterirritants may be used in inflammatory pain; some of these may be helpful for nociceptive pain, while others may increase pain or are contraindicated for open wounds. Neuropathic pain may respond to topical lidocaine or other neuromodulating agents in compounded preparations. Response to topical capsaicin is variable; topical capsaicin may be especially useful in chronic knee pain but requires reapplication multiple times daily and may worsen neuropathic pain. Conditions in which multiple pain mechanisms are active often require a rational combination of therapeutic agents and modalities.

abates through treatment, it is easier to determine where the primary source of pain lies because severe pain spreads temporally and spatially owing to nociceptive processing mechanisms, such as glial activation and central sensitization (discussed in Chapter 2). The parallel pathway model of treating and diagnosing pain in tandem is described in Chapter 4. It is critically important to follow patients with undetermined pain closely in order to ensure that the pain is not an atypical presentation of a life-limiting condition and that the patient is experiencing pain alleviation with treatment.

SUMMARY

Urgent pain problems are those that require prompt evaluation and initiation of treatment. Pain-associated conditions such as migraine, other non-emergency headaches, facial pain, severe low back pain, acute neuropathies, and painful muscle conditions are addressed in this chapter. Systematic assessment and diagnostic approaches are taken in parallel with the initiation of safe treatments so that patients are not enduring unmitigated pain while evaluation progresses.

REVIEW QUESTIONS

1. Which of the following is correct about headaches requiring urgent assessment?
   a. New-onset migraine is uncommon in older adults.
   b. Migraine headaches show strong genetic effects.
   c. Visual loss with headache is correctly explained by migraine.
   d. Tension headache is less common than migraine.

2. Neuropathic pain conditions requiring urgent attention include the following, *except* (choose two options):
   a. Shingles (herpes zoster)
   b. Diabetic amyotrophy
   c. Tension headache
   d. Spinal radiculopathy (pinched nerve)
   e. Myositis

3. Lumbar spine conditions associated with moderate to severe pain persisting for weeks if untreated include the following, *except*:
   a. Lumbar radiculopathy
   b. Disk injury
   c. Myelopathy
   d. Muscle strain
   e. Lateral recess spinal stenosis effecting multiple nerve roots

REFERENCES

1. Stovner LJ, Hagen K, Jensen R, et al. The global burden of headache: a documentation of headache prevalence and disability worldwide. Cephalalgia. 2007;27(3):193–210.
2. Migraine. The International Classification of Headache Disorders (3rd ed.). Accessed February 25, 201.at https://www.ichd-3.org/1-migraine/.
3. Brennan KC, Pietrobon D. A systems neuroscience approach to migraine. Neuron. 2018;97(5):1004–1021.
4. Temporal arteritis. Accessed February 25, 2019 at: https://medlineplus.gov/ency/article/000448.htm.
5. Maleszewski JJ, Younge BR, Fritzlen JT, et al. Clinical and pathological evolution of giant cell arteritis: a prospective study of follow-up temporal artery biopsies in 40 treated patients. Mod Pathol. 2017;30(6):788–796.
6. Chen J, Wall M. Epidemiology and risk factors for idiopathic intracranial hypertension. Int Ophthalmol Clin. 2014;54(1):1–11. doi: 10.1097/IIO.0b013e3182aabf11.
7. Temporomandibular joint disorder. Accessed February 25, 2019 at: https://medlineplus.gov/temporomandibularjointdysfunction.html.
8. John AR, Canaday DH. Herpes ZOSTER IN THE OLDER ADULT. Infect Dis Clin North Am. 2017;31(4):811–826. doi: 10.1016/j.idc.2017.07.016.
9. Bowsher D. The effects of pre-emptive treatment of postherpetic neuralgia with amitriptyline: a randomized, double-blind, placebo-controlled trial. J Pain Symptom Manage. 1997;13(6):327–331.
10. McGreevy K, Bottros MM, Raja SN. Preventing chronic pain following acute pain: risk factors, preventive strategies, and their efficacy. Eur J Pain Suppl. 2011;5(2):365–372.

11. Jensen MC, Brant-Zawadzki MN, Obuchowski N, et al. Magnetic resonance imaging of the lumbar spine in people without back pain. N Engl J Med. 1994;331:69–73.
12. Freemont AJ, Peacock TE, Goupille P, et al. Nerve ingrowth into diseased intervertebral disc in chronic back pain. Lancet. 1997;350(9072):178–181.
13. Freemont AJ, Watkins A, Le Maitre C, et al. Nerve growth factor expression and innervation of the painful intervertebral disc. J Pathol. 2002;197(3):286–292.
14. Gruber HE1, Hoelscher GL, Ingram JA, Hanley EN Jr. Genome-wide analysis of pain-, nerve- and neurotrophin -related gene expression in the degenerating human annulus. Mol Pain. 2012;8:63.
15. Canavan C, West J, Card T. The epidemiology of irritable bowel syndrome. Clin Epidemiol. 2014;6:71–80. doi: 10.2147/CLEP.S40245.
16. Statin induced myopathy. Accessed January 27, 2019 at: https://neuromuscular.wustl.edu/msys/myoglob.html#lovastatin.
17. Link E, Parish S, Armitage J, et al.; SEARCH Collaborative Group. SLCO1B1 variants and statin-induced myopathy: a genomewide study. N Engl J Med. 2008;359(8):789–799.

16 Common Chronic Pain Problems

Beth B. Hogans

Passion is the bridge that takes you from pain to change.
—Frida Kahlo

LEARNING OBJECTIVES

At the completion of this chapter, the learner should be able to discuss:

- Headache as a major cause of chronic pain, including common headache types, key characteristics, examination findings, and first steps in diagnostic assessment and treatment
- Musculoskeletal (inflammatory and nociceptive) pain, which is the most common cause of chronic pain worldwide, including multiple modalities of treatment and how surgical intervention may play a critical role in pain relief in osteoarthritis
- How neuropathic pain can arise from different levels of the nervous system and how some areas are more common as pain generators
- Properties of some common neuropathic pain conditions, including radiculopathy and sciatica, and the multiple modalities of treatment that are appropriate for treating neuropathic pain
- Ways to balance pharmacologic management, using local and systemic agents, and nonpharmacologic management for effective chronic pain management

CASE SCENARIO

A 61-year-old woman presents with an acute episode of neck pain superimposed on a background of chronic neck pain of 10 years' duration. She reports that 1 week prior, she awoke from sleep with severe pain in her neck, radiating into her right shoulder.

She was seen by her primary care physician that day and evaluated for ominous causes, such as heart or lung disease, and then referred to your clinic to address the pain. She typically is quite active and works 40 hours a week at a paint store. She is normally able to lift 5-gallon paint cans (56 pounds) but has not been able to do this since the pain started 1 week ago. She notes that the pain is 7/10 at rest, worsens to 9/10 with movement, and radiates as a deep sensation to her outer shoulder (deltoid insertion) area. On examination, this is a slender, slightly anxious woman. Her general exam is normal. There is no atrophy, fasciculations, swelling, or tenderness in the muscles of the shoulder. There is no limitation in passive or active movement with the arm itself, but she is not able to provide full resistance to downward pressure on the outstretched elbow or resist the examiner from extending the flexed elbow on the right side. The reflex at the right brachioradialis is decreased compared with the left, but not absent. She does have some tenderness and taut bands (knots) in the muscles of the trapezius and neck strap muscles bilaterally. Her physician ordered magnetic resonance imaging (MRI), which shows degenerative cervical spine changes but no disk herniation or operable disease.

1. Do you think the cervical spine MRI was needed?
2. What additional information would lead you to consider MRI justified?
3. How will you use the information from the MRI that has already been performed?
4. What will you order for this patient next?
5. What elements would you counsel this patient to include in her pain self-management plan?
6. Are there medications that you might use to help control pain in this patient?

INTRODUCTION: COMMON CHRONIC PAIN-ASSOCIATED CONDITIONS

Chronic pain is remarkably prevalent around the globe. Although chronic pain is more common in older adults, there are younger adults and children as well who suffer from chronic pain conditions. Some of these conditions are addressed here with the common conditions, and others are addressed in the subsequent chapters, including the "extremes of pain." In the conditions addressed in this chapter, there is a variable degree of central pain perpetuation, with chronic migraine demonstrating clear pain perpetuation processes and other conditions demonstrating features consistent with peripheral processes, extrinsic to the nociceptive system, as major drivers of chronicity.

Pain is defined as chronic when it outlasts the time normally expected for healing. There has been debate as to whether a fixed time limit should be utilized in this definition; however, normal time for healing depends on the type of injury, trauma, or cause of pain as well as the type of patient. Age, stresses, and comorbidities can contribute to prolonged healing times. One type of chronic pain after trauma, complex regional pain syndrome (CRPS), is discussed in Chapter 17.

The most common chronic pain problems include chronic tension headache, migraine, low back pain, neck pain, and shoulder, knee, and hip pain.[1] Taken together, these sources of chronic pain account for the large majority of reported pain in cross-sectional studies and support a large market for over-the-counter (OTC) pain relievers. Most people manage mild to moderate chronic pain utilizing their own resources, often demonstrating excessive reliance on medication-based strategies geared toward immediate relief. Consistent reliance on short-term analgesia to the exclusion of a coordinated plan of exercise and planned pain self-management skills is a strategy that likely contributes to the large number of joint replacement procedures occurring every year in the United States. Coordination of multidimensional evidence-based pain self-management plans is needed in many healthcare settings, including primary care. Recent systematic reviews support the use of nonpharmacologic therapies, and one of the themes of this book is skillful incorporation of multiple modalities, recognized as effective for specific conditions and tailored to the patient's preference.[2] Figure 16.1 presents the model introduced in Chapter 8 and also provides specific examples of therapies that can be incorporated in a coordinated manner. This model provides an essential roadmap for clinicians managing and supporting patients with chronic pain. Some patients will quickly adopt the approach, whereas other will need to be guided through the elements of the roadmap in a step-by-step manner. Nonetheless, it is valuable for the provider to have a vision of what coordinated care looks like. For several of the chronic pain-associated conditions in this chapter, specific examples of tailored roadmaps are provided. Clearly, interprofessional collaboration is essential to the realization of coordinated pain management and self-management plans.

Older adults are especially prone to chronic pain.[2] In part this is a due to degenerative joint processes and the attendant biomechanical dysfunction. Other causes include psychosocial factors associated with aging such as decreased work engagement and social isolation, but age-associated changes in pain signaling also contribute. Management of chronic pain in older adults is more complicated because of the high prevalence of comorbid conditions, such as impaired renal function and

(a)

Physical activity and PT
Daily aerobic activity
Strengthening - home exercise program
Flexibility
Balance
Focus on self-efficacy

Safe medication use
OTCs
Time-based use
Safe disposal
Suicide screening and monitoring
Dosing and backup planning

Psychological support
Cognitive behavioral
Reframing
Stress reduction
Acceptance commitment
Pain flare planning
Scheduled pleasant activities

Environment and productivity
Ergonomics
Modified work schedule
Disability support
Caregiver education
Home safety
Nutrition

Integrative therapies
Acupuncture
Tai chi
Massage
Yoga
Meditation
Mindfulness

Pain modulation
Pain-active antidepressants
Gabapentinoids
Other anticonvulsants
Local anesthetics - topical
Counterirritants - topical

Rescue Interventions
Surgery

Sleep
Sleep hygiene
OSA treatment
Sleep readiness
Relaxation and routine
Out-of-bed/AM routine

FIGURE 16.1 Roadmap for coordinated multimodal evidenced-based pain care with examples, see Figure 8.3 or 12.2 for visual guide to care coordination roadmap". **A,** Overview of the pain management roadmap. Some elements are self-directed by the patient and require patient engagement and commitment; these are "active strategies." Other elements are more passive in nature. Active pain self-management is associated with better long-term outcomes in chronic pain. **B,** Examples of specific therapies and activities that can be incorporated into a pain management and self-management plan. (OSA = obstructive sleep apnea; OTC = over the counter; PT = physical therapy.)

cardiovascular risk factors that increase the hazards of popular OTC pain relievers. Assessment and management of pain in older adults is covered in detail in Chapter 19, but specific conditions are addressed here. Despite this, older adults many have additional resources that can be directed toward pain self-management, such as increased time, reliable access to therapy and durable equipment, and level of psychological determination to age healthfully. These resources, through education, can be more effectively committed to effective long-term strategies, resulting in less utilization of pills as the principal pain management approach.

CHRONIC TENSION HEADACHE

Tension headache is the most common cause of headache worldwide; however, owing to the responsiveness of tension headache to OTC analgesia, it is less commonly seen in clinical practice settings.[2] Tension headache is now classified into several subtypes based on the frequency and chronicity of headaches as well as the presence or absence of cranial and pericranial tenderness.[3] For both chronic tension and migraine headache, it is important to consider whether diagnostic testing is required as part of the care plan; consultation with a neurologist or other headache specialist may be appropriate; however, guidelines are available to support decision-making in this area (see the following box).[4]

Any evidence of neurologic abnormality or deficit in association with headache requires evaluation for harmful conditions. Onset of new headache in older adults especially should be approached with caution. Evaluation for causes such as stroke, infection, or tumor are often warranted based on context, before adopting a chronic symptom-focused approach.

Tension headache is often described as having a dull or pressure-like quality.[3] The region involved is the bilateral frontal region of the head or band-like region around the head. It is generally moderate in severity but can range from mild to severe in intensity. Tension headaches often worsen as the day goes on so that afternoons are the worst time of day. Tension headaches can be associated with stressful events and can worsen when stress is unrelieved. The infrequent, episodic tension headache will be responsive to standard analgesia. Chronic tension headache is less responsive to standard analgesia. Daily taking of OTC pain medication can lead to chronic daily headache, a separate syndrome. Some chronic tension headaches are associated with tenderness in cranial and pericranial muscles.

Examination of those with headache includes a screening neurologic exam with special attention to cranial nerves but also including symmetry of strength, gait, and balance. Muscles such as the temporalis, masseter, pterygoid, and cervical scalene muscles, posterior cervical strap muscles (splenius), trapezius muscles, or sternocleidomastoids may exhibit changes that contribute to headache perpetuation. All of these muscles may be palpated for the presence of trigger points, which can be appreciated as firm knots or taut bands in the muscle; caution must be used when palpating the sternocleidomastoid because the carotid body is nearby and pressure over the region may lower the pulse reflexively. Bilateral pressure to the carotid region can result in bradycardia and syncope, so clinical skills training is essential and

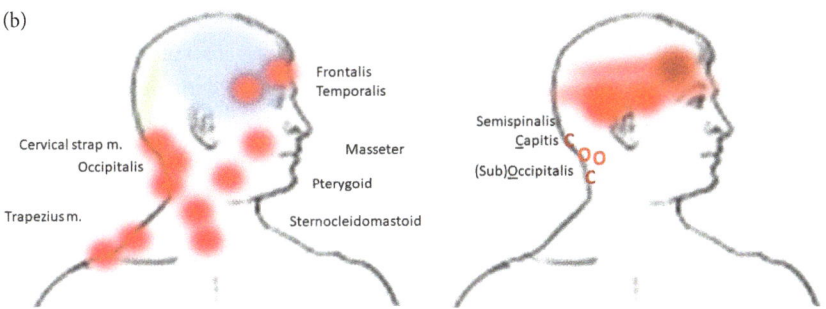

FIGURE 16.2 Examination of patient with chronic headache: palpation of the head and neck for pain-associated findings. **A,** *Red areas* show approximate location of muscles that should be palpated for the presence of trigger points. Muscles are present bilaterally but should be palpated one side at a time, especially over the sternocleidomastoid to avoid syncope. The *blue area* illustrates allodynia that may be observed with chronic migraine headache. The *green area* illustrates the potential area of tenderness relating to compression of the greater occipital nerve. **B,** Trigger-point location and associated pain pattern of the suboccipitalis muscle is shown in *bright red*, and that of the semispinalis capitis muscle is shown in *dark red*. Trigger points in these muscles can produce band-like tightness mimicking tension-type headache. Other muscles are associated with periorbital or hemicranial pain patterns.

unilateral palpation necessary. Locations for palpation in patients with headache are illustrated in Figure 16.2. Trigger points are associated with pain patterns located at a distance from the muscle itself, likely through fascia or tendinous connections. For example, trigger points in the posterior cervical muscles can produce pain in a band-like distribution anteriorly on the head.[4] Patients can learn to identify and manage trigger points with self-massage and stretching. Because muscle trigger points are prevalent and contribute widely to chronic pain perpetuation, it is valuable to be familiar with these techniques.[5]

Treatment of chronic tension headache is multidimensional and includes combining pharmacologic and nonpharmacologic strategies. Treatment of muscle trigger points may be undertaken through skilled physical therapy (PT) and may reduce the occurrence of frequent or chronic headache through unknown mechanisms. Patients can be trained to recognize and manage these muscle changes with manual therapy which may foster a sense of self-efficacy. Patients may also benefit from relaxation techniques, mindfulness-based deep breathing and cognitive behavioral approaches to stress management. It is important to assess and manage perturbations in sleep and eliminate or minimize substances of dependence, such as alcohol and tobacco.

A recent systematic review of chronic pain conditions included chronic tension headache as a musculoskeletal pain-related condition. That study found that few nonpharmacologic therapies have been proven effective for this condition at a moderate or high level of evidence.[2]

CHRONIC MIGRAINE HEADACHE

Chronic migraine headache can be highly disabling and a cause of lost productivity. Acute migraine is highly prevalent and is the most common headache seen in clinical practice as evidenced by prevalence in International Classification of Diseases (ICD) coding events.[1] Chronic migraine poses exceptional challenges because of the severe pain that characterizes migraine headache as well as the usual observation that activity worsens the pain, leading patients to avoid exertion and seek dark, quiet spaces.[3] In addition, some patients with migraine, and also those with chronic migraine, experience transient neurologic symptoms that may include nausea and vomiting, visual obscurations, and motor, speech, or balance impairments.[6] As noted previously, chronic headaches may be due to serious causes that must be excluded before focusing on symptom management, with periodic follow-up and monitoring to ensure patient safety. Imaging may be appropriate for those patients demonstrating atypical features or evidence of neurological abnormality.[7]

Migraine is classically distinguished by throbbing hemicrania of severe intensity that lasts for 4 hours to 3 days.[3] Distinct from the typical acute migraine, chronic migraine may evolve to manifest with pain bilaterally present. Nonetheless, official criteria for chronic migraine include migraine-like qualities present either during or at the start of the extended headache period. To be considered chronic, headaches must be present for more than 15 days a month for 3 or more months.

Exam findings in patients with chronic migraine may be minimal. Novice providers are often struck by how few observable behavioral cues to severe pain can be perceived. Patients wearing sunglasses indoors (photophobia) or broadbrimmed hats or large scarves may be demonstrating genuine sensory sensitivity. Because of the central pain processing events that occur in migraine, patients may develop allodynia, or sensitivity to normally nonpainful stimuli over parts of the head and neck during migraine, as illustrated in Figure 16.2. Examination includes those features of the exam noted previously for appraisal of patients with chronic tension headache. Note that many patients with migraine and chronic migraine are sensitive to light and sound (photophobia and phonophobia), so having a dimmable light in the exam room is one feature of a "headache-informed" office space. At the time of examination, it is ideal to ask permission before shining lights into the pupils because this may be intensely aversive for someone with active migraine. Chronic migraine should be distinguished from occipital neuralgia, a nerve compression syndrome associated with chronic head pain, and there may be evidence of tenderness to palpation over the nerve in the occipital scalp region (Figure 16.2). Chronic migraine can produce an allodynia syndrome that manifests with pain to normally non-painful light touch, brushing, or pressure over areas of the face and scalp, this will not be limited to regions overlying the occipital nerve, as is more characteristic of occipital neuralgia.

Chronic migraine typically requires a comprehensive pain management plan that incorporates both pharmacologic and nonpharmacologic strategies. If the patient is amenable to taking medication daily for migraine prophylaxis, a number of medications have been shown to reduce the severity and frequency of migraine attacks, including tricyclic antidepressants, calcium channel blockers, and some anticonvulsants. The choice of agent should depend on local practice patterns and experience with the side-effect and efficacy profiles of these medications. All of the migraine prophylaxis medications carry side effects that may be serious, although relatively infrequent. Antidepressants carry black box warnings for suicidal ideation and suicide; anticonvulsants may have negative effects on liver, electrolytes, or bone marrow; and calcium channel blockers can produce dose-limited cardiovascular

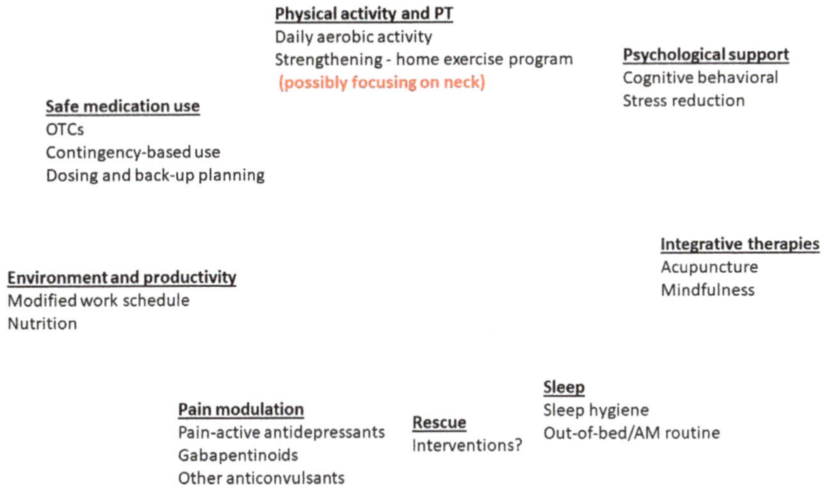

Safe medication use
OTCs
Contingency-based use
Dosing and back-up planning

Physical activity and PT
Daily aerobic activity
Strengthening - home exercise program
(possibly focusing on neck)

Psychological support
Cognitive behavioral
Stress reduction

Environment and productivity
Modified work schedule
Nutrition

Integrative therapies
Acupuncture
Mindfulness

Pain modulation
Pain-active antidepressants
Gabapentinoids
Other anticonvulsants

Rescue
Interventions?

Sleep
Sleep hygiene
Out-of-bed/AM routine

FIGURE 16.3 Example roadmap for management of pain associated with chronic headache. Both active and passive strategies are incorporated. Active self-management is associated with positive long-term outcomes. (OTC = over the counter; PT = physical therapy.)

effects such as low blood pressure. Some patients may obtain relief from occipital nerve blocks, which should be performed only by those with advanced training in the procedure. Other therapies include cranial transcutaneous electrical nerve stimulation (TENS), such as the Cefaly device; acupuncture or acupressure; migraine diet protocols; mindfulness-based stress reduction; and psychological approaches. Lifestyle modifications, such as making changes to a highly stressful occupational setting or avoidance of triggering odorants, may be necessary. Persons with chronic migraine may benefit from PT if there is evidence of musculoskeletal dysfunction that is contributing to lowering the headache threshold (e.g., musculoskeletal sequelae of cervical spondylosis may perpetuate headache); this may be elicited on examination. Patients should be engaged in developing a treatment plan and should be encouraged to learn about their condition (Figure 16.3). A headache diary can be indispensable in aiding the provider and patient in identifying headache patterns and potential responses to therapy. Finally, patients may require support to take intermittent time off from work or other adjustments to work and school life.

CHRONIC NECK PAIN

Chronic neck pain can be resistant to treatment and associated with substantive disability and decreased quality of life. More refractory forms are typically associated with cervical spine degeneration (spondylosis) with either central or lateral spinal stenosis. Central spinal stenosis can cause symptomatic cord compression (i.e., cervical myelopathy), which in addition to spasticity and incontinence can lead to weakness and chronic, treatment-refractory pain. Myelopathic pain is described as deep, diffuse, and highly distressing. Psychologically, some of these patients have led extremely active lives and find the adjustment to persistent disability quite difficult. It can be important to connect these patients with clinical psychology for structured brief therapy or in-depth work, through cognitive behavioral therapy (CBT) or acceptance commitment therapy (ACT), to identify and adhere to lifestyle changes that will increase meaningful engagement and diminish stress and frustration. Pharmacologic treatments may be necessary, but reliance on medications for pain relief is typically met with limited efficacy and ever-increasing side effects that may include respiratory suppression common to several of the antispasticity and pain agents as well as depression, dependence, and addiction. Cervical radicular pain is also deeply felt and distressing to patients, so it is important to evaluate patients with radicular symptoms for evidence of nerve root compression. Typically, an MRI is needed to assess the potential for neurologic structural compromise. If an operable lesion is not identified or the patient is determined to decline surgical management for a noncritical compression, physical therapy and appropriate home exercise programs are essential. Interventional management of cervical root compression may in some cases be viewed as appropriate; however, this often provides only transient relief, with long-term outcomes unchanged. In the event that immediate short-term pain relief will allow an otherwise reticent patient to participate in PT, this may be helpful. The risks of epidural steroid injections in the cervical region are increased compared with those in the lumbar region because cervical nerve roots are very short and the distance to the spinal cord is much less. As with the other chronic pain conditions discussed here, comprehensive pain management incorporating pain self-management strategies is very important in chronic neck pain. Lifestyle adaptations may include modified commuting arrangements, frequent use of heating, cooling, massage, or acupuncture, self-management of trigger points, and topical counterirritant analgesia (e.g., Biofreeze, Tiger Balm, or Bengay). In many respects, the management of chronic neck pain is similar to that of chronic low back pain (Figure 16.5).

CHRONIC LOW BACK PAIN

Chronic low back pain has recently been identified as a leading cause of work-related disability. Some recent studies have identified chronic low back pain as the most common cause of years lost to disability globally. There is considerable controversy over the causes of low back pain, but it is important to recognize that diverse causes can contribute to chronic low back pain. Factors that contribute to low back pain include spinal degeneration (e.g., spondylosis), disk degeneration, radiculopathy, sciatica, and sacroiliac (SI) joint disease; obesity, chronic widespread pain syndromes such as fibromyalgia, and affective disorders contribute to a lesser extent to persistent low back pain. A large number of patients with low back pain have just that—chronic low back pain without clear causation—although the formal recommendations and guidance to refrain from imaging of acute low back pain, except in circumstances of clear hazard (e.g., cancer, infection, progressive severe neurologic deficits) has resulted in fewer patients having access to information about underlying anatomic limitations.

The prevalence of low back pain means that many patients will present for evaluation of "acute" low back pain against the backdrop of existing chronic low back pain. For this reason, it is important to remain vigilant for low back red flags even in those patients with a long history of low back pain.[8] These include concomitant signs and symptoms of neoplasm, infection, or neurologic impairment.

For an overview of low back pain diagnosis, see Appendix V.

Red Flags for Low Back Pain

Trauma
Age >70 years and osteoporosis
Immunosuppression, fever, chronic steroid use, organ transplantation, AIDS, or untreated HIV
Cancer, history of cancer, or recent significant weight loss
Substance use disorder, including illicit substances and alcohol
Pain at night or with recumbency
Neurologic deficit

After red flag–associated low back pain conditions are excluded or appropriately evaluated, it is important to consider the differential diagnosis of chronic, persistent, or waxing and waning low back pain in light of the features of the low back pain. The previous box highlights some of the key features of various low back pain conditions. Location provides essential clues to diagnosis, such as centralizing pain (pain that worsens prominently to the midline with movement), which is most typically associated with disk injury or degeneration. Lateralizing pain by contrast is characterized by the extent and location of lateralization. For example, lateralization of the close paraspinal area at the L5 level is more likely SI joint dysfunction; lateralization to the buttock is more likely piriformis/sciatic syndrome; and lateralization of pain to below the knee is more likely an L5 or S1 radiculopathy (see the following box).

Key Features of Various Chronic Low Back Pain Conditions

Centralizing versus lateralizing
Centralizing low back pain: often disk-related
Lateralizing chronic low back pain: radicular, sciatica, SI joint, postherpetic neuralgia, muscular
Acute severe bouts: spondylolisthesis (spinal instability), SI joint
Insidious with walking limitation: lumbosacral stenosis
Persistent, moderate, unilateral: leg-length discrepancy or hip degeneration

Examination of patients with chronic low back pain includes a focused appraisal of potential causes of the pain. Because of the remarkable prevalence of low back pain, there is an extensive literature oriented toward validating and streamlining the exam process. Basic exam elements are very useful for distinguishing causes of chronic low back pain that critically require referral. A structured screening exam may be especially helpful, please see Appendix I for an examination template. Asymmetric loss of reflexes, muscle mass, or sensation merits evaluation for radiculopathy by imaging or referral, or both. Diagnostic presence of increased pain on straight leg raise also supports a potential diagnosis of radiculopathy and merits evaluation. Radiculopathy is a common cause of low back pain associated with a specific condition. Degeneration of the spine is also commonly identified in persons with chronic low back pain. This can be appraised by range of motion of the spine, especially forward flexion. Spine extension or "backward flexion" may be particularly diminished in patients with facet joint degeneration (Figure 16.4). The hallmark of stenosis is progressive limitation of

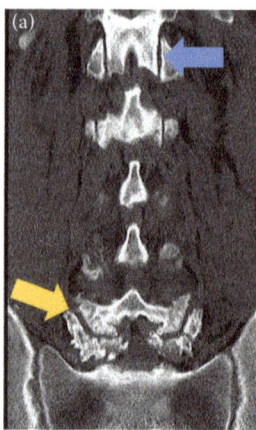 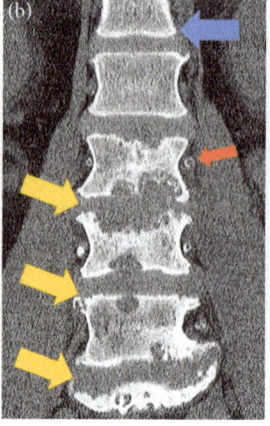 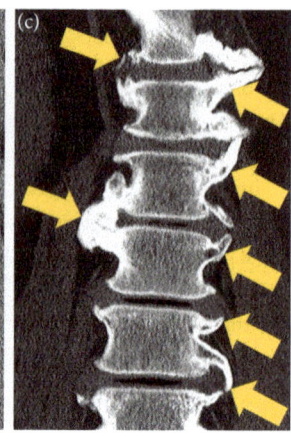

FIGURE 16.4 Degenerative spine states associated with chronic low back pain, selected severe examples. **A,** Facet joint degeneration is associated with chronic pain and limitation in spine extension. In this coronal computed tomography scan of the lumbosacral spine, a facet with minimal osteoarthritic change (joint space narrowing) is observed, *blue arrow*; severely degenerated facet joints are observed at the L5–S1 level, *yellow arrow*; and there is enlargement (overgrowth), destruction of the articular surface, and abundant bone pitting. **B,** Vertebral bones and disks form joints, and these are subject to acute and chronic trauma. In this coronal computed tomography scan of the lumbosacral spine, there is evidence of mild degeneration, *blue arrow*; minimal loss of disk height and mild osteophyte formation (note that the vertebral bone is not rectangular but has sharpened corners) and severe degeneration, *yellow arrows*; demonstrating exuberant overgrowth (osteophyte formation), severe loss of disk height, and degeneration of bone integrity (sclerosis). Calcification of atherosclerotic vertebral arteries is observed, *red arrows*. This patient has chronic unremitting back pain and may not be a surgical candidate. **C,** Multiple exuberant calcified disk osteophytes. Although medically stable, the extensive, multilevel nature of this patient's degeneration was not felt amenable to surgery. This veteran, unaware of his injuries likely sustained while parachuting during military service, now experiences chronic disruptive pain and will benefit from coordinated nonpharmacologic therapy as a complement to pharmacologic treatment. Although the radiographic findings in these patients are dramatic, the occurrence of spinal degeneration in older adults is not uncommon.

walking distance relieved by sitting or forward flexion. The patients will often demonstrate a forward station due to chronic adaptation to facilitate walking despite the limitations of stenosis. Older adults will often have multilevel spinal deterioration (Figure 16.4). In summary, strength, sensation, reflexes, range of motion, and gait should all be assessed as well as selected diagnostic maneuvers based on index of suspicion (e.g., straight leg raise for suspected lumbosacral radiculopathy). A diagnostic overview of low back pain is found in Appendix V.

Chronic low back pain requires comprehensive pain management that is both pharmacologic and nonpharmacologic and centered on the patient's needs and interests (Figure 16.5). Many patients are interested in nonpharmacologic approaches. Patients often ask about dietary supplements and modifications to eating that might be helpful for their pain-associated condition. In low back pain especially, it is critically important to promote healthful lifestyle choices such as having a daily exercise plan including some daily aerobic and daily strengthening exercise. Psychological therapies should be considered and incorporated, whether as CBT, ACT, mindfulness, pacing, or values-oriented approaches. Mind–body therapies such as Qi gong, Tai chi, and yoga have shown good efficacy in clinical trials. The benefits should be explained

Physical activity and PT
Daily aerobic activity
Flexibility
Focus on self-efficacy

Safe medication use
OTCs
Time-based use
Safe disposal
Suicide screening and monitoring
Dosing and backup planning

Psychological support
Reframing
Acceptance commitment
Pain flare planning

Environment and productivity
Ergonomics
Disability support
Caregiver education
Home safety

Integrative therapies
Massage
Mindfulness

Pain modulation
Pain-active antidepressants
Gabapentinoids
~~Local anesthetics - topical~~
Counterirritants - topical

Rescue
Interventions?
Surgery?

Sleep
Sleep readiness
Out-of-bed/AM routine

FIGURE 16.5 Example roadmap for management of pain associated with chronic low back pain. The pain care roadmap is useful for promoting patient understanding of the extent of lifestyle change that is necessary to successfully manage complex conditions such as chronic low back pain. (OTC = over the counter; PT = physical therapy.)

to patients, and incorporation of these activities, consistent with patient values and choice, should be recommended. Training in trigger point self-massage may provide durable relief as the patient acquires skills in self-management[5]. Sleep optimization is essential for long-term success in managing chronic pain for many reasons. There is evidence that poor sleep is associated with worse pain modulation and contributes to obesity, suggesting both direct and indirect effects of good sleep work to improve low back outcomes. Medication safety is important, as is designing a safe and effective pharmacologic plan. Finally, environmental factors come into play in chronic low back pain because pain can discourage patients from maintaining vital social connections, and beyond this, maintaining a safe home environment free from trip and fall hazards and enhancing ergonomics for frequent tasks are useful to patients and appropriate for providers to recommend to patients. Patients with chronic low back pain may have flairs and periods of worsened pain, so intermittent medical leave from work may be needed, and some occupation roles may not be appropriate for those with chronic low back pain.

CHRONIC HIP PAIN

Chronic hip pain is highly prevalent and most commonly associated with hip osteoarthritis. Although there are nonarthritic causes of chronic hip pain, hip joint replacement, often considered the definitive treatment for severe endstage osteoarthritis-related chronic hip pain, is occurring at record levels in the United States. According to the American Joint Replacement Registry, joint replacements are expected to increase in the years ahead. The Registry reports that patients undergoing a first hip replacement are typically in their late 60s, but this can range widely depending on circumstance. Hip osteoarthritis arises from both environmental and genetic factors. It can limit mobility and interfere with sleep, productive activity, and quality of life. Long-term management with standard analgesia leads to increasing risks for gastric bleeding and acceleration of renal dysfunction, which increase in older patients, possibly explaining in part the prevalence of joint replacement procedures in the older adult population. Exercises that strengthen the hip muscles, especially abductors, are important to reduce accelerated wear on the joints, as is education in proper techniques for sitting and standing (see the following box). Side sleepers may experience symptoms of sleep disruption early in the course of hip osteoarthritis, which will worsen as the condition progresses. Addition of a cushioning mattress topper may help resolve this, as may the use of supporting pillows to distribute weight away from the greater trochanter. Chronic hip pain may also be due to bursitis, sciatica, or iliotibial band syndrome, so orthopedic and/or physical therapy consultation may be helpful.

Daily Exercises to Prevent Hip and Knee Pain

1. *Quadriceps strengthening.* The quadriceps muscle weakens reflexively with the onset of knee pain. To counteract this, do the following: while lying down, place a pillow under one knee. Press down on the pillow for 3 seconds and release. Repeat this 20 times daily, building up to 50 times daily on each side.
2. *Gluteus/hip external rotation.* Hip strengthening helps prevent falls and protect the hip joint. Lying on the side with the legs extended straight, bend the knees without flexing the hip so that the feet are behind. Perform modified clamshells in this position, lifting the knees with the feet held together. Repeat 20 times daily, building up to 50 times daily on each side.

Consult your local PT for more exercises.

CHRONIC KNEE PAIN

Chronic knee pain has in previous years been described as the most prevalent cause of chronic pain worldwide. More recently supplanted by chronic low back pain, knee pain remains highly prevalent and associated with prominent levels of disability and decreased quality of life. Knee replacement remains a common final pathway for the management of chronic unresolved knee osteoarthritis with pain; however, there are several measures that can contribute to management of less advanced knee degeneration. Weight loss is especially recommended for knee pain because the knee joint receives forces equal to several multiples of the body weight with each step. Strengthening of the quadriceps muscle may provide substantial relief from mild to moderate knee pain due to early osteoarthritis. Interestingly, the pain associated with early joint arthritis may contribute to quadriceps weakening due to a relaxation reflex from the spinal cord, meaning that it is all the more important to consciously and consistently engage in focus quadriceps strengthening. Proper footwear and correction of podiatric misalignment through orthoses, taping, or bracing may improve persistent knee pain, so podiatric referral may be appropriate for patients with increased pain after running or walking. Physical therapy may extend the primary care assessment and aid the patient by providing additional exercises to counteract muscle laxity or weakness (see the following box).

Three Daily Stretches to Prevent Chronic Joint Pain

1. *Iliopsoas:* subject to chronic contraction with sitting. Shortened iliopsoas prevents correct alignment of the spine and increases low back, hip, and knee pain. Stretch the iliopsoas with the forward lunge or modified Warrior II yoga pose.
2. *Hamstrings:* shortens with prolonged knee flexion, such as with sitting. Tight hamstrings interfere with normal range of motion of the hip and pelvis, preventing forward bending and increasing the risk for back pain. Stretch with extended leg while lying on back; pulsing contractions may help to loosen the muscle.
3. *Pectoralis:* shortens with chronic forward posture as hands are at work on keyboard or other tasks. Trigger points and shortened fibers contribute to chronic neck, shoulder, and upper back pain. Stretch with doorway or corner stretches. Hold arms out from sides with elbows flexed. Gently lean into doorway or corner so that pectoralis is stretched.

Consult your local PT for details and instruction.

CHRONIC SHOULDER PAIN

Chronic shoulder pain can markedly attenuate quality of life and workplace and school productivity (see the following box). The use of upper extremities is central to many workplace activities, from typing to managing materials. Unfortunately, the productivity demands of modern society are such that people at many levels of employment and activity feel compelled to wring many hours of work out of each day, and work often means performing repetitive tasks with the shoulders in a hunched-forward position. Although the most common causes of chronic shoulder pain are musculoskeletal, the shoulder girdle is complex and consists of not only the shoulder joint but also the acromioclavicular joint, several muscles that are prone to injury, and many nerves innervating locally and large nerves of passage (i.e., the brachial plexus, which supplies the distal arm and hand). Supplied by nerves originating from the middle and caudal cervical levels, as well as the rostral-most thoracic spinal levels, the innervation of the shoulder girdle is complex. Injuries to peripheral structures, such as muscles and joints, can result in central sensitization in which benign physical sensations in response to normally nonpainful forms of touch change owing to a cascade of molecular events and become excruciatingly painful. Some patients with central sensitization cannot stand a light brushing stroke of the skin because this can produce a searing painful sensation; others cannot tolerate cold air from an airduct in summer; and still others cannot endure the sharp pain that arises from holding their shoulders in position to type for more than 20 minutes. For people with chronic shoulder pain, the experience of severe pain in response to normal daily stimuli becomes a major psychosocial burden. In these circumstances, it is critically important to engage patients in developing their own self-care plan—a plan that should include working with an experienced psychotherapist because adaptations to overcome the difficult challenge of managing chronic shoulder pain can be painful in themselves as patients struggle to adapt work and home tasks to the physical limitations of the injured shoulder complex. Comprehensive pain management planning is indispensable because complex pharmacologic regimens must dovetail with equally complex nonpharmacologic routines of stretching, strengthening, psychological exercises, sleep hygiene training, and environmental adaptations. Patients often require intermittent medical leave for extended periods of time during the chronic pain management process.

Selected Causes of Chronic Shoulder Pain

Fracture/fracture repair
Postoperative effects
Rotator cuff injury
Arthritis
Frozen shoulder (especially in patients with diabetes)
Cervical spine degeneration
Brachial plexus inflammation
Postherpetic neuralgia

PAINFUL DIABETIC PERIPHERAL NEUROPATHY AND DISTAL SYMMETRIC POLYNEUROPATHY

Painful diabetic peripheral neuropathy (PDPN) and distal symmetric polyneuropathy (DSPN) are distinguished from the other conditions in this chapter by having clear neuropathic character. While the other conditions in this chapter may respond at least briefly or partially to standard OTC analgesic medications, the failure of neuropathic pain conditions such as PDPN to respond to nonsteroidal anti-inflammatory drugs (NSAIDs) or acetaminophen may be a useful clinical clue when diagnosis is not yet established. Diabetes has high and increasing prevalence in our society, and diabetic peripheral neuropathy is present in many patients with diabetes, with occurrence depending on age, degree of diabetic control, and duration of diabetes. Not all diabetic neuropathy is painful: some patients describe numbness or a loss of sensation; others describe a bothersome but not frankly painful band-like tightness around the foot and a sense of having socks bunched under the toes. About half of patients with diabetic neuropathy experience pain. For these patients, evaluation and treatment is critically important to maintain sleep and exercise patterns that are essential to the lifestyle aspects of diabetic control.

PDPN often begins insidiously but usually with a pattern of painful burning in the toe that progresses more proximally over months to years. Symptoms are often most bothersome at night but may be noticeable anytime a patient is not distracted or mentally occupied. Some patients with these symptoms do not have diabetes; of these, about half will be found to have impaired glucose tolerance, and other potential conditions in the differential diagnosis include Lyme disease, metabolic neuropathies, vitamin deficiencies, and autoimmune conditions.[9] A series of tests may be considered in evaluating these patients (see the following box). In almost all patients, the feet are involved before the hands have symptoms; this is because these conditions generally affect the nerves in a length-wise manner, and the nerves to the foot are the longest in the body.

Evaluation of Distal Symmetric Peripheral Neuropathy

Complete blood count and erythrocyte sedimentation rate
Chemistries including renal and liver function studies
Two-hour glucose tolerance test with 0- and 2-hour values, 75-g glucose bolus
Vitamin B_{12} and D
Thyroid function studies
Lyme disease and syphilis screen
Antinuclear antibodies and rheumatoid factor
Electromyogram/nerve conduction studies for evaluation of large nerve fiber involvement
Skin biopsy for epidermal nerve fiber density for small-fiber neuropathy

---

Examination of patients who present with painful distal symmetric polyneuropathy should include a general neurologic exam with special attention to strength, sensation, and reflexes of the distal extremities. In PDPN and DSPN more generally, sensory loss is usually the most prominent, easily recognized exam abnormality; however, sensation may not be obviously impaired in those with early degeneration and pain. This is because in some patients, pain-sensing nerves will be activated by the degenerative process and signal the pathology earlier in the process than evidenced by sensory or motor loss. Motor loss is generally late in the disease process. Reflex drop-off, in which the ankle reflex is markedly decreased relative to the knee reflex, is an intermediate stage of nerve degeneration. In most early-stage patients, the feet will appear completely normal aside from mild hair loss and atrophic nail changes. It is useful to have a bedside test that supports the diagnosis and is consistent with known pathology. One special feature of the smallest nerves (C fibers) that are especially susceptible diabetic stress is that C fibers demonstrate the psychophysical property of windup. Windup is a form of hyperalgesia in which the repeated application of a painful stimulus leads to a progressively stronger perceived pain; something that is mildly painful on the first exposure may be quite painful with repeated stimulation. One key feature of windup is that the stimulus must be presented repeatedly and separated by a short amount of time, from milliseconds to about 1 second. The clinical application of this is that in testing patients with DSPN with a sharp probe (a wooden stick broken with a sharp tip or a Neurotip testing probe is preferred to standard safety pins, which are prone to causing damage to the skin and bleeding), when a tapping procedure is used, presenting the painful sharp sensation quickly and repeated, it is often possible to elicit markedly increased pain (i.e., hyperalgesia) not observed in unaffected patients. The affected patient may reflexively pull the foot away from the noxious tapping stimulation.

The treatment of PDPN rests on the cornerstone of optimizing diabetic control. There is well-validated evidence that strict diabetic control has been shown to reduce the pain associated with PDPN. A coordinated treatment plan is also essential (Figure 16.6). It is important to optimize gait mechanics with a podiatry consultation and treatment so that walking and other forms of exercise can continue because this is essential to diabetes control. Patients with PDPN experience increased pain in the setting of warming of the feet, so wearing sandals or well-ventilated footwear is helpful. Pharmacologic strategies for control of pain in PDPN and DSPN include the use of gabapentinoids, pain-active antidepressants, and selected topical agents. Treatment with gabapentin or pregabalin may begin with a modest dose at bedtime and then

Physical activity and PT
Daily aerobic activity

Psychological support
Stress reduction
Scheduled pleasant activities

Safe medication use
~~OTCs~~
Time-based use
Suicide screening and monitoring

Integrative therapies
Trial of Tai chi

Environment and productivity
Footwear
Foot checks
Home safety – fall prevention
Nutrition

Sleep
Sleep study
OSA treatment

Pain modulation
Pain-active antidepressants
Gabapentinoids
Local anesthetics - topical
~~Counterirritants - topical~~

Rescue
N/A

FIGURE 16.6 Example roadmap for management of pain associated with chronic peripheral neuropathy. Competency in interprofessional approaches to pain management are useful in delivering coordinated care and supporting patient engagement in multimodal pain self-management. (OSA = obstructive sleep apnea; OTC = over the counter; PT = physical therapy.)

taper up according to need to levels limited by prescribing guidelines and individual patient tolerance. Dizziness is a prominent side effect in some patients, and this, in combination with the loss of balance that occurs with DSPN, may represent a critical drug–disease interaction in some patients. Pain-active antidepressants, including duloxetine, may also be effective for PDPN. A tapering approach to therapy is usually most appropriate so that patients can be monitored for side effects; these agents as a class carry black box warnings for suicidality, and patients must be screened and counseled for suicidal ideation before use. Finally, topical agents preferred for use in PNDN are not the same as those used in musculoskeletal disorders. Although capsaicin preparations have been widely promoted for chronic pain, many patients with PDPN will experience worse pain with capsaicin. Lidocaine may provide relief and is available as cream, a compounded topical agent, or a patch. Patients must be counseled about proper use because exceeding dosing guidelines has, rarely, been associated with cardiac effects and even death. Nonetheless, topical lidocaine generally is safe and potentially effective for pain over a limited area.[10]

CARPAL TUNNEL SYNDROME AND ULNAR NEUROPATHY

Carpal tunnel syndrome (CTS) and ulnar neuropathy are chronically painful compressive neuropathies of the upper extremity.[11] CTS involves compression of the median nerve in the wrist, at the base of the hand. This compression arises from repetitive use injury, diabetes, pregnancy, or other conditions that result in local edema or enlargement of the soft tissues surrounding the median nerve as it transits the carpal tunnel en route from the forearm to the hand. Ulnar neuropathy is a common but often unrecognized condition of compression of the ulnar nerve at the medial elbow. Usually a result of external pressure on the median elbow (e.g. resting elbows on the table) or pursuant to excessive flexion of the elbow, as may occur from holding a phone to the ear for prolonged periods or sleeping with the arms acutely flexed, ulnar neuropathy can result in severe weakness of the hands in addition to pain. Typically viewed as benign, these conditions can result in chronic pain and progressive weakness if not recognized, evaluated, and managed. From a pain perspective, an interesting feature of CTS is that pain is often felt in the forearm. Otherwise, the pain of CTS demonstrates neuropathic features of nighttime worsening, exacerbation following periods of increased activity, and stinging, zinging, and burning qualities. CTS is more prevalent in pregnant women, who have increased plasma volumes that may contribute to the pathophysiology, and in those with diabetes, who are at increased risk for compressive neuropathies. Sensation may be reduced in those with these neuropathies. The CTS pattern involves the thumb and first finger most consistently, whereas ulnar neuropathy involves the fourth and fifth digits most consistently. Ulnar neuropathy in particular may produce hyperalgesia or allodynia when neuropathic injury is mild to moderate, so patients may report increased painful sensations in response to light brushing of the skin in the ulnar-innervated forearm area. CTS weakness leads to reduction in thumb abduction (moving the thumb away from the palm), and atrophy may be observed over the thenar eminence of the palm. As ulnar neuropathy progresses, weakness is observed in the interosseus muscles of the hand (resulting in poor abduction, or spreading apart, of the fingers) as well as atrophy in the intrinsic hand muscles and in the first dorsal interosseus muscle (webspace between the thumb and index finger). Referral for nerve conduction studies is essential for diagnosis, and treatment of mild compressive neuropathies may be conservative with bracing; however, more severe forms may require interventional management.

SUMMARY

Chronic pain occurs commonly and is highly prevalent in some populations, especially older adults. Strategies to manage chronic pain should be coordinated into comprehensive treatment plans that are founded on evidence-based effectiveness and patient safety. Treatment plans should include both nonpharmacologic and pharmacologic elements. A mechanism-based model that classifies conditions as primarily nociceptive, inflammatory, or neuropathic can help guide treatment, particularly in the early phases when testing is ongoing or diagnosis is yet to be established.

REVIEW QUESTIONS

1. Which of the following pairings is correct?
    a. Chronic tension headache: pressure-like, bilateral
    b. Chronic migraine: unilateral, throbbing
    c. Chronic low back pain: muscle sprain
    d. PDPN: pain and weakness of one hand

2. Which of the following are not red flags for acute on chronic low back pain?
    a. New onset of incontinence of bowel and bladder
    b. Radiation of pain into the buttock
    c. New weakness of foot or leg
    d. Weight loss
    e. Immunosuppression

3. Which of the following is considered an active pain self-management strategy
   a. Massage
   b. CBT
   c. Acupuncture
   d. Time-based medication management
   e. Steroid injection

REFERENCES

1. Global Burden of Disease Study 2013 Collaborators. Global, regional, and national incidence, prevalence, and years lived with disability for 301 acute and chronic diseases and injuries in 188 countries, 1990–2013: a systematic analysis for the Global Burden of Disease Study 2013. Lancet. 2015;386(9995):743–800.
2. Skelly AC, Chou R, Dettori JR, et al. Noninvasive nonpharmacological treatment for chronic pain: a systematic review [Internet]. Rockville, MD: Agency for Healthcare Research and Quality (US); 2018.
3. International Classification of Headache Disorders (3rd ed.). Accessed at: https://www.ichd-3.org/ https://www.ichd-3.org/2-tension-type-headache/.
4. Simons DG, Travell JG, Cummings BD. Travell and Simons' Myofascial Pain and Dysfunction: The Trigger Point Manual (2-Volume Set) (2nd ed.). Philadelphia: Lippincott Williams & Wilkins; 1998.
5. Davies NCTMB, Clair, Davies CMTPT LMT, Amber, et al. The Trigger Point Therapy Workbook: Your Self-Treatment Guide for Pain Relief (A New Harbinger Self-Help Workbook) Sep 1, 2013. Oakland, CA.
6. Headache and other craniofacial pains. In: Adams and Victor's Principles of Neurology (10th ed., pp. 168–197). New York: McGraw-Hill Education; 2014.
7. AAN and AHS Patient and Provider Shared Decision-Making Tool. Imaging: do I need an imaging study for my headache? Accessed February 18, 2019 at: https://www.aan.com/siteassets/home-page/policy-and-guidelines/quality/quality-improvement/patient-handouts/14headacheimagingsdmtool_pg.pdf.
8. Murinson BB, Fowler I. Red flags for low back pain. Joint Pain Education Project (VA/DoD), 2015. Accessed February 18, 2019 at: http://www.dvcipm.org/clinical-resources/joint-pain-education-project-jpep.
9. Murinson BB. Painful neuropathy. In: Griffin JW, Johnson RD. Current Therapy in Neurological Disease. St. Louis: Mosby; 2006.
10. Baron R, Allegri M, Correa-Illanes G, et al. The 5% lidocaine-medicated plaster: its inclusion in international treatment guidelines for treating localized neuropathic pain, and clinical evidence supporting its use. Pain Ther. 2016;5(2):149–169.
11. O'Brien M. Aids to the Examination of the Peripheral Nervous System (5th ed.). Philadelphia: Saunders Ltd., 2010.

17 Extremes of Pain

Beth B. Hogans

You are so brave and quiet I forget you are suffering.
—Ernest Hemingway

LEARNING OBJECTIVES

At the completion of this chapter, the learner should be able to discuss:

- Selected pain conditions that represent the extremes of chronic pain, including complex regional pain syndrome (CRPS), postherpetic neuralgia (PHN), phantom pain, and trigeminal neuralgia
- Recent genetic insights into selected pain conditions that illuminate pathophysiologic mechanisms, including erythromelalgia and congenital insensitivity to pain
- The literature suggesting that aggressive, early pain management decreases the likelihood of chronic pain

CASE SCENARIO

A 37-year-old man presents for admission to the hospital. Sixteen years ago, during military service, he was on patrol with a heavy backpack when he stepped into a 1-foot-deep hole in the dark and badly fractured his ankle. Because of the circumstance, medical evacuation was delayed for several hours. At the time, nerve blockade in the field was not common practice, but he received morphine with partial relief of the associated pain. The ankle was casted, but severe swelling developed and the cast was removed. There was evidence that the peroneal nerve had been damaged either by the fall or by the cast. The foot remained swollen for an extended period of time with erythema, occasional purpura when dependent, and increased temperature in the foot to touch. The pain was moderate to severe initially but worsened over the ensuing weeks to become severe and continuous. Multiple medications were tried with only partial response. Even opioids to 300 morphine mg/day did not relieve the pain sufficiently to permit rehabilitation of the ankle. The foot became very sensitive to touch and cold air. Over the ensuing months the foot gradually became paler, cool to the touch, and atrophic so that it was visibly smaller than the contralateral foot; however, the pain did not remit. After several years of excruciating pain despite all available therapies, the patient was isolated, depressed, and considering amputation. He was admitted for pain management and multidisciplinary consultation.

1. What is the diagnosis?
2. What mechanisms do you think are at work?
3. What allied health professions would you involve in this patient's care?

INTRODUCTION

One of the themes threaded through the book is the idea of the mechanism-based approach to pain: the view that pain conditions can be understood as primarily nociceptive, inflammatory, neuropathic, or a combination of two or more of these basic mechanisms. Some of the conditions described in this chapter are not yet fully understood but represent important challenges to our thinking about pain and, because of the extreme and persistent nature of the pain associated, also deeply challenge our ability to approach patients with profound empathy and sensitivity toward suffering and to never give up hope. Conditions such as erythromelalgia and congenital insensitivity to pain have been characterized mechanistically by concerted investigation, and yet the optimal management of these and other conditions remains to be explored. The contents of this chapter are not an exhaustive catalog of conditions producing severe, intractable, or persistent pain but are intended to represent the impact of some conditions, not vanishingly rare, that illustrate key mechanisms and insights into pain. It is sometimes the case that pain education in a medical context (e.g., medical schools and pain specialty conferences) has placed too much emphasis on some of these conditions, certainly out of proportion to the actual prevalence of most of these, but the high healthcare utilization and frequency of these patients in academic referral-center pain clinics has likely contributed to the overrepresentation of these conditions in medical education related to pain.[1,2] To meet the needs of general practitioners and primary care providers, education needs to refocus on highly prevalent conditions such as back pain and headaches. This chapter provides content intended to sharpen the focus of students considering the variety of pain mechanisms.

Conditions associated with decreased pain sensation are few in number. Although there are a large number of patients with decreased protective sensation in the distal extremities due to poorly controlled diabetes and other forms of peripheral neuropathy, genuine insensitivity to pain is an exceptionally rare condition.

CONGENITAL INSENSITIVITY TO PAIN
Context and Prevalence

Congenital insensitivity to pain is a very rare condition that arises from genetic mutations affecting the sensory pathways.[3] Some patients have simultaneous, disparate mutations that result in disfunction of a particular gene; other cases may arise from consanguinity.

Mechanisms and Preclinical Studies

These conditions are characterized by varying degrees of autonomic and central nervous system effects and may involve NGF-pathway signaling defects or other genetic mutations. One form is associated with mutations in the *SCN9A* gene, which encodes a specific sodium channel form expressed in small neurons of the dorsal root ganglion.[3]

Clinical Features

These patients cannot experience pain normally and suffer from recurrent mutilating injuries and sometimes death because they lack protective pain sensation. Although the *SCN9A* patients have normal strength, cognition, and preserved autonomic function, they lack epidermal nociceptive nerve endings. Another mutation of *SCN9A* is associated with erythromelalgia.

Treatment and Relevance

Patient education is necessary to prevent unintended injuries. Congenital insensitivity to pain is important to understanding normal function and utility of an intact pain processing system. The absence of protective pain sensation leads to increased risk for devastating injury and infection and decreased reproductive fitness.

Many conditions are associated with increased pain perception; in some conditions, this is primarily due to increased activity of the peripheral pain-sensing afferents (pain generator in the periphery). However, in several conditions the primary pathology is deep in the central nervous system, and in some cases the pathophysiologic origin of pain is not established.

TRIGEMINAL NEURALGIA
Context and Prevalence

Trigeminal neuralgia is an uncommon condition of the trigeminal nerve. It is important because of the profound pain sensations that are produced. Because the presentation demonstrates prominent neuropathic features, the condition often responds well to treatment.[4]

Mechanisms and Preclinical Studies

The most commonly proposed mechanism for trigeminal neuralgia is vascular compression of the trigeminal nerve in the skull base; the compression of the nerve by the adjacent artery results in focal demyelination and ephaptic transmission in which closely apposed demyelinated axons exhibit aberrant electrical excitation due to the loss of myelin. Myelin serves to facilitate conduction of rapid action potentials along large axons but also serves to prevent cross-talk between axons. When myelin is destroyed, an active axon can essentially induce action potentials in a neighboring axon that would otherwise be at rest. This ephaptic transmission leads to profound bolts or shocks of pain as multiple damaged axons are co-excited in an abnormal manner. Because pain-sensing (nociceptive) and touch-sensing axons are together in nerves, this is how light touch or brushing can excite action potentials in light-touch axons, which then cross over at points of demyelination to excite the axons of pain-sensing neurons. Pudendal neuropathy, a syndrome of painful neuropathy in the genital area, may also have vascularly induced mechanism of abnormal excitation.

Clinical Features

Trigeminal neuralgia presents most often in middle-aged women or men with hallmark features of neuropathic pain occurring as shocks or lancinating pains stimulated by touch or brushing. The bouts of pain are brief, lasting seconds to a few minutes, but are profound in intensity. The syndrome may worsen over time. Most often unilateral, the pain radiates from the ear area into the face. Stress and trigger sensations will worsen the syndrome.

Treatment and Relevance

Carbamazepine is effective in 70% of patients with trigeminal neuralgia; therefore, a treatment trial should begin as soon as the diagnosis is suspected. Carbamazepine may be associated with idiosyncratic side effects, so complete blood count with white blood cells, serum sodium, and hepatic function should be assessed initially and monitored periodically. Most patients tolerate this medication well, but a lower starting dose may increase patient acceptance of the medication, which can produce some gastric upset, with increased dose after 1 to 2 weeks as needed to improve efficacy. Some patients require other medications, and surgery or interventional management may be appropriate in some patients. Referral for evaluation is warranted if medical therapy is not completely effective.

POSTHERPETIC NEURALGIA
Context and Prevalence

PHN is a painful neuropathic syndrome that develops in a minority of patients following a bout of shingles. In PHN, the syndrome can last of months or years following an eruption of herpes. It is most common in older adults but can occur in middle-aged or susceptible younger persons. Vaccination with shingles vaccine has reduced both the incidence and severity of PHN; however, efficacy is not complete, and not all persons who develop shingles will have met criteria for vaccination, leaving some at risk. Vaccination, requiring two shots, is recommended by the Centers for Disease Control and Prevention in those 50 years and older.[5]

Mechanisms and Preclinical Studies

PHN ensues from partial injury to the nerve at the level of the dorsal root ganglion. The virus is dormant there, often for decades, until reactivated. Studies of skin biopsies in persons with PHN indicate that skin innervation is often still present but reduced, consistent with the findings in other models and clinical scenarios that partial nerve injury, or in the converse, partially preserved innervation, is associated with neuropathic pain.[6] Patients with PHN often note that pain is less during periods of reduced stress, consistent with the complex interaction of supratentorial and spinal pain-signaling mechanisms.

Clinical Features

PHN pain is often described as deep, burning, unbearable, and unrelenting. It is typically more intense in the dermatome associated with the shingles eruption, but spatial spreading (perception of pain in an area larger than the original insult) can occur. Mirror pain, perception of pain on the opposite side, has been reported and may reflect spinal-glial modulation of pain or other modulation. Patients often report sensitivity to light touch (allodynia) as well as increased pain to normally painful stimuli (i.e., hyperalgesia). Scars may be evident, subtle, or not appreciable.

Treatment

PHN typically requires neuromodulating medications and a coordinated nonpharmacologic treatment plan as well, emphasizing pain self-management, including the full range of options. Nonpharmacologic measures may and when necessary should incorporate sleep optimization; clinical psychological methods such as cognitive behavioral therapy or acceptance commitment therapy; modulation of stress; control over the work environment; and scheduling of pleasurable activities. Patients will typically require baseline treatment with a gabapentinoid, as well as a pain-active antidepressant, and should also have a rescue medication available. Topical agents may also be effective; however, capsaicin may exacerbate pain dramatically and should be used with caution. Even lidocaine, which may be beneficial, can also produce a transient increase in pain as the drug works by blocking open channels, meaning that pain may be perceived as nociception-transducing channels open and then diminish as the pain-sensing channels are blocked by the drug. Opioids, which increase inflammatory mediators and are associated with tolerance, dependence, and lower pain tolerance, are not ideal for management of this persistent pain condition.

PHANTOM LIMB PAIN
Context and Prevalence

Phantom limb pain was once believed to be a rare concomitant of limb amputation. In modern experience, phantom limb sensations are recognized as far more prevalent than previously surmised.[7,8] Phantom limb pain is an extreme manifestation of sensory perturbances after limb amputation, and a number of environmental factors contribute to the development and severity of phantom limb pain. It is important to differentiate phantom limb pain and sensations from those that arise from the proximal amputation site whether from neuroma formation, mechanical, or musculoskeletal causes.

Mechanisms and Preclinical Studies

The mechanisms of phantom limb pain are thought to relate to changes in the central nervous system, especially the somatosensory cortex before and after amputation.

Cortical reorganization has been demonstrated phenomenologically with aberrant sensory percepts (i.e., stroking of the face eliciting the perception of touch of an amputated hand) as well as with magnetic resonance imaging (MRI). Alterations in the spinal cord are also observed when the loss of afferent input results in altered inhibition of nociceptive neurons, with spontaneous and elicited activation of these neurons leading to pain sensations. In addition, the process of cutting the axons during the amputation will initiate a process of axonal disintegration and neuronal cell death in some neurons, with more proximal amputations being associated with higher rates of neuronal cell death, a process that contributes to deafferentation or the loss of normal sensory inputs. In summary, multiple mechanisms—cortical reorganization, spinal reorganization, neuronal cell death, axonal degeneration, and deafferentation—likely all contribute to phantom limb pain.

Clinical Features

Phantom limb pain produces variable degrees of discomfort, with many patients experiencing mild to moderate pain. The sensation may be described as aching, burning, or deep and hard to describe. The pain will wax and wane with environmental stressors and can be worse in cold, damp weather.

Treatment

The treatment of phantom limb pain includes multiprofessional coordination of novel and established therapies. One new therapy involves using a mirror apparatus to activate the cortex associated with the amputated limb but creating the illusion that the limb is moving and functioning. Treatment with oral agents may be only partially effective and may include gabapentinoids, N-methyl-D-aspartate (NMDA) antagonists (ketamine), and other agents. It is important to distinguish and address the concomitant pain arising from focal neuromas, prosthesis issues, and musculoskeletal adaptations and ergonomic factors that can and will contribute to pain after amputation. These other factors often produce more distress and may be highly amenable to treatment. Proximal limb (stump) neuromas arise from the growth processes associated with transected axons and may be detected by judicious palpation of the proximal stump site. When identified, they may respond to focal treatments, application of topical agents, adjustment of prosthesis, or gabapentinoid. Extended-release gabapentin may be especially helpful.

COMPLEX REGIONAL PAIN SYNDROME
Context and Prevalence

CRPS is, fortunately, not highly prevalent, but because of the severe and persistent nature of pain with the condition, these patients demonstrate high healthcare utilization and are seen occasionally in specialty pain clinics.[1] For this reason, the perceived importance of CRPS by pain specialists is disproportionate to the relatively low prevalence. An American physician, Silas Weir Mitchell, provided the first detailed, longitudinal descriptions of CRPS following the US Civil War and published follow-up studies several years later (see the later box about Mitchell). At that time, Mitchell noted that CRPS was somewhat heterogeneous and also that an injury could be relatively mild compared with the degree of pain. CRPS has been recognized to consist of two forms: One including nerve injury, and the other without evident nerve injury. The form of the condition without evident nerve injury is CRPS I, whereas the form with evident nerve injury is termed CRPS II.

Mechanisms and Preclinical Studies

Preclinical models do not generally recapitulate all the features of CRPS, especially because intense subjective suffering is difficult to measure in animal models. Nonetheless, studies have included nerve and partial nerve transection as well as immobilization, both of which broadly demonstrate some features of CRPS, including early swelling, erythema, and calor, followed later by atrophy, bone demineralization, behavioral change consistent with increased pain perception, and cooling of the limb. The proposed mechanisms of CRPS include neural and inflammatory processes. In some forms of CRPS, cytokine production may be prominent, and this has been demonstrated by the relief of pain behavior following pentoxifylline injections and other treatments impacting autonomic function.

Clinical Features

CRPS is characterized by phasic changes to the affected limb consistent with variable autonomic activation. Early features include edema, erythema, and warmth. Pain is prominent and progressively worsens. The limb is typically painful to light touch (i.e., mechanical allodynia), and pain may result from exposure to puffs of cold air. Over the course of several weeks to months, even as the pain persists and worsens, there are changes in the appearance of the limb. The late-phase appearance is usually characterized by atrophy, coolness, pallor, and bone demineralization. Many patients will wrap or swaddle the limb, which is generally felt to perpetuate or worsen the sensory abnormalities. It is important to consider alternatives to this diagnosis as an explanation for severe, persistent pain (Table 17.1).

Treatment

Treatment of CRPS is especially challenging and typically requires multiple combined therapies.

Consistent with other syndromes in which central mediation and perpetuation of pain is prominent, multiple medications are often combined in an effort to reduce side effects while capitalizing on pain reduction that may occur by virtue of approaching the pain processing system from multiple angles. For example, gabapentin may decrease the entry of afferent input from peripheral structures, which can continue to transduce and transmit pain signals peripherally. Whereas pain-active antidepressants may utilize descending pain modulatory mechanisms, topical anesthetics may also dampen peripheral inputs, and anticonvulsants or, where appropriate, cannabinoids may further modulate central pain processes. Historically utilized to a greater or lesser extent, opioids may act at multiple sites in the pain processing system; however, these medications as a class are subject to rapid tachyphylaxis and intense reinforcement of

Table 17.1 Features of Selected Extreme Pain Conditions

Condition	Sentinel Clinical Feature(s)	Treatment Pearls	Prevalence
Complex regional pain syndrome	Severe pain with allodynia, edema/erythema, and calor followed by atrophy and pallor	Sympathetic block, ketamine, or lidocaine infusion may transiently relieve pain	Rare but high utilization, so occasionally seen in specialty pain centers
Trigeminal neuralgia	Lancinating face pain in paroxysms	Majority respond initially to carbamazepine; vascular compression may require procedural management	Rare but high utilization so occasionally seen in specialty pain centers
Erythromelalgia	Paroxysmal redness and pain of feet and sometimes hands	Patient may use ice bath to seek relief Genetic mutation may be present	
Ehlers-Danlos syndrome	Frequent and devastating musculoskeletal strains and compressive neuropathies	Hypermobility of joints, patients accumulate musculoskeletal injuries and experience poor healing and persistent pain	Rare
Congenital insensitivity to pain	Multiple inadvertent injuries due to lack of protective sensation	Protective measures and training; due to genetic mutation	Very rare
Phantom limb pain	Perception of painful distal part of limb that is no longer present	Mirror therapy may be beneficial	Not rare after amputation

reward–addiction pathways, and they may demonstrate proinflammatory features, all of which suggest suboptimal outcomes. A full spectrum of nonpharmacologic therapies should be offered to these patients, and therapies such as water exercise, yoga, Tai chi, and Qi gong may prove useful, depending on the patient's psychological reserves. Clinical psychological support and some sensitive physical therapy environments may provide the patient with necessary support.

Silas Weir Mitchell was an American physician with an interest in disorders of nerves as well as the broad modulation of pain at all levels. He is credited with characterizing CRPS, phantom limb pain, and erythromelalgia, all before the discovery of DNA, nerve conduction studies, or modern microscopy. He wrote of pain: "This mystery of pain is still for me the saddest of earth's disabilities. After all is said that can be said on its values as a safeguard, an indicator of the locality of disease, after the moralist has considered it from the disciplinary view, and the theologian cracked his teeth on this bitter nut, and the evolutionist accounted for its existence, it comes at last to the doctor to say what shall be done with it. I wish it came to him alone. Civilized man has ceased to torture, but nature, relentless still, has in store possibilities of utmost anguish, which seem to fall alike on the guilty and the innocent, the poor and the rich, and in largest proportion on the gentler sex."[9]

PERIPHERAL NERVE VASCULITIS
Context and Prevalence

Peripheral nerve vasculitis is a rare cause of extreme pain, most often associated with progressive loss of sensation and weakness.[10] Nerve vasculitis is often associated with other conditions, including hepatitis with cryoglobulins, systemic lupus erythematosus, rheumatoid arthritis with rheumatoid factor, and vasculitides such as Wegener syndrome, Churg-Strauss syndrome, and polyarteritis nodosa. Thus, when a patient presents with severe progressive pain associated with unexplained weakness, referral for neurologic evaluation is essential.

Mechanisms and Preclinical Studies

Peripheral nerve vasculitis requires nerve biopsy for diagnosis. Patients with isolated peripheral nerve vasculitis do not have other conditions such as noted previously. They may have elevated sedimentation rate. The biopsy may demonstrate evidence of increased immune cells, especially $CD4^+$ and $CD8^+$ T cells and macrophages. The vasculitis primarily effects small vessels, and the nerve biopsy will show dramatic loss of axons, which is variable in different parts of the nerve, consistent with the patchy nature of the pathologic process. Understanding of the underlying mechanisms is limited.

Clinical Features

Patients affected by isolated peripheral nerve vasculitis are typically of later middle age but may range from early adulthood to advanced age. The condition is progressive and features pain in the limbs and progressive loss of sensation and motor strength in a patchy nerve-specific pattern or, when advanced, in a more widespread pattern. Presenting with prominent pain and occasionally with autonomic changes mimicking early CRPS, vasculitis is diagnosed based on nerve biopsy findings of transmural vasculitic infiltration and associated peripheral nerve microischemia.[11]

Treatment

Treatment of peripheral nerve vasculitis includes immune-modifying treatments, sometimes with prednisone, but other disease-modifying medications are used. These therapies require advanced training to use safely, and biopsy is required to establish diagnosis as appropriate for long-term immunosuppressive treatment; thus, referral to a neuromuscular specialist is advised.

FIBROMYALGIA
Context and Prevalence

Fibromyalgia (FM) is among the more prevalent extreme pain syndromes. Previously defined according the American College of Rheumatology "tender points" description, criteria for FM have changed to include more systemic symptoms of fatigue, cognitive clouding, and sleep disturbance . . . , in addition to widespread chronic pain.[12] Widely believed to be more prevalent among women, there is one population-based study in which genders were more closely balanced, suggesting that there may be some ascertainment bias that arises from clinical cohort-based studies.[13] The explanation may be that there are men who experience symptoms that, taken collectively, meet criteria for FM but who do not seek care to specifically address the aggregate symptoms as such.

Mechanisms and Preclinical Studies

There is considerable controversy over the precise mechanism or mechanisms of FM and it seems likely that there may be two or more distinct pathophysiologic aberrations underlying the current syndromic condition of FM. Most practitioners consider FM to be a consequence of abnormal central pain processing. Alternative explanations have been proposed.

Clinical Features

FM is characterized by widespread bodily pain and associated general symptoms of fatigue, unrefreshed sleep, and cognitive difficulty as well as other symptoms, such as nausea, bowel and urinary disturbances, rashes, sensory perturbations, and depression. It is often a condition of middle age but can also affect adolescents, teens, and older adults. The condition must be present for at least 3 months and the symptoms, particularly the pain, not explainable by other conditions.

Treatment

Treatment of FM has become increasingly evidence based. The importance of frequent moderate exercise has been recognized and is supported by systematic review. The recommendations are for 30 minutes of moderate exercise at least 3 days weekly. Pharmacologic therapies may include tricyclic antidepressants, selective serotonin/norepinephrine reuptake inhibitors, and cyclobenzaprine; however, guarding against overreliance on pharmacotherapy and moderation of expectations for effectiveness of medication are advised. Opioids should be stringently avoided because long-term outcomes for treatment of FM with opioids are bleak.

ERYTHROMELALGIA
Context and Prevalence

Erythromelalgia is a very rare condition of extreme episodic pain and marked erythema of the distal extremities in response to various stimuli, such as exposure to warming, standing, and exercise.[14] First described by Weir Mitchell, for many years the syndrome was known to experts in select academic medical centers, but the sporadic and extreme nature of the syndrome meant that some were skeptical of the genuineness of the pathology.

Mechanisms and Preclinical Studies

Erythromelalgia, inherited as a dominant condition, was found to be associated with point mutations in the *SCN9A* gene conferring a gain-of-function that increased activation of sodium channels in nociceptive fibers in response to slow depolarization. The function of the *SCN9A* sodium channels is to amplify the distal generator potentials, and the gain-of-function mutation means that smaller stimulations are amplified and activate the pain system vigorously. The syndrome may also occur as a sporadic, mosaic, and polymorphism mutations.

Clinical Features

Erythromelalgia is characterized by sporadic episodes of severe pain in the legs and hands, associated with pronounced reddening of the affected area. Onset of symptoms may be in the first decade with worsening as the patient ages.

Treatment

Treatment of erythromelalgia relies on scrupulous avoidance of trigger stimuli. Episodes may respond partially to aspirin. Cooling of the limbs is often utilized by patients who will plunge their arms and legs into ice water during attacks. Other topical agents have been utilized.

EHLERS-DANLOS SYNDROME
Context and Prevalence

Ehlers-Danlos syndrome is an eponymous label for a heterogeneous group of heritable collagen disorders.[15] The Ehlers-Danlos collagen disorders may be inherited through dominant or recessive patterns. The hallmark features vary from type to type.[15] The type most relevant in terms of needs for pain management and recognition as a possible cause of lifelong, frequent, and recurrent pain episodes is the hypermobility variant, termed *hEDS* according to the National Organization for Rare Diseases, formerly known as EDS III.[15]

Mechanisms and Preclinical Studies

Mutations in collagen structure lead to suboptimal properties of connective tissue and variable features of hyperelastic skin, frequent joint dislocations, tendon and muscle ruptures, and vascular (aortic) dilatation. In another variant, pneumothorax is observed.

Clinical Features

Patients with hEDS present often in midlife with recurrent joint dislocations, which are often painful unless reduced immediately. Recurrent injuries and progressive compressive neuropathies occur as laxity of connective tissue leads to a loss of protected space for the passage of nerves, and the degeneration of joints may also contribute to chronic pain and nerve compression syndromes. These patients may live a life of nearly continuous pain before recognition of the disorder and the introduction of necessary precautions with activity. Patients with hEDS may endure substantive pain and are also noted to have high prevalence of affective disorders and psychological features, perhaps secondary to unremitting pain and frequent injury.

Treatment

Patients with hEDS require counseling for lifestyle management and support for increasing a sense of self-efficacy in the face of a sometimes inscrutable heritable disorder. Support through the ordering and optimization of orthotics, whether to maintain nerve-compression sparing postures of feet, hands, and arms or to prevent subluxation and dislocation, will reduce pain. Meticulous attention to injury occurrences and prevention is important, as is sympathetic support and engagement of the patient in defining all available nonpharmacologic measures, including clinical psychology support and mindfulness techniques. Yoga should be avoided unless the instructor is well-experienced with adapting poses and postures to patients with potentially harmful hypermobility.

STIFF-PERSON SYNDROME
Context and Prevalence

Stiff-person syndrome (SPS) is a rare neuroimmunologic condition associated with episodic bouts of extreme axial stiffness with profound muscle contractures that are perceived as painful unless managed with immunomodulation and symptomatic measures.[16] Initially described by Moersch and Woltman at the Mayo Clinic in the 1950s, a pathognomonic antibody to GAD65 was identified in the 1990s. The precise mechanism or role of these antibodies is not yet established; however, the antibodies are present at very high concentrations. Thus, SPS can be distinguished from GAD65 in association with diabetes, in which GAD65 is a common autoantigen but at much lower serum titers compared with SPS. SPS is a very rare condition that manifests with GAD65 antibodies present at very high titer (1,000–10,000 times higher in some studies).[16] There is a slight female predominance; thus, the former name of "stiff-man syndrome" is not preferred. A rare form of SPS is associated with breast cancer and antibodies to amphiphysin, a presynaptic nerve terminal protein involved in vesicle fusion events. GAD65 in SPS has not shown an association with cancer.

Mechanisms and Preclinical Studies

The precise pathogenic role of the antibodies is not known. GAD65 is a rate-limiting enzyme in the production of gamma-aminobutyric acid (GABA), a major inhibitory neurotransmitter. Although it seems reasonable that high-titer antibodies to the enzymatic production pathway of GABA would lead to impairment in spinal cord inhibitory function and thus to profound muscle spasms, this has not been demonstrated clearly in the preclinical context.

Clinical Features

SPS typically begins insidiously and worsens over weeks to months. Patients may not be explicitly aware of motor abnormalities but may perceive a sense of profound anxiety, particularly when crossing large spaces unsupported, termed *agoraphobia*. Patients are observed to fall readily and with a stiff, unnatural posture (tinman-like, log-like), when symptoms are not well controlled. The typical age of diagnosis is in the middle to late 40s, with symptom onset variable weeks to years prior. Symptoms are relieved by sleep. Before the discovery of the antibodies, patients with SPS were frequently diagnosed by psychiatrists, who suspected biological causes in these patients and referred them for evaluation of anxiety and functional syndromes. Diabetes is common and may be of the latent adult-onset immune form, which will require insulin; autoimmune thyroid disease is also observed. There is a female predominance, but this is not overwhelming because about 60% of patients are female.

Treatment

Treatment of SPS should avoid opioids, which do not correct the underlying immune disturbance or the severe muscular contractions but merely tend to mitigate pain with a clear biological precipitant. Instead, immunomodulation with intravenous immunoglobulin (IVIG), or plasmapheresis or rituximab if IVIG is not possible, and muscle relaxant symptom management with benzodiazepines with or without baclofen is one reasonable approach. It is recommended to avoid tricyclic antidepressants because they have been noted to worsen spasms. Exercise may trigger spasms, and when immunomodulation is not effective, physical therapy, touch, startle, and loud noises may all induce profound bouts of axial and appendicular rigidity.

ENDOMETRIOSIS
Context and Prevalence

Endometriosis is a distressingly common cause of pelvic pain in women of childbearing age. Beginning with menarche, endometrial tissue may become implanted outside of the uterus and with hormonal fluctuations may produce symptoms of severe and cyclic pain. Estimates of prevalence range from 2 to 10% of the population at risk.

Mechanisms and Preclinical Studies

Mechanisms by which endometrial tissue becomes established outside the uterus are not clearly known. Posited mechanisms include retrograde flow through the fallopian tubes, developmental seeding, and hematogenous spread. Early menarche and rapid menstrual cycling have been associated with increased likelihood of endometriosis.

Clinical Features

Endometriosis is associated with increased pain at the time of menstruation as well as variable occurrence of pain with intercourse, pain with urination, pain with defecation, and pain during the intermenstrual period. Endometriosis is graded according to the type, location, and number of sites of endometrial tissue localization.

Treatment and Relevance

Endometriosis treatment varies with the severity of the condition. It may be possible to address mild disease with analgesia; however, hormonal therapy is used frequently. More invasive therapies are used in some cases of severe disease or in the event of intractable pain or complications. Heavy bleeding and infertility may be observed in endometriosis and are additional indications for treatment. Endometriosis is distinct from the other extreme pain conditions discussed in this chapter because it is not clearly neuropathic in nature.

SUMMARY

Extreme chronic pain can also arise from other causes such as stroke in the brainstem or basal ganglia, transverse myelitis, spinal cord injury, polytrauma, or other conditions. It is important to appraise patients reporting severe pain carefully. A careful clinical history should be obtained and parsed for consistency with specific patters. Particularly useful is evidence of neurologic deficits that may correlate with the description of pain; this can provide clues to aid with diagnosis. It may be necessary to refer the patient to multiple specialists in order to identify the causative process because the first specialist may not recognize the condition. Although most pain is caused by musculoskeletal conditions, many of the extremes of pain are caused by neurologic conditions; thus, a neurologist or pain medicine specialist can be helpful. Several of the extremes of pain are benefited by disease-modifying treatments in concert with pain-relieving therapies so that obtaining a credible diagnosis is valuable for the patient. Finally, because living with an extreme pain-associated condition is highly stressful, it is important to ensure that the patient has appropriate psychological support; clinical psychology has many techniques and therapeutic approaches that can help patients live better despite pain and can reduce suffering.

REVIEW QUESTIONS

1. CRPS is characterized by all of the following, *except* (choose 2):
    a. Early erythema, increased temperature, and swelling
    b. Late pallor, coolness to touch, and atrophy
    c. Involvement of axial structures such as tongue and abdomen.
    d. Involvement of peripheral structures such as hands and feet
    e. Immediate treatment response after condition is recognized and correct medication started

2. SPS is rare, and the key features include:
    a. Antibodies to a glycine-producing enzyme
    b. Antibodies to a glutamate-producing enzyme
    c. Antibodies to a GABA-producing enzyme
    d. Antibodies to a dopamine-producing enzyme

3. Which of the following is not recognized as a neuropathic condition?
   a. CRPS
   b. Endometriosis
   c. PHN
   d. Trigeminal neuralgia
   e. Erythromelalgia

REFERENCES

1. Global Burden of Disease Study 2013 Collaborators. Global, regional, and national incidence, prevalence, and years lived with disability for 301 acute and chronic diseases and injuries in 188 countries, 1990–2013: a systematic analysis for the Global Burden of Disease Study 2013. Lancet. 2015;386(9995):743–800.
2. McMahon SB, Koltzenburg M, Tracey I, Turk D. Wall and Melzack's Textbook of Pain (6th ed.). Philadelphia: Saunders; 2013.
3. Pestronk A. Congenital inability to experience pain. Accessed February 18, 2019 at: https://neuromuscular.wustl.edu/time/hsn.htm#painexp.
4. National Institutes of Health. Trigeminal neuralgia fact sheet. Accessed February 18, 2019 at: https://www.ninds.nih.gov/Disorders/Patient-Caregiver-Education/Fact-Sheets/Trigeminal-Neuralgia-Fact-Sheet.
5. Centers for Disease Control and Prevention. Shingles vaccine factsheet for providers. Accessed February 18, 2019 at: https://www.cdc.gov/shingles/downloads/shingles-factsheet-hcp.pdf.
6. Petersen KL, Rice FL, Farhadi M, Reda H, Rowbotham MC. Natural history of cutaneous innervation following herpes zoster. Pain. 2010;150(1):75–82.
7. Desmond DM, Maclachlan M. Prevalence and characteristics of phantom limb pain and residual limb pain in the long term after upper limb amputation. Int J Rehabil Res. 2010;33(3):279–282.
8. Hsu E, Cohen SP. Postamputation pain: epidemiology, mechanisms, and treatment. J Pain Res. 2013;6:121–136.
9. Mitchell SW. Doctor and Patient (3rd ed.). Philadelphia: JB Lippincott; 1901. Accessed February 18, 2019 at: http://www.gutenberg.org/cache/epub/15004/pg15004-images.html.
10. Isolated peripheral nerve vasculitis. Accessed January 26, 2019 at: https://neuromuscular.wustl.edu/antibody/pnimax.html#pnvasc.
11. Ramchandren S, Chaudhry V, Hoke A, et al. Peripheral nerve vasculitis presenting as complex regional pain syndrome. J Clin Neuromuscul Dis. 2008;10(2):61–64.
12. Wolfe F, Clauw DJ, Fitzcharles MA, et al. 2016 Revisions to the 2010/2011 fibromyalgia diagnostic criteria. Semin Arthritis Rheum. 2016;46(3):319–329.
13. Wolfe F, Walitt B, Perrot S, Rasker JJ, Häuser W. Fibromyalgia diagnosis and biased assessment: sex, prevalence and bias. PLoS One. 2018;13(9):e0203755.
14. Pestronk, A. Erythromelalgia. Accessed February 18, 2019 at: https://neuromuscular.wustl.edu/sensory-pain.html#erythromelalgia.
15. Ehlers-Danlos syndrome. Accessed January 24, 2019 at: https://rarediseases.org/rare-diseases/ehlers-danlos-syndrome/.
16. Murinson BB, Butler M, Marfurt K, et al. Markedly elevated GAD antibodies in SPS: effects of age and illness duration. Neurology. 2004;63(11):2146–2148.

18 Basics of Pediatric Pain Management

Tommy Rappold, Matthew Digiusto, and M-Irfan Suleman

All through the world, there is a special league of those who have known anxiety and physical suffering. A mysterious bond connects those marked by pain. They know the terrible things man can undergo; they know the longing to be free of pain. Those who have been liberated from pain must not think they are now completely free again and can calmly return to life as it was before. With their experience of pain and anxiety, they must help alleviate the pain and anxiety of others, insofar as that lies within human powers."
—Albert Schweitzer (1875–1965)

LEARNING OBJECTIVES

At the completion of this chapter, the learner should be able to discuss:

- Methods for evaluating pain in neonates, school-aged children, and adolescents
- Common causes of acute and chronic pain in pediatric populations
- Key concepts in nonpharmacologic pediatric pain management
- Basic principles of opioid analgesia in pediatric populations

CASE SCENARIO

A 2-year-old otherwise healthy child presents to the pediatric emergency department crying. His father says that about an hour ago he heard both of his two children laughing and playing in another room, and all of sudden his son started to scream, holding his leg and saying "ouch, ouch." On examination you note that the child is developmentally normal; he interacts with toys and his parents. Neurologic exam seems normal except that the child refuses to walk and retracts his leg when touched.

1. How do you assess the cause of pain in a child who can only form two- to three-word phrases?
2. How do you best communicate with the father about his son's pain?
3. If no serious injuries are identified, what can the father do to manage his son's pain if you send them home today? What pharmacologic and nonpharmacologic approaches will you recommend?

INTRODUCTION

Pain is a common problem in the pediatric population. Pediatricians routinely manage pain for patients covering a wide range of not only ages but also neurocognitive, social, and physical development. These differences make pain management of pediatric patients more nuanced and complex. Only a few decades ago was it thought that young children did not perceive noxious stimuli nor experience pain. Through the advancement of technology and research, we now know this paradigm was false. But how do we manage pain in neonates or adolescents who are unable to communicate, especially in the hospital setting where pain may be one of many acute physiologic processes affecting behavior and comfort?

Recognizing the overlaps and many differences in pediatric versus adult pain management is crucial in helping treat pain in children. In this chapter we explore the basic tools and approaches to managing pediatric pain. We discuss pain assessment in an age-appropriate fashion as a first and necessary step. The etiology of pediatric pain is also an important focus; children are generally healthy and resilient, so acute or chronic pain can be a sign of serious illness. Last, we introduce management practices specific to children, including nonpharmacologic therapies.

BASIC APPROACH TO PAIN ASSESSMENT IN CHILDREN
Neonates and Infants

Assessment of pain in neonates and infants is challenging because routine interviewing through verbal communication is often not possible. The idea that these patients do not experience pain is antiquated; there are several studies demonstrating pain and long-term memory development from these experiences. Although there are studies that suggest a cry's acuity, rhythmicity, and pitch can delineate whether a child is in pain or not, overall, crying is nonspecific in this age group because it may indicate hunger, tiredness, need for affection, or other wants.[1]

Researchers have developed more than 40 neonatal and infant pain assessment instruments and pain scales in the past several decades, focusing on various aspects of pain. These instruments were developed in a variety of patient populations, including premature and term infants, children younger than 3 years unable to verbalize pain, ventilated infants, and postprocedural children. Because pain affects behavioral, physiologic, contextual, and biologic domains of functioning, we may observe and interact with patients in pain and assess a variety of relevant features and characteristics. Although many of the published pain assessment instruments are most relevant in a research context, knowledge of specific instruments can serve as a guide to structure a clinically useful pain assessment As illustrated in Table 18.1, which provides the details of selected pain assessment instruments, several features and characteristics can be observed or measured.

Table 18.1 Examples of Multidimensional Pain Assessment

Standard Clinical Assessment: QRSTUVW	IMMPACT Consortium Recommendations for Pain Research
Quality: Query: What does the pain feel like? Rationale: Pain quality often provides clues to mechanistic basis for pain; for example, nociceptive pain is often sharp, whereas neuropathic pain may be tingling or burning **Region:** Query: Where is the pain? Does it radiate? Rationale: Pain location is an important feature to guide the differential diagnosis. Pain is often but not always located at the site of the pain generator (primary afferent nerve ending) that responds to injury; sometimes pain is perceived in a location distant to the pain pathology. **Severity:** Query: How intense/strong/bad is the pain? Rationale: Pain severity has a major impact on function and biopsychosocial effects of pain. Pain severity may affect clinical decisions, especially in acute pain management settings where algorithms sometimes drive analgesic dosing. **Timing:** Query: When did the pain start? Is it getting better/worse? Rationale: Pain timing provides essential diagnostic information and may help guide decisions regarding advancing or tapering treatments. **Usually associated symptoms:** Query: What else is going along with this? Rationale: Associated symptoms provide essential clues to diagnosis and may necessitate adjustments to therapy if due to side effects of treatment, e.g., itching due to opioids **Very much alleviating:** Query: What makes the pain better? Rationale: Knowing what alleviates pain can guide treatment and may be useful diagnostically. It is essential for chronic pain to know what treatments be been used successfully in the past.	Recommendations that provide guidance for the design of clinical and preclinical trials Includes engagement of device and pharmaceutical manufacturers Emphasizes research utility and impact of pain study outcome measures Includes: • Pain intensity • Effects on physical functioning • Effects on emotional function • Participant impression of change • Side effects and adverse events • Study participant disposition **Personal pain history:** additional potentially relevant features of the pain narrative

Table 18.1 Continued

Standard Clinical Assessment: QRSTUVW	IMMPACT Consortium Recommendations for Pain Research
Worsening factors: Query: What makes this pain worse? Rationale: Understanding what makes a problem worse can guide both diagnosis and treatment. For example, pain that is abruptly worse with activity may signal a fracture or other acute injury.	• Prior pain experiences • Family history of pain • Prior experience of adverse events

Preschool- and School-Aged Children

By age 3 years, normally developing children can follow three-part commands, construct sentences with five or six words, tell stories, be understood by strangers, and understand comparison words like "same" and "different." For these reasons the primary mode of pain assessment in this population is self-report. However, because of variation in development and temperament, observational reports by guardians and physiologic parameters are also important. To aid pediatric pain assessment and guide appropriate therapy, multiple scales and tools are available to clinicians.

The Initiative on Methods, Measurement and Pain Assessment in Clinical Trials (IMMPACT, http://www.immpact.org) identified a framework for pain assessment (Table 18.1) in children that enables providers to understand the dimensions of a pain presentation (e.g., intensity, location) and the functional impact as reported by the patient as well as guardians and other caregivers (e.g. day-care provider or school teacher). Pain location in children can be challenging, particularly if there are multiple sources of pain. There are multiple methods for eliciting location, including pointing to "all parts of pain," completing a body diagram with parental assistance, or using a doll or manikin.[2]

Depending on age, language development, and temperament, eliciting dimensional pain components may be difficult or not possible. In this instance, practitioners can gain an overall sense of the patient's pain with the Faces Pain Scale (FPS) (Figure 18.1). This is analogous to the numeric rating scale used in the adult population. The FPS

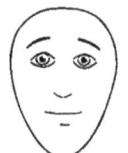 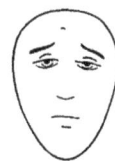 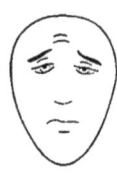 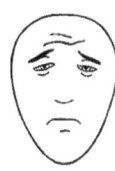 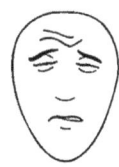 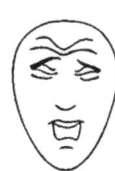

FIGURE 18.1 Faces Pain Scale—Revised (FPS-R). The FPS-R is a scale that can be used with children to assist in pain assessment. Instructions in about 40 languages are available at http://www.iasp-pain.org/FPSR. Reproduced from Hicks CL, von Baeyer CL, Spafford PA, van Korlaar I, Goodenough B. The Faces Pain Scale—Revised: toward a common metric in pediatric pain measurement. Pain. 2001;93(2):173–83, Copyright © 2001. This figure has been reproduced with permission of the International Association for the Study of Pain [IASP]. The figure may NOT be reproduced for any other purpose without permission.

presents a patient with a series of faces and allows children to pick which face most represents their current state.[3] This can be asked in various ways: "Which of these faces is you right now?" "Which face best represents your pain?" "Tell me how you feel with these faces."

Children Aged 8 Years and Older

Validated tools like the visual analog scale can be used in children 8 years and older. At this age, children have a better sense of pain quality, although it may be difficult for children to communicate. The Adolescent Pediatric Pain Tool (APPT)[4] contains 67 pain quality descriptors that encompass four dimensions: sensory, affective, evaluative, and temporal. Depending on the patient's age, these can be completed independently or with the help of a guardian or practitioner. Keep in mind that this tool can be used in patients younger than age 8 years; however, it has undergone validation in patients ages 8 to 17 years old.

Summary of Pain Scales in Children

Examples of validated *self-report pain intensity measures and pain quality tools* for children ages 3 years and older include[5]:

1. Faces Pain Scale
2. Faces Pain Scale—Revised
3. Pieces of Hurt tool
4. Oucher—Photographic
5. Oucher—Numeric Rating Scale
6. Wong-Baker FACES Pain Scale
7. Visual Analog Scale
8. Adolescent Pediatric Pain Tool (APPT)

Examples of validated *observational* (behavioral) pain measures in children include[6]:

1. Face, Legs, Arms, Cry, Consolability Scale (FLACC)
2. Children's Hospital of Eastern Ontario Pain Scale (CHEOPS)
3. COMFORT Scale (for nonresponsive patients)
4. Procedure Behavior Check List (PBCL)
5. Procedure Behavioral Rating Scale—Revised (PBRS-R)

COMMON CAUSES OF PAIN IN PEDIATRIC PATIENTS
Acute Versus Chronic Pain

Distinguishing acute versus chronic pediatric pain is an important distinction that must be made. Acute pain has a sudden onset, usually from nociceptor stimulation to soft tissues, bone, skin, or viscera. Often there is an identifiable cause, and with appropriate management it will resolve in less than 3 months. Chronic pain is defined as lasting longer than 3 months, with a healing time of 6 months or longer. Distinguishing between these categories is important for diagnostic and treatment purposes, but also for understanding the functional impacts of pain. For example, children with chronic abdominal pain report lower quality-of-life scores and have higher rates of school absence.[7]

Neonates and Infants

In the inpatient and outpatient setting, the most common cause of pain in neonates and infants is tissue damage by way of needle sticks (e.g., heel sticks for laboratory draws, thigh sticks for vaccine administration). This is a form of acute pain that may resolve within minutes to hours. Some neonates in the neonatal intensive care unit may receive as many as five to six heel sticks per day with varying levels of premedication.

Chronic pain in this population is rare; however, practitioners should be aware of specific populations where chronic pain is common. Neonates and infants who may have chronic pain include: (1) patients who require removal of bowel, sometimes referred to as "short-gut babies"; (2) patients who are unable to tolerate enteric nutrition; (3) patients with osteogenesis imperfecta or other bony abnormalities; (4) infants with sickle cell disease and associated pain crises; (5) patients with malignant tumors; and (6) those who have had repetitive heel lances and resulting scarred heels.

School-Aged Children and Adolescents

As children learn to walk, explore their surroundings, and shed dependence on their caregivers, they may seek treatment for a varying range of acute, chronic, or acute-on-chronic pain presentations. In the hospital and clinic setting, injections for intravenous therapy, lab collections, and vaccinations continue to be common causes of acute pain. Oral pain associated with dental caries persists from childhood and into adulthood. Headache, abdominal pain, and musculoskeletal pain are common presentations in children older than 8 years. Many of these ailments are managed by primary care practitioners, who generally will consult subspecialty practitioners if conservative management is not effective.

As in neonates and infants, there are special patient populations who will likely have chronic pain throughout their lives, and their care may require the help of advanced-level pain providers. Patients living with sickle cell disease often have sickle cell pain crises that increase in severity and frequency with age as well as genotype. Classic initial presentation is dactylitis, a swelling of the hands and fingers. Into adolescence and adulthood, pain presentations can be in the limbs, lower back, chest, or any other part of the body. It is important to know that these patients often live with daily, chronic pain.[8] Other special pediatric populations include those with juvenile idiopathic arthritis, juvenile rheumatoid arthritis, and pain associated with primary tumor or malignancy.

PEDIATRIC PAIN MANAGEMENT
Key Concepts

Goals of pain management include reducing, controlling, and preventing pain. Pain management consists of both pharmacologic and nonpharmacologic interventions to include cognitive, behavioral, and supportive therapies. Safe and effective pharmacologic management of pain requires an understanding of drug distribution and metabolism. Clearance of medications can be slower in younger children compared with adults because of immaturity of renal function. Regular pain assessments are important to guide pain management decisions. Multimodal pain management is the combined use of several types of analgesic drugs with different mechanisms of actions in order to decrease the adverse side effects of any one medication as well as target various receptors at different points along the pain pathway. Pediatric patients may be more likely to suffer from dose-limiting side effects of certain medications, necessitating multimodal pain management.

Nonpharmacologic Pain Management Strategies

Nonpharmacologic strategies are essential for managing acute and chronic pain, reducing the stress of painful procedures, and decreasing medication requirements. Stephens et al. described a simple five-part model on techniques to comfort children during stressful procedures: (1) preparing the child and parent/caregiver for the procedure and for their role during the procedure; (2) inviting the parent/caregiver to be present; (3) utilizing the treatment room for stressful procedures; (4) positioning the child in a comforting manner; and (5) maintaining a calm, positive atmosphere.[9] Assessing what techniques in the past have helped a child can also assist in reducing distress.

Distraction interventions may be cognitive, behavioral, or sensory and can be adapted to age and developmental level. Active distractions involve child participation such as using a toy or tablet, and passive distractions may include music, swaddling, virtual reality technology, or toys with lights or sounds.[10] Child life therapists may be available in a hospital to assist with distraction techniques.

For management of pediatric chronic pain, other nonpharmacologic approaches, in addition to distraction techniques mentioned previously, can be successfully utilized. Although more research is needed to identify the most effective nonpharmacologic techniques in children, strategies and programs tailored to developmental level and age group should be routinely implemented.

Nonpharmacologic Pain Management Strategies for Children

1. *Distraction techniques* (active and passive)
2. *Interprofessional collaboration*[13]
3. *Diaphragmatic breathing* (with simple imagery for younger children such as blowing a pinwheel or bubbles, blowing out candles, rocking or rhythmic techniques)
4. *Mindfulness meditation* (may be more applicable to older children and adolescents, younger children may respond to guided imagery)
5. *Hypnosis* (using calming imagery and therapeutic suggestions)
6. *Acupuncture or acupressure*[11]
7. *Psychological and cognitive behavioral therapies*[12]
8. Physical therapy and *rehabilitation* strategies
9. *Yoga* activities or programs

Mnemonic: DID'M HAPPY

Pediatric Pain Rehabilitation and Interdisciplinary Programs

Children who suffer from chronic pain may be best served by a specialized pediatric pain clinic with access to an interdisciplinary team.[13] This team may consist of a pain physician, psychologist, nurse, social worker, physical therapist, and/or occupational therapist. These clinics may offer different treatment settings, including outpatient, intensive outpatient, and inpatient services depending on each individual circumstance to best serve the child and the family.

Pediatric Pain Specialist

The pediatric pain specialist may prescribe medications to help with difficulties with sleep, anxiety, and depression in addition to medications to decrease pain and inflammation. The pain specialist may also be able to perform interventional procedures such as nerve blocks to help decrease and diagnose certain types of pain.

Psychological Treatment

Psychologists will screen pediatric patients for depression and anxiety because these symptoms may exacerbate pain. They will work with the child on coping skills, pain reduction strategies, and other behavioral techniques, offer support, and collaborate with parents and caregivers on how to communicate about pain with their children. Cognitive behavioral therapy is often employed along with biofeedback (a process whereby electronic monitoring of a normally automatic bodily function is used to train someone to acquire voluntary control of that function, e.g., heart rate and temperature). Pain clinics may also provide support groups for pediatric patients with chronic pain to encourage social interaction.

Occupational and Physical Therapy

Physical and occupational therapists will work with patients to improve their overall physical fitness level and conditioning. They will help make activities of daily living more manageable through various different interventions such as working on flexibility, using heat and cold to alleviate pain, and utilizing electrostimulation to decrease pain.

Pharmacologic Pain Management in Children

The World Health Organization has published recommendations to guide medication management of pediatric pain.[14] This includes a two-step strategy for pharmacologic selection based on pain severity. Mild pain is initially treated with acetaminophen or nonsteroidal anti-inflammatory drugs (NSAIDs), and moderate to severe pain is treated with opioids. Additionally, pain should be treated at regular intervals and not only on an as-needed basis.

Mild pain treatment begins with acetaminophen and ibuprofen. Ibuprofen is the most extensively studied NSAID in regard to its safety and efficacy profile in the pediatric population. Both medications should be dosed based on age and weight to avoid toxicity (Table 18.2).

Table 18.2 Oral Medication Dosing for Selected Standard Analgesic Agents, by Age Group

Drug Name	Dose for Neonates	Dose for Infants 1–3 mo	Dose for Infants 3–12 mo	Children 1–12 yr	Maximum Daily Dose
Acetaminophen	5–10 mg/kg every 4–6 hours*	10 mg/kg every 4–6 hrs*	10–15 mg/kg every 4–6 hr*	10–15 mg/kg every 4–6 hr*,†	4 doses/day
Ibuprofen			5–10 mg/kg every 6–8 hr	5–10 mg/kg every 6–8 hr	Children: 40 mg/kg/day
Selected **oral** opioid doses are for opioid-naïve patients					
Morphine Immediate release		80–200 µg/kg every 4 hr	80–200 µg/kg every 4 hr	1–2 yr: 200–400 µg/kg every 4 hr 2–12 yr: 200–500 µg/kg every 4 hr	For children 2–12 yr: the maximum dose is 5 mg
Oxycodone Immediate release		50–125 µg/kg every 4 hr	50–125 µg/kg every 4 hr	125–200 µg/kg every 4 hr	5 mg/dose
IV opioid doses are different because of bioavailability; please consult your local practice manual.					

*Children with poor nutritional status at risk for toxicity due to lack of metabolic glutathione function.
†Maximum single dose is 1 g.
Adapted from WHO guidelines on the pharmacological treatment of persisting pain in children with medical illnesses. World Health Organization. 2012:37.

Additional medications such as muscle relaxants, antidepressants, and anticonvulsants may be beneficial for some age groups and in certain pain states.

Opioid Analgesics

Moderate to severe pain should be treated with opioid analgesic medications. In addition to opioids, as part of a multimodal pain management plan, children should continue to receive scheduled acetaminophen and ibuprofen for their opioid-sparing effect or their ability to decrease the dose of opioid needed to achieve pain control. Opioid sparing potentially reduces the risk for opioid-induced respiratory depression.

Opioids are most commonly used in the pediatric population to treat acute pain such as after surgery or trauma. Chronic pain conditions, in general, are managed by a team utilizing many different approaches to pain management in order to avoid or minimize the use of chronic opioids. Specific chronic disease exceptions where opioids are more commonly used include cancer and sickle cell disease. Opioids are best avoided in the pediatric population to treat pain related to headaches and functional abdominal pain. Side effects and risks for addiction and diversion must be evaluated (see Chapter 20).

Morphine is well established as an initial opioid for pain management in children. Initial dosing and schedules are listed in 18.2 for commonly used opioids in the pediatric population. The optimal dosing is one where pain is consistently well-managed between scheduled dose and frequency. After pain has been managed for a 24-hour period, the total opioid requirement can be calculated, and a long-acting opioid may be used for pain management. An additional, as needed, short-acting opioid may be used for breakthrough pain or sudden, severe pain that lasts for short periods of time. This pain "breaks through" the baseline pain medication but should not be confused with procedural pain, pain related to movement, or pain that begins to escalate before the next scheduled dose of medication. Breakthrough pain dosing may be set to 10% of the 24-hour total opioid requirement. If more than three doses of breakthrough pain medication are needed in a day, then a new 24-hour opioid requirement can be calculated and long- and short-acting opioid dosages adjusted.

Opioid rotation is the practice of switching to an alternate opioid due to inadequate analgesic effect or to dose-limiting side effects. Morphine has long been thought of as the gold standard for initiation of pediatric pain management, but some studies have demonstrated that patients on morphine are more likely to have inadequate analgesia and pruritis compared with patients on hydromorphone.[15] While definitive data demonstrating superiority of one opioid over another are lacking, if a patient has inadequate analgesia despite escalating dosages or significant adverse effects, it may be helpful to change opioid agents. When switching opioids, extreme care must be given to properly calculating equianalgesic dosing, with possible dose reductions, so that respiratory depression is not precipitated by giving a larger dose than intended.

Contraindications: Codeine and Tramadol

The US Food and Drug Administration (FDA) issued contraindication warnings on the use of the pain medications codeine and tramadol in children younger than 12 years of age.[16] Both of these medications utilize the enzyme P450 2D6 (*CYP2D6*) for metabolism to their active metabolites. Some children are considered ultrarapid metabolizers of these drugs because of genetic differences and can have a quick accumulation of active metabolites. In these ultrarapid metabolizers, there were a number of reported incidents of respiratory depression as well as death. Because of these complications, codeine and tramadol are contraindicated in all children younger than 12 years and in adolescents 12 to 18 years for treating pain after a tonsillectomy or adenoidectomy. A warning was also placed on both medications against the use in adolescents 12 to 18 years with obstructive sleep apnea or compromised respiratory function.

SUMMARY

The goal of this chapter is to illustrate the "tip of the iceberg" in understanding pediatric pain assessment, etiology, and management. The various tools to assess pain are guides, many of which have been studied and validated in respective age groups. We encourage clinicians to incorporate parental or caregiver intuition into their evaluations, especially when a scale does not correlate with caregivers' assessments and concerns. Obtaining a detailed history that will allow clinicians to classify pain as acute versus chronic is imperative; categorizing the pain will help develop a differential diagnosis appropriate for various age groups. Knowing common pain etiologies of various age groups may help diagnose pathology more quickly, forego unnecessary testing, and put patients on the path to relief sooner.

Pain management in children can be complex, and successful treatment affects not only physical development but also social, psychological, and neurocognitive development. Poorly managed pediatric pain can have profound implications on a child into adulthood. Understanding the various modalities, their mechanistic properties, how to advance therapies, and how to use them in combination is necessary for all practitioners. We encourage our readers to consistently address pain with patients and families in all clinical settings. Having an open discussion about what is and is not working in a patient's pain management plan is important for building trust and ensuring successful treatment outcomes.

REVIEW QUESTIONS

1. You are rotating on the pediatric pain service and are called to evaluate a 6-month-old for pain management. What instrument will you use to appraise pain in this patient?
    a. Numeric rating scale
    b. Faces Rating Scale
    c. FLACC scale
    d. Pieces of Hurt tool

2. A 2-year-old presents to the emergency department with acute abdominal pain and blood work. An intravenous catheter placement is needed, but the patient is inconsolable and extremely frightened. All of the following are best next-step strategies to allow for obtaining the blood sample, *except*:
    a. Distract with light-up toys.
    b. Ask the parents to leave to minimize stress.
    c. Hold the patient tightly in his parent's arms.
    d. Convince the patient to blow bubbles.

3. Chronic pain conditions in children where chronic opioids should be avoided include all of the following, *except*:
   a. Chronic migraine headaches
   b. Menstrual pain
   c. Sickle cell disease
   d. Functional abdominal pain

REFERENCES

1. Corwin MJ, Lester BM, Golub HL. The infant cry what can it tell us. Curr Probl Pediatr. 1996;26(9):324–334.
2. von Baeyer CL, Uman LS, Chambers CT, Gouthro A. Can we screen young children for their ability to provide accurate self-reports of pain? Pain 2011;152(6):1327–1333. doi: 10.1016/j.pain.2011.02.013.
3. Hicks CL, von Baeyer CL, Spafford PA, van Korlaar I, Goodenough B. The Faces Pain Scale—Revised: toward a common metric in pediatric pain measurement. Pain. 2001;93(2):173–183.
4. Savedra MC, Holzemer WL, Tesler MD, Wilkie DJ. Assessment of postoperative pain in children and adolescents using the Adolescent Pediatric Pain Tool. Nurs Res. 1993;42:5–9
5. Stinson JN, Kavanagh T, Yamada J, Gill N, Stevens B. Systematic review of the psychometric properties, interpretability and feasibility of self-report pain intensity measures for use in clinical trials in children and adolescents. Pain. 2006;125(1-2):143–157. doi: 10.1016/j.pain.2006.05.006.
6. von Baeyer CL, Spagrud LJ. Systematic review of observational (behavioral) measures of pain for children and adolescents aged 3 to 18 years. Pain. 2007;127(1-2):140–150. doi: 10.1016/j.pain.2006.08.014.
7. Assa A, Ish-Tov A, Rinawi F, Shamir R. School attendance in children with functional abdominal pain and inflammatory bowel diseases. J Pediatr Gastroenterol Nutr. 2015;61(5):553–557. doi: 10.1097/MPG.0000000000000850.
8. Dampier C, Ely B, Brodecki D, Oneal P. Characteristics of pain managed at home in children and adolescents with sickle cell disease by using diary self-reports. J Pain. 2002;3(6):461–470. doi: 10.1054/jpai.2002.128064.
9. Stephens BK, Barkey ME, Hall HR. Techniques to comfort children during stressful procedures. Adv Mind Body Med 1999;15(1):49–60.
10. Villacres S, Chumpitazi CE. Acute pediatric pain management in the primary care office. Pediatr Ann. 2018;47(3):e124–e29. doi: 10.3928/19382359-20180222-01.
11. Brown ML, Rojas E, Gouda S. A mind–body approach to pediatric pain management. Children (Basel). 2017;4(6). doi: 10.3390/children4060050,
12. Fisher E, Law E, Dudeney J, Eccleston C, Palermo TM. Psychological therapies (remotely delivered) for the management of chronic and recurrent pain in children and adolescents. Cochrane Database Syst Rev. 2019;(4):CD011118. doi: 10.1002/14651858.CD011118.pub3,
13. Liossi C, Johnstone L, Lilley S, et al. Effectiveness of interdisciplinary interventions in paediatric chronic pain management: a systematic review and subset meta-analysis. Br J Anaesth. 2019 Feb 28. [Epub ahead of print]. doi: 10.1016/j.bja.2019.01.024.
14. World Health Organization. WHO guidelines on the pharmacological treatment of persisting pain in children with medical illnesses. World Health Organization. 2012:37.

15. DiGiusto M, Bhalla T, Martin D, et al. Patient-controlled analgesia in the pediatric population: morphine versus hydromorphone. J Pain Res. 2014;7:471–475. doi: 10.2147/JPR.S64497.
16. US Food and Drug Administration. FDA restricts use of prescription codeine pain and cough medicines and tramadol pain medicines in children; recommends against use in breastfeeding women. Drug Safety Communications. https://www.fda.gov/drugs/drug-safety-and-availability/fda-drug-safety-communication-fda-restricts-use-prescription-codeine-pain-and-cough-medicines-and. Accessed September 10, 2019.

19 Pain in Older Patients

Staja Q. Booker and Keela A. Herr

You must never think of anything except the need and how to meet it.
—Clara Barton

LEARNING OBJECTIVES

At the completion of this chapter, the learner should be able to discuss:

- The prevalence and major causes of pain in older patients
- The importance of coordinating pain therapy with other pharmacotherapy given the prevalence of polypharmacy in older patients
- The impact of decreased cognitive function on standard pain assessment tools and the importance of proactive pain assessment in the elderly
- Strategies for counseling older patients and the role of caregivers

CASE SCENARIO

You are asked to see a 69-year-old woman with lifelong severe scoliosis that has progressively worsened, and she now has a nonhealing pressure ulcer on the left paraspinal region at about T6. She has been diagnosed with antibiotic-resistant *Pseudomonas aeruginosa*, which has limited her ability to participate in the water-based therapy and exercise that you recommended for her. She has arm and leg contractures, is wheelchair bound, and experiences constant pain from her hips, legs, and the pressure ulcer over her back. What strategies can you use to improve this patient's pain management?

INTRODUCTION

Although pain is not a normal physiologic phenomenon of aging, it is common, with nearly 30% of older adults in each age group, 60 to 69, 70 to 79, and 80 years and older, reporting persistent pain.[1] While changes in pain transmission, tolerance, threshold, and interpretation may result in a slowed pain response, aging does not decrease sensitivity to pain,[2] but pain sensitivity may, in fact, increase with age.[3] Frailty can also lower physiologic threshold, making older adults more vulnerable to persistent pain conditions.

More concerning is that subgroups of older adults are at increased risk for persistent pain, and these include racial and ethnic minorities; war veterans; lesbian, gay, bisexual, transgender, and questioning (LGBTQ); prisoners; frail elders experiencing frequent transitions; elders at the end of life; and older adults with cancer pain. For example, a recent study of older prisoners revealed that 39% have severe persistent pain, while an astounding 75% reported any pain.[4] When persistent or acute pain is inadequately managed in older adults, it is a major source of discomfort and distress, resulting in a cascade of deleterious consequences, including accelerated physiologic deconditioning (e.g., frailty), impaired executive function, psychosocial issues (e.g., depression, delirium), loss of independence, sleep deprivation, and socioeconomic hardships (e.g., inability to afford pain medications, increased medical visits, job absenteeism).[5,6] The imperative to provide compassionate pain management is urgent; therefore, this chapter provides best practice recommendations for comprehensive pain management in older patients.

PAIN ASSESSMENT TECHNIQUES

Pain assessment appears to be an easy and obvious task, yet assessment and reassessment in older adults are often absent or inconsistent.[7,8] Nearly 30% of older adults in emergency departments did not receive pain assessments, while only 59% were assessed using self-report measures,[9] the gold standard for those able to self-report. Accurate pain assessment is the foundation for pain treatment and evaluation, and its accuracy depends on the healthcare providers' ability to accommodate for older adults' sensory and motor deficits and simultaneously cue in on idiosyncrasies that affect pain assessment, collaborate with patients and families, and utilize evidence-based (i.e., reliable and valid) practice techniques.

Pain assessments can be comprehensive or focused, in which a comprehensive assessment is typically completed upon initial or first-time visits with providers or when there is a change in health status, and a focused assessment is an abbreviated assessment that can be performed at the bedside or during follow-up clinic visits. In severe, acute pain, a focused assessment can facilitate rapid pain treatment, followed by a more thorough evaluation.

Comprehensive Assessment

Pain is a complex phenomenon that affects every aspect of life and should be incorporated into a comprehensive geriatric assessment to evaluate an older adult's medical history, pain story, function, psychological state, social support and physical environments, and health-related legal affairs (Figure 19.1).[10]

Medical History. Review the medical history and physical exam in order to understand the etiology and sequence of events contributing to pain. Comorbidities and multimorbidities, such as cancer, diabetes, cardiovascular disease, and musculoskeletal disorders, are common pathologic sources of chronic, acute, neuropathic, nociceptive, and visceral pain. Laboratory and diagnostic tests, cultural practices, and past and current review of medications are also important to ascertain. Providers should ask about

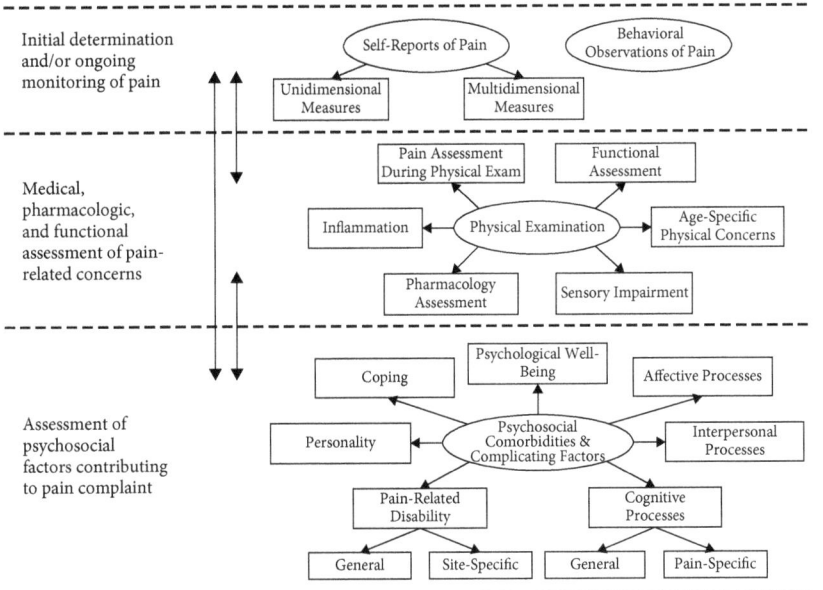

FIGURE 19.1 Domains included in a comprehensive pain assessment. (From Hadjistavropoulos T, Herr K, Turk DC, et al. An interdisciplinary expert consensus statement on assessment of pain in older persons. Clin J Pain. 2007;23[1 Suppl]:S5.Used with permission from Wolters Kluwer Health/Lippincott Williams & Wilkins.)

the types and dosage of medications and natural/herbal therapies because these may potentiate or decrease the effectiveness of pain medications. Moreover, older adults may be less willing to add medications for the treatment of pain; therefore, patient preference for assessment and treatment should be elicited.

The Pain Narrative. In the past few years, patient-centered assessment, such as the Clinically Aligned Pain Assessment (CAPA), have focused on gathering key information about the patient's comfort, function, sleep, change in pain, and perceived pain control.[11] This conversation allows patients to discuss what really matters to them. The process of gathering a pain history begins with several minutes of uninterrupted listening to build rapport, and as the patient speaks, the provider is attuned for the (1) cardinal features of pain described during the conversation, (2) healthcare-related values that may influence preferences for treatment (e.g., favors home remedies over medications), and (3) prior pain experiences and how they responded, surgeries, injuries, illnesses, treatments, and side or adverse effects. After assessing pain history, also ask about present pain, including intensity, frequency, pattern, location, duration, and precipitating and relieving factors, see also Key Pain Characteristics, in Chapter 6. In some situations, however, characteristic pain symptoms of acute illness may present atypically, such as in silent myocardial infarctions and painless intra-abdominal acute problems or intracranial tumors.[12] Pain with these conditions may be masked by symptoms such as fatigue, and clinicians should consider ways to effectively treat atypical symptoms and pain while minimizing treatment burden (i.e., polypharmacy).

Particular cultures may prefer not to discuss or express pain openly to family or providers, particularly when rapport and trust have not been established. Some older patients may deny pain or report that pain medication is effective because they believe this is the "right" thing to say[13]; they may also deny pain for fear of painful diagnostic tests or the diagnosis itself. It may be challenging for the older adult to isolate the location and severity of pain or understand how pain affects psychosocial health. Providers can ask about specific areas that may be painful,[13] given common pain disorders and locations such as arthritis that may affect multiple locations. Particularly in acute care, providers must emphasize to older adults to report not only acute pain but also chronic pain problems that need consideration in the treatment plan.

Function. Assess function and ability to complete basic and instrumental activities of daily living (ADLs). Pain may cause older adults to be less active and more prone to gait impairments and falls. Recent studies show that pain is a risk factor for and predictor of falls in older adults.[14,15] Pain also affects sleep quality and quantity, and impaired sleep is a risk factor for development of persistent pain. Impact and interference of pain on function are essential in goal setting and treatment planning.

Example Assessment Tools for Pain-Related and General Function:

- Brief Pain Inventory (BPI)
- Pain, Enjoyment, and General Activity (PEG) Scale
- Katz Index of Independence in ADLs
- Lawton Instrumental ADLs

Example Assessment Tool for Sleep:

- Pittsburgh Sleep Quality Index (PSQI)

Psychological State. Evaluate cognitive status (e.g., mild cognitive impairment, dementia, delirium) and mental health (e.g., depression, anxiety, suicidal ideation, post-traumatic stress disorder [PTSD]). Cognitive impairments affect a large proportion of older adults and are a major risk factor for underassessment and lack of treatment of pain,[7] despite similar rates in self-report of pain.[16] It is often assumed that persons with cognitive issues are less sensitive to pain, but transmission of pain stimulus to the brain remains intact.[17] People with persistent pain are shown to have some degree of impaired executive function,[18] which may further decrease self-report and decision-making ability in persons with existing dementia. While there may be issues with recalling, interpreting, appraising pain intensity level, and articulating pain, those with mild to moderate cognitive impairment may still be able to self-report, and self-report should always be attempted.[8]

Other cognitive alterations, such as depression and delirium, also limit report of pain, making treatment more complicated. Although pain and depression comorbidity are common, 75% of older patients with depressive symptoms either denied pain or self-reported no pain.[9] Delirium and agitation are especially challenging because either can be triggered by pain, undermedication or overmedication for pain, or other processes such as infection, change in environment, adverse drug effects, and anesthesia. Hodgson et al. found that pain was associated with the number of behavioral symptoms in those with dementia and concluded that pain is a risk factor for behavioral and neuropsychological symptoms, necessitating proper assessment and treatment.[19] At times, it is difficult to differentiate between dementia- and delirium-related behaviors and pain-related behaviors. When older adults are unable to self-report pain, a multifaceted assessment approach should be incorporated (Figure 19.2).

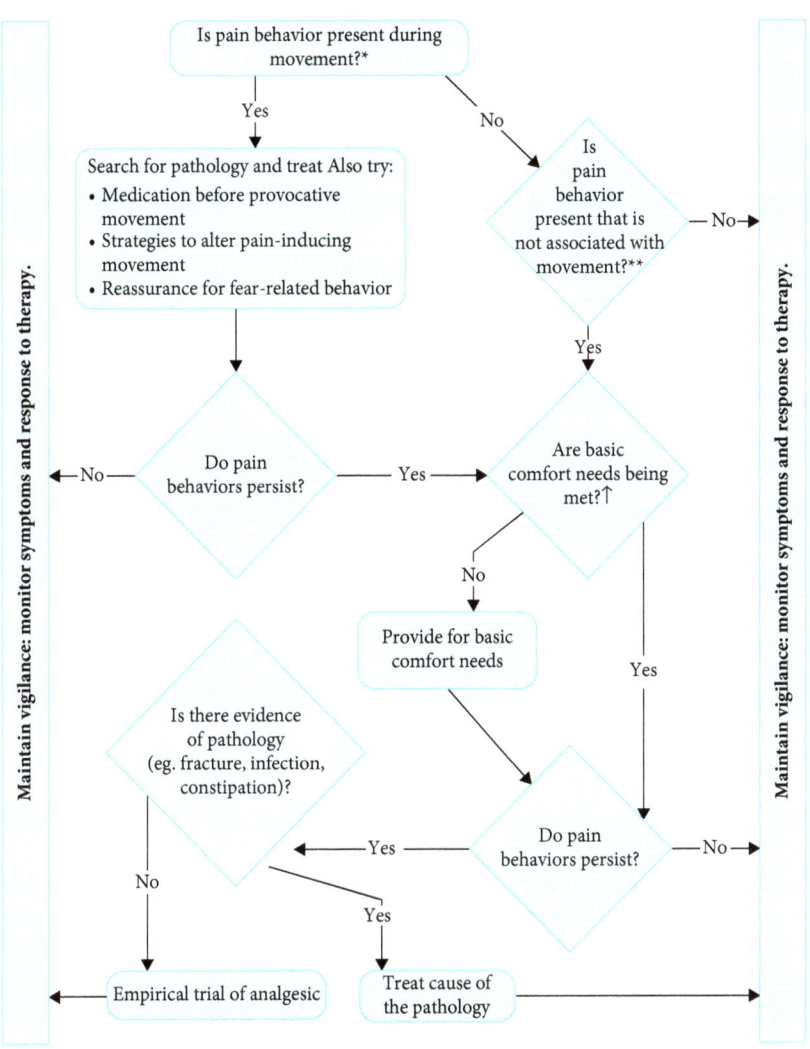

* Examples: grimacing, guarding, combativeness, groaning with movement; resisting care

** Examples: agitation, fidgeting, sleep disturbance, diminished appetite, irritability, reclusiveness, disruptive behavior, rigidity, rapid blinking

†Examples: toileting, thirst, hunger, visual or hearing impairment

FIGURE 19.2 Algorithm for Pain Assessment in Cognitively Impaired Older Adults.[27] (Used with permission from American Geriatrics Society.)
Source: Reuben DB, Herr KA, Pacala JT, Pollock BG, Potter JF, Semla TP. Pain. In: Reuben DB, Herr KA, Pacala JT, Pollock BG, Potter JF, Semla TP, eds. *Geriatrics at your fingertips*. 17th ed. New York, NY: American Geriatrics Society, 2015:234.

Example Assessment Tools for Cognition:

- Mini-Cog
- Brief Interview for Mental Status (BIMS)

Example Assessment Tools for Depression:

- Patient Health Questionnaire (PHQ-9 or PHQ-2)
- Geriatric Depression Scale (GDS)

Example Assessment Tool for Delirium: Confusion Assessment Measure (CAM)
Example Assessment Tool for Anxiety: Geriatric Anxiety Inventory (GAI)
Example Assessment Tool for PTSD: Horowitz's Impact of Event Scale

Social Support. Persistent pain may decrease socialization with family and friends, potentially leading to isolation. Considering that many older adults rely on family members or other social support as caregivers, assessment of pain should be a patient-centered and collaborative process between patients, families, and providers, particularly in those with cognitive challenges. It is essential to determine patients' and families' support needs for pain education; educational, financial, and emotional ability to follow pain management plan (i.e., health literacy and finances); and coping skills.[20] Nonetheless, caregiver burden, caregiver role strain, anxiety, and sense of helplessness are major issues that can influence effective management of pain in older adults[21]; thus, caregivers must also be evaluated for their ability to assess pain and safely and consistently implement the treatment plan. Pain is rarely discussed in terms of advanced directives, but this is an equally important component of pain assessment providing direction on how pain should be treated at the end-of-life or during times when the older adult is unable to make decisions.

Example Assessment Tools for Caregivers

- Modified Caregiver Strain Index
- Preparedness for Caregiving Scale

Focused Assessment

Pain is generally assessed by asking: "Are you hurting or having any pain right now? On a scale of 0 to 10, with 0 being no pain and 10 being the worst pain, how would you rate your pain right now?" While these are two very important questions, they represent only a partial picture of how older adults experience pain. Recommendations suggest that tolerability, function, and mood also be assessed during the bedside pain assessment (Table 19.1).[20] When an older adult is unable to report pain because of communication or cognitive alterations, different approaches to recognize potential pain problems are needed (Figure 19.2).

MULTIMODAL PAIN TREATMENT: ANALGESIA AND NONDRUG THERAPIES

Because there are numerous ways to treat pain in older adults, evidence-based strategies to control pain, prevent pain escalation or breakthrough pain, and maintain or improve function and mood should be explicit and appropriate based on patient needs, values, and cultural preferences. Pain should be treated in a timely manner, but for many older adults, this is an issue. A recent study found that the average initial time to pain treatment in the emergency department was 73 minutes for older adults compared with 52 and 54 minutes for children and young/middle-aged adults, respectively.[7] Delays in treatment are harmful to older adults, causing undue suffering and making it more difficult to effectively reduce pain. This reflects the larger issue

Table 19.1 Steps for Focused Pain Assessments in Older Adults

Cognitively Intact and/or Able to Self-Report	Cognitively Impaired and Unable to Self-Report
Step 1: Determine willingness, ability, and reliability to provide self-report pain by observing coherence of verbal communication, using a pain screen test,[29] assessing conceptual understanding on how to use a pain scale by asking where mild pain and severe pain are represented on a 0–10 pain scale,[8] and/or administering a mini-mental status exam (MMSE). Older adults who score 18 or above on MMSE can usually reliably self-report pain.[30]	**Step 1:** Same step for those able to self-report and note whether there is a diagnosis of cognitive impairment or dementia. Some older adults with mild to moderate dementia remain able to self-report; in these situations, refer to left column. If unable to self-report, continue with steps 2–6 in this column.
Step 2: Determine presence/absence of pain by asking older adults if they are experiencing pain "right now" or "at this moment." Alternative descriptors, such as ache, sore, hurt, and discomfort, should be used if "pain" is denied. Older adults may have difficulty explaining characteristics of the pain, such as location, quality, and duration.	**Step 2: Search for possible etiologies of pain** such as history of pain conditions, pathologic (e.g., chronic diseases, infections), procedural (e.g., postoperative pain, blood pressure cuff pain, wound care), accidental (e.g., skin tears), trauma (e.g., falls, concussions, elder abuse), and emotional causes (e.g., depression, anxiety, post-traumatic stress disorder).
Step 3: Measure self-reported pain intensity using a valid, reliable, and preferred pain scale such as the Faces Pain Rating Scale–Revised (FPS-R), Iowa Pain Thermometer (IPT and IPT–Revised), Verbal Descriptor Scale (VDS), or Numeric Rating Scale (NRS).[8] Pain scale preference by race: • African and Hispanic Americans: Defense and Veterans Pain Rating Scale (DVPRS), IPT—Revised, and FPS-R • Asian Americans: verbal NRS • Caucasian Americans: NRS, VDS, and IPT—Revised[31,32] Older adults may have difficulty with a verbally administered request for pain intensity rating, and a printed reference of the tool should be provided.	**Step 3: Observe for potential pain behaviors using an appropriate pain behavior observation tool.** While pain is a subjective experience, close observation of facial expressions, verbalizations/vocalizations, body movements, changes in interpersonal interactions, changes in activity patterns or routines, and mental status changes may help confirm pain. When there is a change in older adults' behavior, it is a rule of thumb to consider pain as an etiology. There are many pain behavior observation tools, and the Pain Assessment in Advanced Dementia Scale (PAINAD) and Pain Assessment Checklist for Seniors with Limited Ability to Communicate (PACSLAC-II) are recommended for long-term care residents[33]; other pain behavior tools may be appropriate and clinically usable for different populations, settings of care, and languages.

(Continued)

Table 19.1 Continued

Cognitively Intact and/or Able to Self-Report	Cognitively Impaired and Unable to Self-Report
Step 4: Assess impact of pain on function to determine pain tolerability and interference with life activities. Different patients will find different pain intensities more tolerable. Use established measures such as the BPI or Functional Pain Scale.[34]	**Step 4: Obtain proxy reporting from family or caregivers** (e.g., nurse, certified nursing assistant) about older adult's usual behavior, communication style, functional patterns, and mood. Proxies need recent knowledge of pain problem, activity level, and normative behavior to pick up on subtle changes that may otherwise go unnoticed.
Step 5: Assess (a) interference of pain on sleep by simply asking patients how pain affects ability to fall and stay asleep and the average number of hours of sleep obtained at night or use the Pittsburgh Sleep Quality Index (PSQI) and **(b) emotional stability** using the Patient Health Questionnaire (PHQ) or Geriatric Depression Scale (GDS) for depressed mood and Geriatric Anxiety Index for anxiety. Mood and function may improve before significant reductions in pain intensity are observed.	**Step 5: Initiate analgesic trial** if (a) pain is the suspected cause of behaviors as demonstrated by a pain behavior observation tool, (b) behaviors do not respond to nondrug interventions, or (c) etiology known to be painful and other causes ruled out. The type of pain suspected (e.g., nociceptive or neuropathic), comorbidities, and contraindications determine the stepped approach taken. The trial length can range from 1–7 days. Example analgesic trials are presented as follows: *Suspected Nociceptive Pain*: Option 1—If patient does not have an order/prescription or is taking a low dose of acetaminophen, give oral acetaminophen 500–1,000 mg acetaminophen every 8 hr (maximum dose 3 g/day). Option 2—If pain is not responsive to acetaminophen and localized inflammatory pain suspected, try topical nonsteroidal anti-inflammatory drugs or lidocaine. Option 3—If no response to above, try oral morphine sulfate 5 mg every 12 hr or buprenorphine transdermal patch 5–10 µg/hr. *Suspected Neuropathic or Mixed/Undetermined Pain*: Option 1—Give oral acetaminophen 500–1,000 mg acetaminophen every 8 hr (maximum dose 3 g/day). Option 2—Try pregabalin 25–75 mg every 8 hr (maximum dose 300 mg/day). Improved behavior after administration of an analgesic is support for assuming pain is present; proceed to step 6. If unresponsive to analgesic trial, explore other potential causes and/or consult a pain management specialist.

Table 19.1 Continued

Cognitively Intact and/or Able to Self-Report	Cognitively Impaired and Unable to Self-Report
Step 6: Develop a multimodal treatment plan guided by realistic goals for comfort, function, and mood. Continue to reassess regularly, based on pain severity and type using the same self-report pain intensity scale. See "Multimodal Pain Treatment" section for more information on the multimodal treatment.	**Step 6: Develop a multi-modal treatment plan** guided by attainable goals for continued comfort, function, mood, and behavioral improvement. Continue to reassess behaviors using the same pain behavior observation tool. See "Multimodal Pain Treatment" section for more information on the multimodal treatment.

Used with permission of Booker S, Herr KA. © 2019. The University of Iowa, College of Nursing.

of undertreatment of pain in older adults across settings, including acute care, home care, nursing homes, and hospice.[22,23] Many older adults rely on family or friends as caregivers for daily assistance, so healthcare providers are encouraged to collaborate with the older adult and the family/caregiver to develop a multimodal treatment plan that is individualized, based on best practices for the pain mechanism and severity, and aligned with patient preferences and goals. A multimodal treatment plan includes a combination of complementary and alternative strategies and medications, plus adjuvant medications and interventional techniques if needed (Figure 19.3). Caregivers are integral to supporting and implementing the multimodal pain treatment plan and identifying potential problems with treatment in those unable to advocate for themselves, especially older adults with advanced dementia. Caregivers need to be particularly aware of treatment of coexisting pain comorbidities, such as depression, how these affect pain control, and how to determine whether overall treatment is successful.

Complementary and Alternative Strategies

Complementary and alternative treatments are recommended alongside medications and should always be integrated into a multimodal plan. While there are many complementary and alternative approaches available, interventions should be selected based on safety, evidence of effectiveness, and the older adult's physical and cognitive ability and treatment preferences. Complementary and alternative treatments can be categorized as physical, cognitive, spiritual, or natural/herbal.

Physical interventions may consist of exercise, physical therapy, massage, acupressure, acupuncture, use of assistive devices/orthotics, chiropractic, transcutaneous electrical nerve stimulation, heat/cool compresses, positioning, and sleep hygiene. Physical exercise, aquatic and nonaquatic, has strong evidence for use in older adults, particularly in helping musculoskeletal pain. These exercises focus on strengthening, flexibility, endurance, and balance. An older adult's mobility and gait should be assessed before development of an exercise regimen; frail older adults or those with severe osteoporosis will require carefully implemented and monitored exercise and rehabilitation activities. Additionally, some older adults, such as older African Americans, may prefer group- or faith-based exercise, or older Asian Americans may use tai chi, yoga, or other culturally based exercise routines.

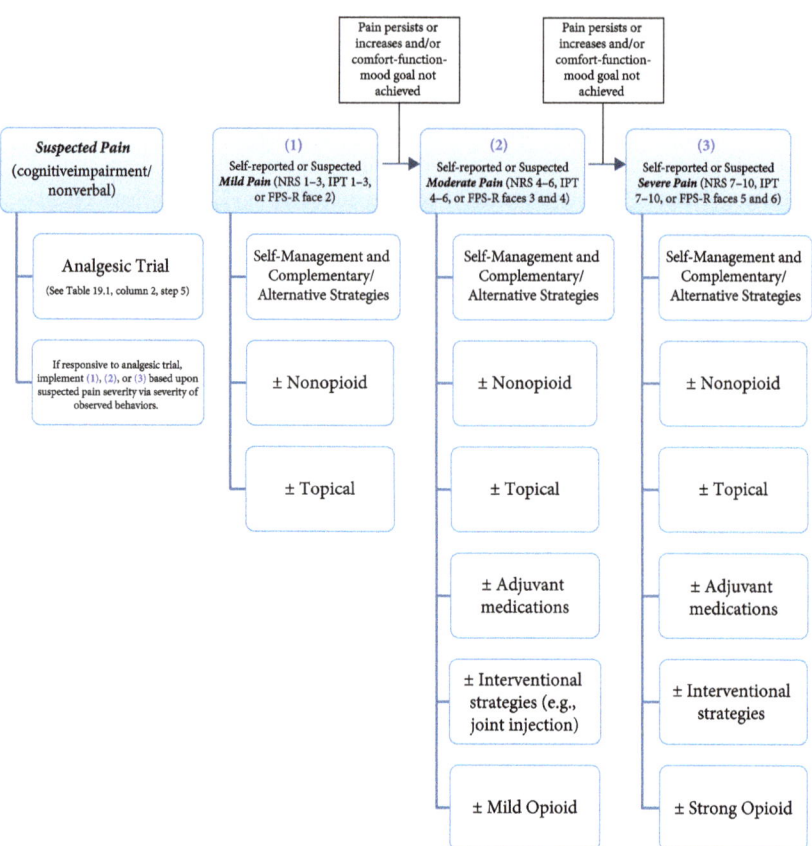

FIGURE 19.3 Hierarchy of multimodal pain treatment in older adults. Note that self-management and complementary/alternative strategies include nondrug approaches. (Used with permission from Booker SQ, Herr KA. © 2019. The University of Iowa, College of Nursing. NRS = numeric rating scale; IPT-R = Iowa Pain Thermometer—Revised; FPS-R = Faces Pain Scale—Revised.)

Cognitive interventions may include cognitive behavioral therapy (e.g., acceptance and commitment therapy), distraction, guided imagery, music, reminiscence therapy, hypnosis, coping skills training, motivational interviewing, and biofeedback. Psychosocial interventions, including various forms of cognitive behavioral therapy, are shown to be effective pain management techniques. These types of therapies must be selected carefully, considering that older adults with cognitive or intellectual disabilities may be unable to use these because of issues with attention/focus, memory, and understanding. Moreover, some ethnic cultures may not be open to applying certain cognitive strategies.

Spiritual strategies are also important complementary and alternative interventions. In fact, spiritual interventions are a primary strategy for treatment of pain and other health conditions in older African Americans,[24] although research evidence on the use and effectiveness of spiritual approaches in the general population of older adults is limited. However, it is important that providers inform patients that spiritual strategies are best used in combination with other complementary and alternative and pharmacologic interventions. A few examples of spiritual strategies are mindfulness meditation, prayer, faith healing, and gospel or spiritual music. Other alternative strategies include energy field therapies (reiki, healing touch, therapeutic touch) and electromagnetic therapies (copper bracelets, spiritual crystal stones).

Natural/herbal therapies are less often utilized and integrated in pain management plans, but strategies such as weight loss can improve musculoskeletal pain. Examples of natural therapies include diets that reduce inflammation or uric acid, glucosamine and chondroitin, fish oil, vitamins, and weight loss. All older adults should be asked about current use of complementary and alternative treatments to evaluate safe use because many herbal therapies can interfere with prescribed medication effectiveness and their willingness to try these therapies.

Medication Selection, Dosing, and Administration Strategies

The selection, dosing, and administration of pain medications require careful attention and continuous evaluation and depend on a number of factors: pain type and severity, interference with function, allergies, polypharmacy, contraindications, comorbidities, cognitive function, medication beliefs and concerns, and risk for adverse effects (See Table 19.2). Careful evaluation of risks and benefits is essential to identify issues with medication tolerance and promote treatment adherence and safe use. Before implementing a pain treatment plan, it is imperative to keep in mind the effect of physical and cognitive abilities, medication tolerance, age-related physiologic changes, weight, and pain type, severity, and interference with function.

Physical and Cognitive Ability. Many older adults have physical impairments that limit their ability to follow the treatment plan. For example, osteoarthritis or rheumatoid arthritis affects manual dexterity to manipulate a patient-controlled analgesic system or medication bottles. Evaluating older adults' ability to swallow (and what medications can be given intravenously, via gastrostomy tubes, etc.) or risk for intravenous collapse or infection from insertion of continuous intravenous medication is rarely considered but important.

Cognitive impairment and fear of taking opioid medications (opiophobia) could reduce adherence to treatments. Those with cognitive impairment may forget to take medications or become confused and take more than recommended, resulting in nontherapeutic levels. When the older adult takes more than recommended, suddenly becomes adherent, or has their medication dose increased, a phenomenon called *adherence toxicity* may occur. Adherence toxicity describes a sudden adherence to medications that leads to higher systemic levels of medication. Older adults with opiophobia or polypharmacy may prefer not to add more medications to their daily medication regimen. and adjustments to the overall medication regimen may be needed.

Medication Tolerance. More often, there are greater risks for overmedication, leading to drug toxicity, delirium, oversedation, falls, and even death. Opioid-tolerant older adults on chronic opioid therapy may require higher doses of opioids compared with opioid-naïve patients. Additionally, older adults with persistent pain may respond differently to medications than older adults with acute pain. It is wise to consider tolerance to past pain medications as well as current medications. Current medications or herbal therapies can potentiate or lower therapeutic effects of pain medication, making the older adult either more or less tolerant. More important, pharmacokinetics and pharmacodynamics of an individual will directly affect medication tolerance.

Table 19.2 Principles of Analgesic Management for Persistent Pain in Older Adults

Drug Class and Dosing	Practical Considerations

Step 1: Treatment of mild pain (score of 1–3 and limited functional impairment), not relieved from nondrug interventions.

Acetaminophen (APAP)	Continue evaluating risk/benefit ratio for prescribing APAP because of recent evidence of uncertain analgesic benefit and increased safety concerns.
	Renal impairment, hepatic dysfunction, and alcohol abuse are known risk factors for ADR.
	APAP in treating persistent mild to moderate musculoskeletal pain with maximal dose of 3 g/d in healthy patients and 2 g/d in frail older adults. Advise against alcohol use; schedule around the clock. Ask about all OTC medications with acetaminophen.
	NOT anti-inflammatory; leading cause of acute liver failure (including accidental overdose); monitor for severe liver injury and acute renal failure.
Nonacetylated salicylates (e.g., salsalate, trisalicylate)	Consider if inflammatory pain. Does not interfere with platelet function.
	Educate regarding salicylism and monitor Cr.
	Avoid in patients with advanced renal disease or hepatic impairment.
Counterirritants	Many available OTC medications with limited evidence to support use.
	Use in localized musculoskeletal pain. May be effective for arthritic pain, but effect limited when pain affects multiple joints. Apply to affected area and monitor for skin injury, especially if used with heat or occlusive dressing.
	Ideal for minor pains because of minimal side effects. Caution when applying near sensitive areas such as the eyes or genitals.
Topical analgesics	Temporary treatment of minor pain associated with muscles and joints due to backache, strains, sprains, cramps, arthritis; pain associated with diabetic neuropathy.
	OTC compounded topical analgesics available, although no evidence to support use.
	Never apply over broken or compromised skin. Wash hands after applying or use glove. Do not use heating pad.
Topical NSAIDs	As effective as oral NSAIDs with fewer systemic and GI adverse effects for chronic localized musculoskeletal pain, particularly hand and knee OA. Lack of clear efficacy data in acute or chronic low back pain, neuropathic pain.
	Don't combine topical plus oral NSAIDs.
	Evaluate serum Cr because of some systemic absorption.
	Diclofenac 1% gel, 1.5% topical sol, 1.3% patch
	Note: Some topical treatments are expensive and insurer may not cover.

Table 19.2 Continued

Drug Class and Dosing	Practical Considerations
	Application: Gel rubbed into skin with dosing card to determine correct amount. Elbow, wrist, or hand: use 2-g dose 4 times daily; knee, ankle, or feet: use 4-g dose four times daily. Maximum amount per day not to exceed 32 g.
	Do not apply heat or occlusive dressing after application.
	Application: Patch applied twice daily to most painful area with intact skin. Reinforce peeling edges with tape. Mesh sleeve or netting can be used. Remove patch during bathing (reduces adhesiveness). Wash hands after applying, touching, or removing patch.
	Application: Sol applied via pump or dropper; typically 40 drops to each painful knee (10 drops per time, and rub in to avoid spillage). Do not apply clothing until totally dry.
NSAIDs/ COX-2 anti-inflammatory drug	Avoid nonselective NSAIDs for chronic use (>6 wk) and in patients with history of gastric or duodenal ulcers, unless other alternatives are not effective, and patient can take gastroprotective agent.[BC]
	Avoid preexisting HTN, CKD, HF, and/or peptic ulcer disease, or those taking concomitant warfarin or corticosteroids.[BC]
	Use NSAIDs with caution in highly selected patients (e.g., acute-on-chronic pain flare or new acute pain problem such as gout in existing persistent pain disorder [e.g., CLBP]) for short-term use (<2 wk) with nonacetylated salicylate, or ibuprofen or celecoxib.
	Use misoprostol or PPI with nonselective NSAIDs to reduce GI bleeding risk. Avoid scheduled use of PPI for >8 wk unless for high-risk patients (e.g., chronic NSAID use).[BC]
	Consider celecoxib for patients who would benefit from anti-inflammatory medication with no cardiovascular risk based on risk/benefit assessment. Long-term use not recommended.
	Avoid in HF.[BC] Avoid in renal impairment (CrCl <30).[BC] Caution in patients with cardiovascular disease or at risk for cardiovascular disease.

Step 2: Treatment of moderate pain (score 4–7 and interference with active function (e.g., exercise, mobility-related), pain not alleviated with nondrug interventions and medicine from Step 1, and/or if pain worsens

Neuromodulating agents	Consider neuromodulating agents, including antidepressants and anticonvulsants, for patients with neuropathic pain or mixed pain syndromes or refractory persistent pain.
	Tailor to pain characteristics/etiology and risk factors.
	Effects may be enhanced when used in combination with other analgesics and/or nondrug strategies.
	Select agents with lowest adverse effect profiles.
	Begin low and titrate slowly; allow adequate therapeutic trial (e.g., 2–3 wk for onset of efficacy).

(Continued)

Table 19.2 Continued

Drug Class and Dosing	Practical Considerations
Short-acting opioids	Patients with moderate to severe pain, pain-related functional impairment, or diminished quality of life due to pain should be considered for treatment with opioids when other recommended approaches prove unsuccessful. Long-term safety of opioid use in persistent pain in older adults has not been established.
	Avoid if history of falls or fracture or concurrent benzodiazepine use; institute fall prevention when starting opioids because of increased risk for fracture in the first 2 wk of short-acting opioid treatment.
	Increased risk for hospitalization relative to NSAIDs, constipation, and other adverse effects impact treatment success.
	Do not prescribe opioid analgesics as first-line treatment for chronic noncancer pain.[CW]
	Do not prescribe opioid analgesics as long-term treatment for chronic noncancer pain until the risks are considered and discussed with the patient.[CW]
	Medications with long half-life or depot effects (e.g., methadone, levorphanol, transdermal fentanyl) should be used and titrated cautiously, with close supervision of effects; duration of effect may exceed usual dose intervals because of reduced metabolism and clearance.
	NEVER start ER formulation before determining needs with short-acting
	Assess for ongoing attainment of treatment goals, adverse effects, and safe and responsible medication use.
	Treatment not resulting in functional improvement should be tapered or discontinued and other options explored.
	Morphine sulfate equivalent dose (MS equiv) provided to use in converting from one opioid to another due to differences in opioid potency. MS equiv = dose of opioid equivalent to 10 mg of parenteral morphine or 30 mg of oral morphine with chronic dosing.

Step 3: Treatment of moderate to severe pain (score 4–10), pain not alleviated with nondrug interventions and medicine from Step 2, and severe enough to impact function and quality of life

Extended-release and long-acting opioids	Avoid if history of falls or concurrent benzodiazepine use.[BC]
	When opioids are indicated, ER products reduce dosing frequency and may be useful in adherence and in those with cognitive impairment.
	Given that the long-term use of opioids is not recommended unless clearly warranted, ER and LA opioids are less often used.
	FDA label indication for ER opioids for management of pain severe enough to require daily, around-the-clock, long-term opioid treatment and for which alternative options are inadequate.

Table 19.2 Continued

Drug Class and Dosing	Practical Considerations
	ER formulation should ONLY be used in opioid-tolerant patients (i.e., those taking at least 60 mg/day of oral morphine, 25 μg/hr of transdermal fentanyl, 30 mg/day of oral oxycodone, 8 mg/day of oral hydromorphone, 25 mg/day of oral oxymorphone, or an equianalgesic dosage of another opioid for ≥1 wk). For opioid-tolerant patients, calculate based on conversion factors. See product information for starting dose for ER products. *Note:* Conversion from any oral immediate-release opioid should be based on conversion ratios; start by administering 50% of calculated total daily dose of ER opioid, and titrate until adequate pain relief is achieved with tolerable adverse effects.
Methadone	Methadone is an option if other long-acting agents are not affordable but should be used with extreme caution and only with expertise and monitoring ability because of highly variable half-life, risk for dose accumulation, and high interpatient variability. Associated with prolonged QTc interval. Acceptable in renal insufficiency. Consult palliative care or pain service. For details on methadone prescribing and monitoring, see geriatricscareonline.org
Abuse-deterrent drugs	These products contain an opioid antagonist intended to decrease misuse and abuse. If the product is taken as intended and taken whole, analgesia is not affected. If the product is altered (e.g., chewed, crushed, dissolved), the opioid antagonist is released and can reverse the analgesic effect. See product information.
Rapid-acting opioids	Do not use in opioid-naïve patients. Use is for breakthrough pain in those on opioid treatment. May be used in oncology and palliative care. Consult package information and consult with palliative care or pain specialist.

ADR = adverse drug reaction; BC = Beer's Criteria; CKD = chronic kidney disease; CLBP = chronic low back pain; COX-2 = cyclooxygenase-2; Cr = creatinine; CrCl = creatinine clearance; CW = Choosing Wisely; ER = extended-release; FDA = US Food and Drug Administration; GI = gastrointestinal; HF = heart failure; HTN = hypertension; LA = long-acting; OA = osteoarthritis; OTC = over-the-counter; NSAID = nonsteroidal anti-inflammatory drug; PPI = proton pump inhibitor.

Adapted from: Reuben DB, Herr KA, Pacala JT, Pollock BG, Potter JF, Semla TP. Pain. In: Reuben DB, Herr KA, Pacala JT, Pollock BG, Potter JF, Semla TP, eds. *Geriatrics at your fingertips*. 20th ed. New York, NY: American Geriatrics Society, 2018:253–263.

Age-Related Physiologic Changes. Declines in function of organ systems affect pharmacokinetics (drug absorption, bioavailability, distribution, metabolism, and excretion) and pharmacodynamics (i.e., what the body does to the drug). Specifically, decreased hepatic blood flow affects first-pass metabolism, resulting in an increased amount of drug in the systemic circulation and placing the older adult at risk for adverse drug effects. Additionally, decreased renal function and benign prostatic hypertrophy impair excretion of drugs, also increasing risk for drug toxicity. Changes in body composition, fat-to-water ratio, organ function, gastrointestinal motility, and blood flow can increase or decrease sensitivity to medications and risk for adverse drug reactions. Frail and malnourished older adults may have lower albumin levels, affecting drugs that bind primarily to proteins.[12]

The effect of pharmacogenetics is less often considered in the treatment of pain in older adults. However, some ethnic groups may be more or less sensitive to medications, and when this occurs, they may need less or more pain medication and be more inclined to use culturally specific nondrug therapies. For example, because codeine is widely ineffective in relieving pain in many ethnic groups, it is not recommended in older adults. One issue, nonetheless, is the lack of research on genetic polymorphisms in older adults. Another issue to consider is the interaction between traditional or cultural therapies (e.g., Ayurveda or Traditional Chinese Medicine) and pharmacodynamics and pharmacogenetic variations.

Weight. Weight is an important factor in the dosing and adjustment of medications. Older adults who are undernourished or frail may be underweight and require lower doses. Older adults with nutrient absorption issues may be at increased risk for drug adverse effects. Resources are available to guide geriatric dosing,[25] but recommendations are often extrapolated from adult guidelines, given limited evidence in frail older adults.[6] Some suggest, however, starting with a 25 to 50% reduction in the adult dose.[26] The general principle of prescribing in older adults is "Start low (i.e., dosing), go slow (i.e., titration), but go (i.e., initiation/administration) and get to therapeutic goal (i.e., therapeutic evaluation)."

Pain Type, Severity, and Interference With Function. Nociceptive pain may be managed with nonopioids and opioids, while neuropathic or mixed pain types often require antidepressants or anticonvulsants. Pain severity and pain interference with function will determine whether the initial medication is nonopioid or opioid. In cases of severe pain that impair physical function, long-acting (extended/sustained release) opioids are used. More advanced delivery systems may be needed when pain is persistent and severe, such as neuraxial blocks, continuous infusions through patient-controlled analgesia systems, transdermal on-body injectors in older adults who are able to manage such systems, and neurostimulators.

Strategies to Reduce Medication Adverse Effects and Risk

All medications are associated with adverse effects, but incorporation of vigilant monitoring and preventive interventions can reduce the risk for bothersome side effects and adverse events and development of addiction or misuse.[27] This is especially important for older adults who have an increased affinity to adverse effects;

thus, risk-reduction strategies for the major types of medications used in pain management are essential.

Nonopioids. Acetaminophen and ibuprofen should be used with caution in those with liver impairment and chronic alcoholism. To prevent acetaminophen-induced liver, daily dosage should not exceed 3,000 mg in healthy older adults and 2,000 mg in frail older adults. Acetaminophen, rather than nonsteroidal anti-inflammatory drugs (NSAIDs), is also recommended for older adults with heart failure. In addition, liver function should be monitored regularly.

NSAIDs. While topical NSAIDs are associated with fewer adverse effects, systemic (oral) NSAIDs must be used with extreme caution and are not recommended as first-line treatments. One issue with oral NSAID therapy is the risk for gastrointestinal irritation and bleeding; therefore, evaluation should include history of heart failure, gastrointestinal ulcers and bleeding, renal disease, and concurrent use of anticoagulants or antiplatelets. Many NSAIDs are contraindicated in older adults, and the Beers Criteria list should be consulted for a full listing of these medications.[28] When NSAIDs are used, prophylactic measures for gastrointestinal protection should be implemented, and these include use of a proton pump inhibitor or misoprostol, time-limited NSAID use, and consumption with food, or use of a cyclooxygenase-2 selective NSAID instead of traditional NSAIDs.

Opioids. Careful selection and monitoring of opioid therapy is essential because older adults, particularly those with frailty and multiple morbidities, have an increased susceptibility to opioid-induced side and adverse effects, such as nausea and vomiting, constipation and impaction, and sedation and respiratory depression. The risk, however, varies with type and strength, dose, and frequency of administration and renal function. Select opioids may be inappropriate to use in older adults with renal impairment.

To prevent opioid-induced constipation prophylaxis, monitor for constipation using a standard bowel movement scale, maintain adequate hydration, encourage fiber-rich foods and supplements, prescribe a stool softener and mild laxative or increase dose of laxative, and encourage mobility and ambulation. When these methods are ineffective in preventing constipation, medications that target opioid-induced constipation, such as methylnaltrexone bromide or naloxegol, may be indicated.

Some older adults become overly sedated, whether owing to overmedication or sensitivity to the sedating properties of opioids. To monitor and counter opioid-induced sedation and respiratory depression, prescribe the lowest effective dose, monitor respiratory rate and sedation level, and incorporate capnography. Tolerance to sedative effects develops typically within a few days to a week. Decreasing dose, changing opioid medication, or administering an opioid antagonist may be indicated to reverse sedation and respiratory depression.

Many find it difficult to conceive of an older adult abusing opioid medications; however, a universal approach to preventing misuse of opioids that includes screening for risk, yearly drug urine test, establishing a monitoring program, and education on safe storage of medications may be appropriate. Risk Evaluation and Mitigation Strategies (REMS) established by the US Food and Drug Administration address education and approaches for use of long-acting or extended-release opioids.[27] Screens are available to assess risk for opioid misuse or abuse (e.g., Opioid Risk Tool [ORT]). Older adults with a history of substance misuse or abuse or who are at high risk for abuse may warrant opioids prepared in abuse-deterrent formulations in order to minimize misuse. Again, the safety and appropriateness of these medications must be determined before prescription.[28]

Education of patients and families about safe analgesic storage and disposal is important but frequently missed. For example, medications should not be placed on the windowsill because the sunlight could decrease their effectiveness. Moreover, keeping opioids in a secure space and ensuring proper disposal can help prevent theft by those who might misuse. A different issue is the growing number of older adults caring for young grandchildren, necessitating that medications are stored and disposed of properly. For example, a child may mistake a transdermal fentanyl patch for a sticker.

SUMMARY

Pain assessment and management are critical to the vitality and quality of life of older adults. Thorough assessment and deliberate individually tailored treatments can ensure effective pain relief in older adults. Healthcare provider collaboration with patients and families can minimize concerns and support development of a realistic treatment plan based on best practices, available resources, provider's clinical expertise, and patient and family/caregiver preferences.

REVIEW QUESTIONS

1. Major causes of pain in older adults include the following, *except*:
    a. Low back pain
    b. Knee pain
    c. Hip pain
    d. Peripheral neuropathy
    e. Hand pain

2. Pain scales may not work well for assessment of pain in patients with cognitive impairment or communication difficulties alternatives include the following, *except*:
    a. Behavioral assessment
    b. Functional assessment
    c. Pharmacologic assessment
    d. Physical exam
    e. Financial assessment

3. Factors that increase the risks of pharmacologic therapy in older adults can include the following, *except*:
    a. Difficulty opening pill bottles because of hand arthritis
    b. Decreased lean muscle mass
    c. Increase tendency toward risk-taking
    d. Decreased renal function
    e. Increased risks for falling

REFERENCES

1. Kennedy J, Roll JM, Schraudner T, McPherson S. Prevalence of persistent pain in the U.S. adult population: New data from the 2010 national health interview survey. J Pain. 2014;15(10):979–984.
2. Cole LJ, Farrell MJ, Gibson SJ, Egan GF. Age-related differences in pain sensitivity and regional brain activity evoked by noxious pressure. Neurobiol Aging. 2010;31(3):494–503.
3. Riley JL 3rd, Cruz-Almeida Y, Glover TL, et al. Age and race effects on pain sensitivity and modulation among middle-aged and older adults. J Pain. 2014;15(3):272–282.
4. Williams BA, Ahalt C, Stijacic-Cenzer I, et al. Pain behind bars: The epidemiology of pain in older jail inmates in a county jail. J Palliat Med. 2014;17(12):1336–1343.
5. Institute of Medicine. Relieving Pain in America: A Blueprint for Transforming Prevention, Care, Education, and Research. Washington, DC: National Academies Press; 2011.
6. American Geriatrics Society. Pharmacological management of persistent pain in older persons. J Am Geriatr Soc. 2009;57(8):1331–1346.
7. Boccio E, Wie B, Pasternak S, et al. The relationship between patient age and pain management of acute long-bone fracture in the ED. Am J Emerg Med. 2014;32(12):1516–1519.
8. Herr K. Pain assessment strategies in older patients. J Pain. 2011;12(3, Suppl 1):S3–S13.
9. Spillman SK, Baumhover LA, Lillegraven CL, et al. Infrequent assessment of pain in elderly trauma patients. J Trauma Nurs. 2014;21(5):229–235.
10. Hadjistavropoulos T, Herr K, Turk DC, et al. An interdisciplinary expert consensus statement on assessment of pain in older persons. Clin J Pain. 2007;23(1 Suppl):S1–S43.
11. Topham D, Drew D. Quality improvement project: replacing the numeric rating scale with a clinically aligned assessment (CAPA) tool. Pain Manag Nurs. 2017;18(6):363–371. doi: 10.1016/j.pmn.2017.07.001.
12. Ferrell BA. Acute and chronic pain. In: Cassel CK, Leipzig RM, Cohen HJ, Larson EB, Meier DE, eds. Geriatric Medicine: An Evidence-Based Approach (4th ed., pp. 323–340). New York: Springer, 2006.
13. Diallo B, Kautz DD. Better pain management for elders in the intensive care unit. Dimens Crit Care Nurs. 2014;33(6):316–319.
14. Lazkani A, Delespierre T, Bauduceau B, et al. Predicting falls in elderly patients with chronic pain and other chronic conditions. Aging Clin Exp Res. 2015;27(5):653–661.
15. Stubbs B, Schofield P, Binnekade T, et al. Pain is associated with recurrent falls in community-dwelling older adults: evidence from a systematic review and meta-analysis. Pain Med. 2014;15(7):1115–1128.
16. Shega JW, Paice JA, Rockwood K, Dale W. Is the presence of mild to moderate cognitive impairment associated with self-report of non-cancer pain? A cross-sectional analysis of a large population-based study. J Pain Symptom Manage. 2010;39(4):734–742.
17. Hadjistavropoulos T, Herr K, Prkachin KM, et al. Pain assessment in elderly adults with dementia. Lancet Neurol. 2014;13:1216–1227.
18. Berryman C, Stanton TR, Bowering KJ, et al. Do people with chronic pain have impaired executive function? A meta-analytical review. Clin Psychol Rev. 2014;34(7):563–579.
19. Hodgson N, Gitlin L, Winter L, Hauck WW. Caregiver's perceptions of the relationship of pain to behavioral and psychiatric symptoms in older community-residing adults with dementia. Clin J Pain. 2014;30(5):421–427.
20. Booker SQ, Bartoszczyk DA, Herr KA. Pain management in frail elders. Am Nurs Today. 2016;11(4):1–9.

21. McPherson CJ, Hadjistavropoulos T, Devereaux A, Lobchuk MM. A qualitative investigation of the roles and perspectives of older patients with advanced cancer and their family caregivers in managing pain in the home. BMC Palliat Care. 2014;13:39.
22. Platts-Mills TF, Esserman DA, Brown DL, et al. Older US emergency department patients are less likely to receive pain medication than younger patients: results from a national survey. Ann Emerg Med. 2012;60(2):199–206.
23. Lapane KL, Quilliam BJ, Chow W, Kim MS. Pharmacologic management of non-cancer pain among nursing home residents. J Pain Symptom Manage. 2013;45(1):33–42.
24. Booker SQ. Older African Americans' beliefs about pain, biomedicine, and spiritual medicine. J Christian Nurs. 2015;32(3):148–255.
25. Semla T, Belzer J, Higbee M. Geriatric Dosage Handbook (20th ed.). Hudson, OH: Lexicomp; 2015.
26. Reuben DB, Herr KA, Pacala JT, et al. Pain. In: Reuben DB, Herr KA, Pacala JT, et al., eds. Geriatrics at Your Fingertips (20th ed., pp. 247–268). New York: American Geriatrics Society; 2018.
27. Arnstein P, Keela H. Risk evaluation and mitigation strategies for older adults with persistent pain. J Gerontol Nurs. 2013;39(4):56–65.
28. American Geriatrics Society 2019 AGS Beers Criteria® for potentially inappropriate medication use in older adults. J Am Geriatr Soc. 2019;67(4):674–694. doi: 10.1111/jgs.15767
29. Buffum MD, Miaskowski C, Sands L, Brod M. A pilot study of the relationship between discomfort and agitation in patients with dementia. Geriatr Nurs. 2001;22(2):80–85.
30. Hadjistavropoulos T. Assessing pain in older persons with severe limitations in ability to communicate. In: Gibson SJ, Weiner DK, eds. *Pain in older persons* (Vol. 35, pp. 135–151). Seattle: IASP Press; 2005.
31. Herr K, Spratt KF, Garand L. Evaluation of the Iowa Pain Thermometer and other selected pain intensity scales in younger and older adult cohorts using controlled clinical pain: a preliminary study. Pain Med. 2007;8(7):585–600.
32. Ware LJ, Herr KA, Booker SS, et al. Psychometric evaluation of the revised Iowa Pain Thermometer (IPT-r) in a sample of cognitively intact and impaired diverse older adults: A pilot study. Pain Manage Nurs. 2015;16(4):475–482.
33. Herr KA, Bursch H, Ersek M, Miller LL, Swafford K. Use of pain-behavioral assessment tools in the nursing home: expert consensus recommendations for practice. J Gerontol Nurs. 2010;36(3):18–29.
34. Arnstein P. Pain assessment. In: Arnstein P. Clinical Coach for Effective Pain Management (pp. 63, 66). Philadelphia: FA Davis; 2010.

20 Opioid Misuse and Addiction Among Patients With Chronic Pain
From Risk Factors to Risk Reduction

Marc O. Martel and Robert N. Jamison

If you end up in an accident and in the hospital and they give you opioids for three days continuously, you will be physically dependent on the opioids; this is very different from addiction, and emerges very rapidly. I speak from experience. I was in a car accident and hospitalized and released with opioids. I didn't want to take them, so I went cold turkey and had physical withdrawal. The withdrawal was very disagreeable and forced me to take one of the pills even though I didn't want to. Addiction, on the other hand, takes much longer to develop. Not everyone getting the drugs will become addicted. A physician seeing that a patient with pain is starting to have symptoms of withdrawal may then describe that patient as addicted when they are not; they have *physical* dependence. And that leads to improper management.
—Nora Volkow MD, Director of the National Institute of Drug Abuse (June 6, 2018 interview with Ricki Rustig, *Knowable Magazine*)

LEARNING OBJECTIVES

At the completion of this chapter, the learner should be able to discuss:

- The terms tolerance, physical dependence, pseudoaddiction, opioid misuse, and opioid addiction

- The factors contributing to an increased risk for prescription opioid misuse and addiction
- Screening tools to identify patients at risk for opioid misuse or addiction

CASE SCENARIO

A 58-year-old former body builder is status post multiple lumbar surgeries and continues to suffer from daily, chronic severe low back pain. He is not a repeat surgical candidate. He has tried multiple interventional, medication, physical therapy, and alternative strategies. He has been taking morphine sustained-release 30 mg three times a day and morphine 15 mg every 6 hours as needed for the past few years. He is unable to work because of pain. He feels the medication helps him to be able to be social with his family and friends and take care of his daily activities. He presents for a prescription refill of his morphine and says he is out of his medication. He looks agitated, sweaty, and uncomfortable. You check the prescription monitoring program and notice that he presents 6 days before when his refills should be due.

1. How do you decide whether or not to fill his prescription early?
2. How can you assess if there is a concern for misuse of his medication?
3. How do you distinguish tolerance versus dependence versus addiction to opioids?
4. Should you fill his prescription early?
5. What role do prescribers play in contributing to rates of opioid addiction in North America and beyond?

INTRODUCTION

The use of opioids for the management of chronic noncancer pain has increased exponentially over the past few decades in North America. Despite the potential benefits of opioids, the rise in the use of opioids has been accompanied by escalating rates of prescription opioid misuse and addiction among patients with chronic pain. Opioid misuse and addiction may lead to numerous adverse consequences, including serious health problems, and may ultimately result in opioid-related overdose death. In this chapter, the prevalence of opioid misuse and addiction in patients with chronic pain will first be presented. The factors that contribute to an increased risk for prescription opioid misuse and addiction will then be discussed, and we will provide an overview of screening tools and strategies that can be used for the assessment and management of patients at risk for problematic opioid use. A brief definition of key terms that will be used in subsequent sections of this chapter is provided in Box 20.1.

PREVALENCE OF PRESCRIPTION OPIOID MISUSE AND ADDICTION

Rates of opioid misuse and addiction among patients with pain treated with opioids have long been assumed to be negligible because of a number of widely cited case reports and observational studies published during the 1980s, in which these problems were claimed to be very low or even nonexistent. Over the past few years, however, many authors have expressed skepticism toward these low estimates, and it is now

Box 20.1 Key Terms Relevant to Long-Term Opioid Therapy

Terms

Tolerance

State of physiologic adaptation manifested by a need for increasing opioid doses in order to maintain the same effects or analgesic benefits over time.

Physical dependence

State of adaptation manifested by physical withdrawal symptoms once opioids are discontinued.

Pseudoaddiction

Transient condition that occurs when patients exhibit drug-seeking behaviors in an attempt to obtain adequate pain relief. Drug-seeking behaviors usually disappear following dose increase.

Aberrant drug behaviors

Refers to a wide range of erratic behaviors exhibited by patients in relation to their prescribed medication. Some of these behaviors may include requesting early refills, losing prescriptions, or hoarding opioid medications. While aberrant drug behaviors may simply be due to error or misunderstanding, they may also be the reflection of more serious problems, such as opioid misuse, addiction, or diversion.

Opioid misuse

Refers to the use of opioids in a manner other than how they are indicated or prescribed. Opioid misuse, also sometimes termed "nonadherence," includes behaviors such as taking higher doses of opioids than prescribed, using opioids for symptoms other than pain (e.g., to improve mood or sleep), and using unsanctioned substances in addition to prescription opioids.

Opioid abuse

Refers to the use of opioids, without the supervision of a physician, for "recreational" or "nonmedical" purposes. A typical example would be an individual who occasionally takes prescription opioids provided by friends or family members solely to experience the pleasurable or euphoric effects of the opioid. The term "abuse" is less used in the medical field because of negative connotations of the term. "Opioid misuse," "opioid use disorder," and "opioid addiction" are more preferred terms.

Opioid use disorder (i.e., opioid addiction)

Refers to a problematic pattern of opioid use leading to clinically significant impairment or distress. The term "addiction" is not formally used for diagnostic purposes. However, it is commonly used when referring to patients meeting diagnostic criteria for an opioid use disorder (OUD). The specific OUD diagnostic criteria that were put forward by the American Psychiatric Association (APA) in the *Diagnostic and Statistical Manual of Mental Disorders* (DSM) are listed in Box 20.2.

well-acknowledged that early estimates of misuse and addiction were far too low. As pointed out by Sullivan,[1] one of the reasons these estimates were too low is that they were derived from unrepresentative populations of chronic pain patients treated with opioids. For instance, early estimates of opioid misuse or addiction were based on studies that excluded "high-risk" patients, such as those with mental health issues or past history of substance use problems. Studies conducted among patients with chronic pain indicate that up to 65% of patients meet diagnostic criteria for one (or more) comorbid psychiatric disorder, with mood disorders, anxiety disorders, and personality disorders being among the most prevalent.[2] Given that these patients are particularly likely to be prescribed opioids in real-life clinical scenarios, it is reasonable to argue that early studies yielded artificially low estimates of prescription opioid misuse and addiction.

To date, there are very few large-scale studies that have been conducted to reliably determine rates of addiction among patients with pain. While rates of aberrant drug behaviors and opioid misuse have been found to be up to 40 to 60% in primary and tertiary care settings,[3] much less is known about rates of opioid use disorder, (i.e. opioid addiction). The best evidence comes from a cross-sectional study conducted by Boscarino et al.,[4] who randomly selected 705 clinic patients and administered structured diagnostic interviews to assess opioid addiction. In this study, it was found that 35% of patients prescribed long-term opioid therapy met *Diagnostic and Statistical Manual of Mental Disorders, fifth edition* (DSM-V) criteria for an opioid use disorder, see Box 20.2). While uncertainty remains about the true rates of opioid use disorder (OUD) among patients with pain, another recent study has provided evidence that OUD may occur in up to 20% of chronic pain patients prescribed long-term opioid therapy.[5]

FACTORS CONTRIBUTING TO AN INCREASED RISK FOR PRESCRIPTION OPIOID MISUSE AND OPIOID USE DISORDER

In the literature and the media, it is often implied that problems such as opioid misuse and OUD are directly caused by the "addictive potential" of opioids. In the 2016 Surgeon General's Report on Alcohol, Drugs and Health, "Facing Addiction in America," it was reported that four out of five new heroin users started with misusing prescription opioid medications. It is pivotal to understand, however, that the determinants of opioid misuse and OUD rest with the user and that many patient-specific factors may increase susceptibility to these problems. The following is an overview of the demographic, psychological, and neurobiological factors known to be associated with an increased risk for opioid misuse and OUD among patients with chronic pain prescribed opioids.

Demographic and Background Factors

Chronic pain patients at increased risk for opioid misuse and/or OUD include those who are (1) younger, (2) single, (3) less educated, and (4) unemployed and those with (5) a personal or family history of substance use problems, such as smoking, heavy drinking, or illicit drug use. Patients with a history of (6) sexual or physical abuse,

> **Box 20.2** DSM-V Diagnostic Criteria for Opioid Use Disorder (i.e., Opioid Addiction)
>
> **DSM-V Diagnostic Criteria**
>
> A problematic pattern of opioid use leading to clinically significant impairment or distress, as manifested by at least two of the following, occurring within a 12-month period:
>
> 1. Opioids are often taken in larger amounts or over a longer period than was intended.
> 2. There is a persistent desire or unsuccessful efforts to cut down or control opioid use.
> 3. A great deal of time is spent in activities necessary to obtain the opioid, use the opioid, or recover from its effects.
> 4. Craving, or a strong desire or urge to use opioids
> 5. Recurrent opioid use resulting in a failure to fulfill major role obligations at work, school, or home.
> 6. Continued opioid use despite having persistent or recurrent social or interpersonal problems caused or exacerbated by the effects of opioids
> 7. Important social, occupational, or recreational activities are given up or reduced because of opioid use.
> 8. Recurrent opioid use in situations in which it is physically hazardous
> 9. Continued opioid use despite knowledge of having a persistent of recurrent physical or psychological problem that is likely to have been caused or exacerbated by the substance
> 10. Opioid tolerance
> 11. Opioid withdrawal
>
> *Note: Opioid tolerance and withdrawal criteria are not considered for individuals taking opioids under appropriate medical supervision. Specify current severity: mild—presence of two or three symptoms; moderate—presence of four or five symptoms; severe: presence of six or more symptoms.*
>
> *From the Diagnostic and Statistical Manual of Mental Disorders, fifth edition (DSM-5). Arlington, VA: American Psychiatric Association; 2013.*

(7) criminal or legal problems, and (8) risk-taking or thrill-seeking behaviors and (9) who are in frequent contact with high-risk individuals or environments are also at increased risk for opioid misuse and OUD.[3,6]

Psychological Factors and Psychiatric Illness

As noted earlier, psychological disturbances and psychiatric disorders are known to be highly prevalent among patients with chronic pain. While a few recent studies have found that personality disorders are associated with an increased risk for prescription opioid misuse,[7,8] the most consistent finding that has emerged from previous studies among patients with pain is the association between symptoms of anxiety and depression (i.e., negative affect) and prescription opioid misuse. Findings from several previous studies have indicated that patients with high levels of negative affect are two to three times more likely to misuse prescription opioids than patients with low levels of negative affect.[9-11] Symptoms of negative affect have also been found to be associated with an increased likelihood of meeting criteria for an opioid use disorder.[12,13] Among patients with pain, other psychological factors have also been found to be associated with an increased risk for prescription opioid misuse and/or OUD, including catastrophizing, somatization, and low self-efficacy. These psychological factors are discussed in Chapter 5.

POTENTIAL PSYCHOLOGICAL FACTORS LINKING NEGATIVE AFFECT TO PROBLEMATIC OPIOID USE

Although the elevated rates of opioid misuse and OUD among patients with high negative affect have been well-documented, the specific factors linking negative affect to problematic opioid use remain elusive. Research and theory suggests that a number of psychological and biological factors might contribute to explaining the elevated rates of opioid misuse and OUD observed among chronic pain patients with high negative affect.

Preexisting Personality Traits

There is reason to believe that patients with high negative affect hold preexisting personality traits that make them prone to misusing opioids or to developing disordered use of opioid medications. For example, some studies have found that individuals with high negative affect are characterized by heightened impulsivity and sensation seeking, two personality traits that have consistently been identified as risk factors for various types of substance use problems.[14]

Self-Medication

The self-medication hypothesis, which was proposed by Khantzian,[15] suggests that certain individuals tend to use medication and other substances to self-medicate their symptoms or to alleviate their problems. Based on this theory, one may speculate that chronic pain patients high in negative affect take higher doses of opioids than prescribed in order to improve their mood, to alleviate their anxiety, or to cope with their pain. Passik[16] used the term "chemical copers" to describe chronic pain patients having a limited repertoire of coping strategies and a tendency to misuse their medications as a way to cope with pain-related distress.

Opioid Craving

Findings from recent studies suggest that opioid craving might also be responsible, in part, for the association between negative affect and problematic opioid use. The concept of craving, which refers to the subjective desire to consume certain substances, has long been invoked in the substance use literature to explain the development and persistence of problems such as alcoholism, smoking, and illicit drug use. Among patients with chronic pain prescribed long-term opioid therapy, negative affect has been associated with heightened reports of opioid craving,[17,18] and craving has been associated with various indices of misuse, including patient reports of opioid misuse,[17,19] physician ratings of opioid misuse behaviors,[18] and abnormal urine toxicology screens.[18,20] In a recent study,[17] opioid craving was found to mediate the association between negative affect and opioid misuse, which suggests that craving might contribute to explaining the increased rates of prescription opioid misuse observed among patients with high levels of negative affect.

POTENTIAL NEUROBIOLOGICAL FACTORS CONTRIBUTING TO PROBLEMATIC OPIOID USE AMONG PATIENTS WITH PSYCHOLOGICAL OR PSYCHIATRIC PROBLEMS

A number of neurobiological factors might contribute to explaining why patients with psychological or psychiatric problems are at increased risk for prescription opioid misuse and OUD. To date, much of our thinking about the neurobiological bases of opioid misuse and addiction in patients with pain derives from basic science research conducted within the field of substance use disorders. It is now firmly established that opioids, like any other drug of abuse, stimulate the release of dopamine within mesocorticolimbic brain pathways, also known as the "reward system," which is primarily subserved by the nucleus accumbens, the ventral tegmentum, the amygdala, the prefrontal cortex, and the anterior cingulate cortex. Dopaminergic activity within mesocorticolimbic pathways has the potential to produce rewarding effects (e.g., euphoria) that may, in some individuals, contribute to reinforcing the use of opioids. Interestingly, some of the key brain regions subserving the reward system receive direct projections from higher order cortical areas involved in the regulation of mood and anxiety,[21] providing a neural basis for the influence of psychological factors on reward processing and the perceived rewarding effects of opioids.

There are other mechanisms beyond the dopaminergic reward system, however, that are likely to account for opioid misuse and addictive behaviors among patients with psychological or psychiatric problems. For example, there is a vast preclinical and clinical literature indicating that repeated opioid use may cause alterations in opioidergic[22] and noradrenergic[23] function. These two neurotransmitter systems are known to play a key role in the pathophysiology of depression and anxiety, which might contribute to explaining the high prevalence of these psychological problems among long-term opioid users. Other studies suggest that abnormalities in serotonergic function might also contribute to explaining why patients with psychological or psychiatric problems are at increased risk for problematic opioid use.

IDENTIFYING PATIENTS "AT RISK" FOR PRESCRIPTION OPIOID MISUSE OR OPIOID USE DISORDER BEFORE INITIATION OF OPIOID THERAPY

Over the past few years, several professional and regulatory organizations have released recommendations and guidelines related to the use of opioids among patients with chronic pain.[24–26] Although certain differences exist across guidelines, they all clearly emphasize the importance of opioid risk assessment before initiation of long-term opioid therapy. In addition to performing a thorough medical history, a review of past medical records, and a medical examination, it is recommended to conduct an opioid risk assessment using validated screening tools. Some of the most common include the Screener and Opioid Assessment for Patients With Pain—Revised (SOAPP-R[20]), the Opioid Risk Tool (ORT[11]), the Diagnosis, Intractability, Risk, and Efficacy (DIRE[27]) scale, and the Screening Instrument for Substance Abuse Potential (SISAP[28]). Scores on any of these tools are not necessarily a reason to deny opioids; rather, they allow clinicians to identify patients who might need close monitoring over the course of therapy in order to minimize the likelihood of opioid misuse and opioid use disorder. A brief description of these tools and their characteristics is provided in Table 20.1.

IDENTIFYING PATIENTS WHO ARE MISUSING OPIOIDS OVER THE COURSE OF OPIOID THERAPY

A number of tools have been developed to identify patients who are misusing opioids over the course of opioid therapy. These tools are grouped into three categories: (1) standardized self-report questionnaires, (2) clinician-based measures, and (3) urine toxicology screening (UTS). As can be seen in Table 20.2A, some of the most common *self-report questionnaires* used to assess opioid misuse include the Current Opioid Misuse Measure (COMM[29]), the Pain Medication Questionnaire (PMQ[30]), and the Prescription Drug Use Questionnaire—patient version (PDUQ-p[31]). *Clinician-based measures* include questionnaires and checklists completed by clinicians, such as the Pain Assessment and Documentation Tool (PADT[32]), the Addiction Behavior Checklist (ABC[33]), and the Opioid Compliance Checklist (OCC[34]). Although less reliable, clinicians may also use pill counts and direct observations of aberrant drug behaviors in order to identify patients who might be misusing opioids. Finally, UTS can be used by clinicians in order to determine whether patients have misused their prescribed opioid medication. UTS can be particularly helpful to identify the presence and quantities of prescription medications and illegal substances and/or the absence of prescribed medications. However, given that UTS is potentially prone to error, the interpretation of UTS results and inferences about opioid misuse should be made while considering patients' overall behavioral patterns and other relevant contextual information.

Although the use of opioid-specific instruments is recommended for identifying patients who are misusing opioids over the course of opioid therapy, other instruments can also be used to monitor opioid misuse. For instance, as can be seen from Table 20.2B, a number of "generic" instruments can be used in order to rapidly screen and/or identify patients with any type of substance use problems. Some of the most commonly used generic instruments include the Drug Abuse Screening Test (DAST-10[35]), the Drug Use Disorders Identification Test (DUDIT[36]), and the CAGE-AID (Brown and Rounds, 1995).* Although these instruments were not specifically developed and validated for patients with chronic pain, they have proved useful in clinical and research settings for the identification of patients with substance use problems. However, similar to the opioid-specific instruments that were described in previous sections (e.g., COMM, OCC), scores on these instruments cannot be used for diagnostic purposes,

---

* Brown RL, Rounds LA. Conjoint screening questionnaires for alcohol and other drug abuse: criterion validity in a primary care practice. Wis Med J. 1995;94(3):135–140.

Table 20.1 Instruments for the Identification/Screening of Patients at Risk for Prescription Opioid Misuse or Addiction

Name	Description	Scoring
Screener and Opioid Assessment for Patients with Pain—Revised (SOAPP-R[37])	• Completed by the patient • 24-item questionnaire • Items designed to capture eight domains, including substance abuse history, psychiatric history, criminal history, medication-related behaviors, doctor–patient relationship, emotional attachment to pain medications, personal care and lifestyle issues, and psychosocial problems	• Any individual who scores 18 or more on the SOAPP-R is considered to be at risk for opioid misuse
Opioid Risk Tool (ORT[31])	• Completed by the clinician • Five-item questionnaire • Items designed to capture patients' background characteristics and psychiatric history	• Scores suggesting risk for misuse or addiction: 0–3 = low risk 4–7 = moderate risk ≥8 = high risk
Diagnosis, Intractability, Risk, and Efficacy (DIRE[35])	• Completed by the clinician • Seven-item checklist designed to predict future opioid-related outcomes and compliance during opioid therapy • Items capture four domains: diagnosis, intractability, efficacy, and risk. Four sub-domains of risk are assessed (psychological, chemical, reliability, social support).	• Scores: ≤13 = unsuitable candidate for opioid therapy ≥14 = good candidate for opioid therapy
Screening Instrument for Substance Abuse Potential (SISAP[1])	• Completed by the clinician • Five-item telephone interview • Items designed to capture patients' substance abuse history	• A positive answer to any of the SISAP questions suggests risk for opioid misuse and need for further assessment

Note: Recent opioid treatment guidelines jointly released by the American Pain Society (APS) and American Academy of Pain Medicine (AAPM) consider all these tools as having good content, construct, and face validity.[24]

Table 20.2A Opioid-Specific Instruments for Identifying Patients Who Might Be Misusing Opioids Over the Course of Therapy

Name	Description	Scoring
Current Opioid Misuse Measure (COMM[7])	• Completed by the patient • 17-item questionnaire designed to assess various types of opioid misuse and aberrant drug behaviors	• A score of ≥9 is used as a cutoff suggesting potential opioid misuse or aberrant drug behaviors
Pain Medication Questionnaire (PMQ[3])	• Completed by the patient • 26 items designed to assess various types of opioid misuse and aberrant drug behaviors	• Higher scores suggest greater likelihood of opioid misuse and/or aberrant drug behaviors
Prescription Drug Use Questionnaire—Patient version (PDUQ-p[14])	• Completed by the patient • 31-item questionnaire designed to assess behaviors indicative of opioid abuse or dependence.	• A score >10 suggests potential opioid use disorder (i.e., abuse or dependence).
Pain Assessment and Documentation Tool (PADT[21])	• Completed by the clinician • 41-item checklist designed to assess/monitor opioid-related outcomes and compliance over the course of therapy	• No cutoff score; PADT used for documentation purposes only
Addiction Behavior Checklist (ABC[10])	• Completed by the clinician • 20-item checklist designed to assess various types of opioid misuse and aberrant drug behaviors as well as behaviors characteristic of addiction related to prescription opioid medications in chronic pain populations	• A score of ≥3 suggests ongoing problematic opioid use and potential prescription opioid addiction. Further assessment needed.
Opioid Compliance Checklist (OCC[19])	• Completed by the patient • Five-item questionnaire to assess opioid compliance	• A positive answer to any of the OCC items suggests ongoing opioid misuse

Table 20.2B Generic Instruments for Identifying Patients at Risk for Substance Use Disorders

Name	Description	Scoring
Drug Abuse Screening Test (DAST-10)	• Self-administered or administered by a trained interviewer • 10 items • Includes yes/no questions about illicit and prescription drug use over the past 12 months. Does not include problems associated with alcohol or tobacco use.	• 1–2 (Low): Monitor and reassess later • 3–5 (Moderate): Further investigation needed • 6–8 (Substantial): Intensive assessment needed • 9–10 (Severe): Intensive assessment needed
Drug Use Disorders Identification Test (DUDIT)	• Self-report questionnaire • 11 items • Designed to screen for drug-related problems. Items are based on the ICD-10 and DSM-IV diagnostic systems for substance abuse and dependence.	• Probable substance use disorder when score >6 for men and >2 for women
CAGE-AID (Brown et al., 1995)	• Self-report questionnaire • Four items • Designed to screen for drug and alcohol problems	• One (or more) positive score on the CAGE-AID requires further evaluation

DSM-IV = Diagnostic and Statistical Manual of Mental Disorders, fourth edition; ICD-10 = International Classification of Disease, tenth revision.

and additional steps must be taken to diagnose patients with a prescription drug use disorder (i.e., prescription drug addiction).

IDENTIFYING PATIENTS WITH OPIOID USE DISORDER IN ASSOCIATION WITH PRESCRIPTION OPIOIDS

While the tools described previously may be useful for identifying patients who are misusing opioids over the course of therapy, the diagnosis of OUD can only be performed based on a clinical interview administered by a trained clinician. The diagnosis of OUD has traditionally been based on the diagnostic criteria put forward by the American Psychiatric Association in the DSM. These criteria, however, have been criticized by many clinicians and researchers within the field of pain. For example, based on the DSM-IV, patients meeting criteria either for "opioid abuse" or "opioid dependence" were diagnosed with an opioid use disorder, and the blurred distinction between these two diagnoses created confusion for many clinicians. More important, only three criteria were needed to diagnose patients with opioid dependence based on the DSM-IV, and two of these criteria could include opioid tolerance and opioid withdrawal. Given that most patients are expected to show tolerance and/or withdrawal as a result of long-term opioid therapy, DSM-IV criteria were not considered suitable for patients with chronic pain prescribed opioids because they could lead to erroneous (i.e., false-positive) diagnosis of opioid use disorder. Because of these criticisms, modifications were made in the fifth version of the DSM (DSM-V) that was published in 2013 for the diagnosis of opioid addiction. In the DSM-V, the distinction between opioid abuse and opioid dependence was abandoned, and diagnostic criteria from these two diagnoses are now combined to form a single disorder (i.e., opioid use disorder) of graded severity (i.e., mild, moderate, severe). Moreover, tolerance and withdrawal symptoms are no longer considered to be diagnostic criteria for individuals taking opioids (or any other substance) under medical supervision. The complete list of DSM-V criteria used for the diagnosis of opioid use disorder can be found in Box 20.2.

MANAGEMENT OF PATIENTS KNOWN TO BE AT RISK FOR OPIOID MISUSE OR OUD

As discussed earlier, patients identified to be at risk for opioid misuse or OUD should not be necessarily denied access to opioid treatment. However, opioid treatment guidelines offer a number of strategies and recommendations in order to minimize the likelihood of problematic opioid use in these patients. Some key elements of these guidelines include (1) documenting patients' baseline risk profile and (2) obtaining a signed opioid treatment agreement from patients before initiating opioid therapy. When patients sign the opioid treatment agreement, they consent to the proposed opioid treatment plan and agree to be compliant to the specific conditions and responsibilities set by the clinic. After opioid therapy is initiated, (3) assessment of opioid effectiveness and (4) monitoring of patient compliance with treatment should be performed periodically. Those at highest risk should be monitored regularly (e.g., on a weekly or monthly basis) because early recognition of opioid misuse and aberrant drug behaviors may prevent the development of more serious opioid misuse behaviors and the progression toward addiction. As discussed previously, monitoring of opioid misuse and/or patient compliance can be performed through the use of self-report measures, prescription drug monitoring programs, or UTS.

MANAGEMENT OF CHRONIC PAIN PATIENTS WHO SHOW SIGNS OF OPIOID MISUSE OR OUD OVER THE COURSE OF OPIOID THERAPY

As previously discussed, rates of opioid misuse and aberrant drug-related behaviors have been found to be fairly high among patients with chronic pain prescribed opioids. Unfortunately, patients who misuse opioids or show aberrant drug behaviors are often discharged from clinics, even when opioids represent the only viable option for managing their pain. While the management of patients with problematic opioid use may be challenging, there is general agreement that tightening the structure of care and other aspects of opioid treatment can be effective for managing these patients. For instance, developing a new treatment plan with clear treatment goals and asking patients to sign a new opioid treatment agreement are recommended to ensure patients know exactly what is expected of them. The structure of care may also be tightened by requesting more frequent clinic visits and by implementing more intense monitoring strategies. Finally, changing the frequency of opioid supply as well as the quantity of opioids released to patients may also be considered.

In the context of multidisciplinary care, clinical psychologists as well as other trained mental health professionals may be useful to help manage chronic pain patients with problematic opioid use. Input from psychologists may be particularly helpful when patients present with psychological features or psychiatric comorbidities that contribute to opioid misuse or behaviors reflective of substance use disorders. For example, cognitive behavioral interventions may be used to help patients manage mood and anxiety symptoms, which, in turn, may contribute to reducing problematic opioid use. Adjunct psychological interventions may also help patients cope with opioid cravings and urges to misuse opioids and may be used to enhance patients' motivation to adhere to the opioid treatment plan. While the potential benefits of psychological interventions for patients with other types of substance use problems have been recognized for decades, there is preliminary evidence indicating that brief cognitive behavioral interventions involving substance misuse education, problem-solving, coping skills training, and motivational counseling may be effective in reducing opioid misuse among high-risk chronic pain patients prescribed long-term opioid therapy.[37] While further clinical treatment research is needed in this area, there is reason to believe that improving prescription opioid compliance among high-risk patients is feasible and that adjunct psychological interventions may contribute to reducing the number of patients being discharged from clinics because of problematic opioid use.

Despite the number of tools and management strategies available to clinicians to manage patients with disordered use of prescription opioid medications, experience tells us that some patients will continue to deviate from the treatment plan and persist in misusing prescription opioids. After repeated violations of the opioid treatment agreement, it may be appropriate to discontinue opioid therapy. If patients have become physically dependent on opioids, they should be tapered off their medication gradually to mitigate the severity of opioid withdrawal. If opioid use disorder is suspected, assessment by an substance use disorder (i.e., addiction) specialist and/or mental health professional should be mandated.

As recommended by the Centers for Disease Control and Prevention (CDC)guidelines for opioid prescribing,[26] medication-assisted treatment with buprenorphine or methadone (in combination with behavioral therapies) should be offered to patients diagnosed with an opioid use disorder. If needed, opioid detoxification in a specialized inpatient or outpatient setting may be considered, but detoxification *alone* is neither the standard of care nor supported by evidence for the management of chronic pain in patients with OUD receiving prescription opioid treatment.

SUMMARY

The use of opioids for the management of chronic noncancer pain has increased substantially over the past two decades in North America. Despite the potential benefits of opioids, concerns have been raised regarding the potential consequences of opioid therapy, including opioid misuse, opioid use disorder, and overdose. Evidence indicates that rates of opioid misuse and OUD are fairly high among chronic pain patients prescribed long-term opioid therapy, but there is consensus that opioids can be safe and effective for carefully selected and monitored patients. Opioid risk assessment, using validated screening tools, is recommended for all patients who are being considered for long-term opioid therapy. For high-risk patients, such as those with high negative affect or psychiatric illness, the structure of opioid therapy may include intensive monitoring, and co-management with healthcare professionals specialized in addiction medicine or mental health may be necessary. While the nature and structure of therapy will vary from patient to patient, close attention to screening, monitoring, and documentation of opioid treatment outcomes will continue to be the gold standard of opioid therapy.

REVIEW QUESTIONS

1. Screening tools for opioid misuse or opioid use disorder in a patient prescribed opioid medications include all of the following, *except*:
   a. Opioid Risk Tool (ORT)
   b. Current Opioid Misuse Measure (COMM)
   c. Addiction Behavior Checklist (ABC)
   d. Drug Abuse Screening Test-10 (DAST-10)
   e. Prescription Drug Use Questionnaire (PDUQ)

2. Risk factors for opioid misuse include all of the following, *except*:
   a. Negative affect
   b. Report of medication withdrawal symptoms
   c. Family history of alcohol use disorder
   d. Young age
   e. Depression and anxiety

REFERENCES

1. Sullivan M. Clarifying opioid misuse and abuse. Pain. 2013;154:2239–2240.
2. Dersh J, Gatchel RJ, Mayer T, Polatin P, Temple OR. Prevalence of psychiatric disorders in patients with chronic disabling occupational spinal disorders. Spine. 2006;31:1156–1162.
3. Turk DC, Swanson KS, Gatchel RJ. Predicting opioid misuse by chronic pain patients: a systematic review and literature synthesis. Clin J Pain. 2008;24:497–508.
4. Boscarino JA, Rukstalis MR, Hoffman SN, et al. Prevalence of prescription opioid-use disorder among chronic pain patients: comparison of the DSM-5 vs. DSM-4 diagnostic criteria. J Addict Dis. 2011;30:185–194.
5. Hojsted J, Nielsen PR, Guldstrand SK, Frich L, Sjogren P. Classification and identification of opioid addiction in chronic pain patients. Eur J Pain. 2010;14:1014–1020.
6. Jamison RN, Edwards RR. Risk factor assessment for problematic use of opioids for chronic pain. Clin Neuropsychol. 2013;27:60–80.
7. Tragesser SL, Jones RE, Robinson RJ, Stutler A, Stewart A. Borderline personality disorder features and risk for prescription opioid use disorders. J Pers Disord. 2013;27:427–441.
8. Wilsey BL, Fishman SM, Tsodikov A, et al. Psychological comorbidities predicting prescription opioid abuse among patients in chronic pain presenting to the emergency department. Pain Med. 2008;9:1107–1117.
9. Edlund MJ, Sullivan M, Steffick D, Harris KM, Wells KB. Do users of regularly prescribed opioids have higher rates of substance use problems than nonusers? Pain Med. 2007;8:647–656.
10. Wasan AD, Butler SF, Budman SH, et al. Psychiatric history and psychologic adjustment as risk factors for aberrant drug-related behavior among patients with chronic pain. Clin J Pain. 2007;23:307–315.
11. Webster LR, Webster RM. Predicting aberrant behaviors in opioid-treated patients: preliminary validation of the Opioid Risk Tool. Pain Med. 2005;6:432–442.
12. Boscarino JA, Rukstalis M, Hoffman SN, et al. Risk factors for drug dependence among out-patients on opioid therapy in a large US health-care system. Addiction. 2010;105:1776–1782.
13. Edlund MJ, Sullivan MD, Han X, Booth BM. Days with pain and substance use disorders: is there an association? Clin J Pain. 2013;29:689–695.
14. Verdejo-Garcia A, Lawrence AJ, Clark L. Impulsivity as a vulnerability marker for substance-use disorders: review of findings from high-risk research, problem gamblers and genetic association studies. Neurosci Biobehav Rev. 2008;32:777–810.
15. Khantzian EJ. The self-medication hypothesis of addictive disorders: focus on heroin and cocaine dependence. Am J Psychiatry. 1985;142:1259–1264.
16. Passik SD, Lowery A. Psychological variables potentially implicated in opioid-related mortality as observed in clinical practice. Pain Med. 2011;12(Suppl 2):S36–42.
17. Martel MO, Dolman AJ, Edwards RR, Jamison RN, Wasan AD. The association between negative affect and prescription opioid misuse in patients with chronic pain: the mediating role of opioid craving. J Pain. 2014;15:90–100.
18. Wasan AD, Ross EL, Michna E, et al. Craving of prescription opioids in patients with chronic pain: a longitudinal outcomes trial. J Pain. 2012;13:146–154.
19. Wasan AD, Butler SF, Budman SH, et al. Does report of craving opioid medication predict aberrant drug behavior among chronic pain patients? Clin J Pain. 2009;25:193–198.

20. Butler SF, Fernandez K, Benoit C, Budman SH, Jamison RN. Validation of the revised Screener and Opioid Assessment for Patients with Pain (SOAPP-R). J Pain. 2008;9:360–372.
21. Volkow ND, Wang GJ, Fowler JS, Tomasi D. Addiction circuitry in the human brain. Annu Rev Pharmacol Toxicol. 2012;52:321–336.
22. Christie MJ. Cellular neuroadaptations to chronic opioids: tolerance, withdrawal and addiction. Br J Pharmacol. 2008;154:384–396.
23. Koob GF. Brain stress systems in the amygdala and addiction. Brain Res. 2009;1293:61–75.
24. Chou R, Fanciullo GJ, Fine PG, et al. Clinical guidelines for the use of chronic opioid therapy in chronic noncancer pain. J Pain. 2009;10:113–130.
25. Dowell D, Haegerich TM, Chou R. CDC guideline for prescribing opioids for chronic pain—United States, 2016. JAMA. 2016;315:1624–1645.
26. Furlan AD, Reardon R, Weppler C. Opioids for chronic noncancer pain: a new Canadian practice guideline. CMAJ. 2010;182:923–930.
27. Belgrade MJ, Schamber CD, Lindgren BR. The DIRE score: predicting outcomes of opioid prescribing for chronic pain. J Pain. 2006;7:671–681.
28. Coambs RE, Jarry JL, Santhiapillai AC, Abrahamsohn RV, Atance CM. The SISAP: a new screening instrument for identifying potential opioid abusers in the management of chronic nonmalignant pain in general medical practice. Pain Res Manage. 1996;1:155–162.
29. Butler SF, Budman SH, Fernandez KC, et al. Development and validation of the Current Opioid Misuse Measure. Pain. 130:144–156, 2007
30. Adams LL, Gatchel RJ, Robinson RC, et al. Development of a self-report screening instrument for assessing potential opioid medication misuse in chronic pain patients. J Pain Symptom Manage. 2004;27:440–459.
31. Compton PA, Wu SM, Schieffer B, Pham Q, Naliboff BD. Introduction of a self-report version of the Prescription Drug Use Questionnaire and relationship to medication agreement noncompliance. J Pain Symptom Manage. 2008;36:383–395.
32. Passik SD, Kirsh KL, Whitcomb L, et al. A new tool to assess and document pain outcomes in chronic pain patients receiving opioid therapy. Clin Ther. 2004;26:552–561.
33. Wu SM, Compton P, Bolus R, et al. The addiction behaviors checklist: validation of a new clinician-based measure of inappropriate opioid use in chronic pain. J Pain Sympt Manage. 2006;32:342–351.
34. Jamison RN, Martel MO, Edwards RR, et al. Validation of a brief opioid compliance checklist for patients with chronic pain. J Pain. 2014;15(11):1092–1101.
35. Skinner HA. The drug abuse screening test. Addict Behav. 1982;7:363–371.
36. Berman AH, Palmstierna T, Kallmen H, Bergman H. The self-report Drug Use Disorders Identification Test: Extended (DUDIT-E): reliability, validity, and motivational index. J Subst Abuse Treat. 2007;32:357–369.
37. Jamison RN, Ross EL, Michna E, et al. Substance misuse treatment for high-risk chronic pain patients on opioid therapy: a randomized trial. Pain. 2010;150:390–400.

Appendix I
Examination Template

GENERAL APPEARANCE: Neat and clean, cooperative   casually attired   unkempt   uncooperative

MOOD: Pleasant   upbeat   sad   irritable   angry   frustrated   briefly tearful w/sad things   labile   unconcerned

MENTAL STATUS:

Awake and alert   sleepy   somnolent   inattentive   unaware   distractible

Oriented to place and time: (note)

Fund of knowledge: **Excellent**   Very good   Good   Fair   Poor

Repetition: **intact**   poor

Follows commands: **Crossed body**   **3 step**   Lateralizing   Midline psychomotor slowing

Language: fluent   dysarthric   slurred   paraphasic errors   word finding

Recall: **3/3 at 5'**   __/3 at 5'   **Naming:**   **intact**   reduced

Parts naming: **intact**   reduced absent

CRANIAL NERVES:

PRRL: ___ => ___ mm   irregular   non-reactive   s/p cataract removal   pinpoint dilated

VFF to FC s ext.   (R) hemi   quadr.   (L) hemi   quadr.

EOMI   no nystagmus   (R) fine coarse   (L) fine coarse   INO ( )   IV ( )   VI ( )

Face symmetrical to LT   RV1 ↓↑   RV2 ↓↑   RV3 ↓↑   LV1 ↓↑   LV2 ↓↑   LV3 ↓↑

Face symm. to sharp   RV1 ↓↑   RV2 ↓↑   RV3 ↓↑   LV1 ↓↑   LV2 ↓↑   LV3 ↓↑

Face moves well to e.c.   R ptosis   L ptosis   R weak   L weak

Face moves well to show teeth   R weak   L weak   R NLF flat.   L NLF flat.

Hearing symmetrical to finger rub   R decreased   L decreased   HOH

Palate: elevates symmetrically   R down   L down   R dec. move.   L dec. move.

Tongue: protrudes midline, moves well   points right   points left   weak   fascics.

Shoulder shrug   **R**   5   5-   4+   **L**   5   5-   4+

Neck: flexion   5   5-   4+   **extension**   5   5-   4+

RIGHT	Delt	Bi	Tri	WE	ADV	FDI	APB	SLR IP	NI Q	R: H	DF	L: PF	EHL		
	5	5	5	5	5	5	5	5	5	5	5	5	5	5	5
	5–	5–	5–	5–	5–	5–	5–	5–	5–	5–	5–	5–	5–	5–	5–
	4+	4+	4+	4+	4+	4+	4+	4+	4+	4+	4+	4+	4+	4+	4+
	4–	4–	4–	4–	4–	4–	4–	4–	4–	4–	4–	4–	4–	4–	4–
	+3–	+3–	+3–	+3–	+3–	+3–	+3–	+3–	+3–	+3–	+3–	+3–	+3–	+3–	+3–
	+2–	+2–	+2–	+2–	+2–	+2–	+2–	+2–	+2–	+2–	+2–	+2–	+2–	+2–	+2–
	10	10	10	10	10	10	10	10	10	10	10	10	10	10	10

LEFT	Delt	Bi	Tri	WE	ADV	FDI	APB	IP	Q	H	DF	PF	EHL		
	5	5	5	5	5	5	5	5	5	5	5	5	5	5	5
	5–	5–	5–	5–	5–	5–	5–	5–	5–	5–	5–	5–	5–	5–	5–
	4+	4+	4+	4+	4+	4+	4+	4+	4+	4+	4+	4+	4+	4+	4+
	4–	4–	4–	4–	4–	4–	4–	4–	4–	4–	4–	4–	4–	4–	4–
	+3–	+3–	+3–	+3–	+3–	+3–	+3–	+3–	+3–	+3–	+3–	+3–	+3–	+3–	+3–
	+2–	+2–	+2–	+2–	+2–	+2–	+2–	+2–	+2–	+2–	+2–	+2–	+2–	+2–	+2–
	10	10	10	10	10	10	10	10	10	10	10	10	10	10	10

MOTOR EXAM

Tone: Nl Inc. Dec. Flaccid **Bulk: Nl** Decreased: generally
focally (see below) **Pronator: no** (R) (L)

SENSORY: LT: **Intact UE and LE** R Hemi L Hemi LE score:
R -1 -2 -3 -4 -5 L -1 -2 -3 -4 -5

Sharp: Normal Absent: (R) ___L4 ___L5 ___S1
  Hyperalgesia: (R) toes feet ankles low calves Ulnar
            (L) toes feet ankles low calves Ulnar

Proprioception: Normal R ___mm L _ mm
  Vibration: R 10 L 10 R ___s L __s
  Temp: Nl decreased:

CEREBELLAR: F-t-N intact R fine trem. L fine trem. R inacc. L inacc.
Heel-shin Nl R poor L poor deferred

  Toe gait normal unsteady v. unsteady R weak L weak **Heel gait** Nl
  unsteady v.unsteady R weak L weak

  Tandem normal unsteady v. unsteady R unstd. L unstd.
  Stands well eyes closed unsteady retropulses

REFLEXES:
  RIGHT Bi2 0 1 3 4 BR2 0 1 3 4 Tri2 0 1 3 4 Pat2 0 1 3 4
  Ank2 0 1 3 4 Toes ↓ ↑ ↕ →
  LEFT Bi2 0 1 3 4 BR2 0 1 3 4 Tri2 0 1 3 4 Pat2 0 1 3 4
  Ank2 0 1 3 4 Toes ↓ ↑ ↕ →

TTP:
Scalp: none
Scalenes: none R middle L middle Pterygoid

Cervical paraspinals: none R: L:

Thoracic paraspinals: none R: L:

Lumbar paraspinals: none R: Lumb 1 L: Lumb 1 mid:Lumb 1
                Lumb 2 Lumb 2 Lumb 2
                Lumb 3 Lumb 3 Lumb 3
                Lumb 4 Lumb 4 Lumb 4
                Lumb 5 Lumb 5 Lumb 5

Sacroiliac: none R L
Piriformis: none R L

Knee: R Nl effusion warm TTP **L Nl** effusion warm TTP

Foot: R Nl pulse 1 0   hairless   purple   red   TTP:
Morton's screen: TTP lat. comp.   TTP over L3-4
intertarsal space

L Nl   pulse 1 0   hairless   purple   red   TTP:
Morton's screen: TTP lat. comp.   TTP over L3-4
intertarsal space

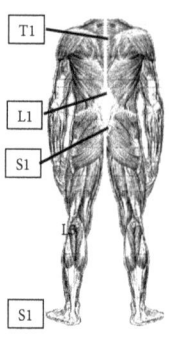 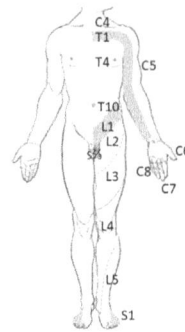 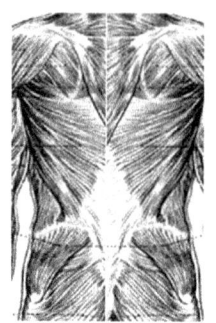 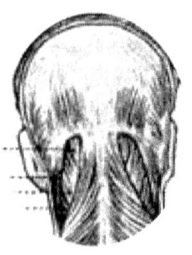 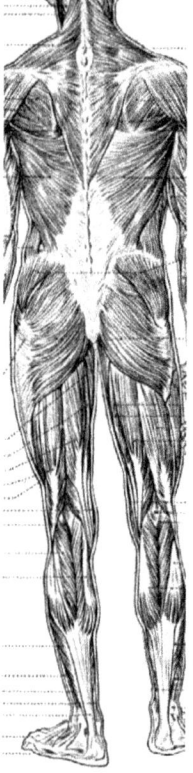

Range of motion:
SLR: R 90 no pain   10 20 30 45 60   pain back only
  pain back rad. to leg
  L 90 no pain   10 20 30 45 60   pain back only
  pain back rad. to leg
Back: Forward flexion   >90   90
  Extension: 20 15 10 5
  Side Bend: R 45 30 20 10   L 45 30 20 10
  Twist: R 45 30 20 10   L 45 30 20 10

Neck: Forward flexion   >90   90
  Extension: 20 15 10 5
  Side Bend: R 45 30 20 10   L 45 30 20 10
  Twist: R 45 30 20 10   L 45 30 20 10

Appendix II
Chemical Structure of Commonly Used Pain Medications

Standard (OTC) analgesics

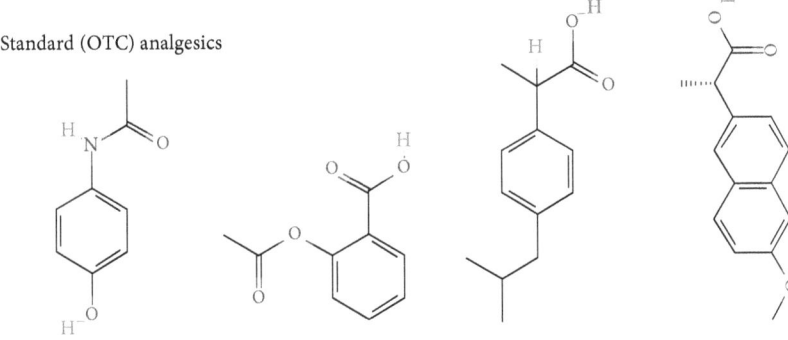

Acetaminophen Aspirin Ibuprofen Naproxen

Gabapentinoids

Pain-active antidepressants

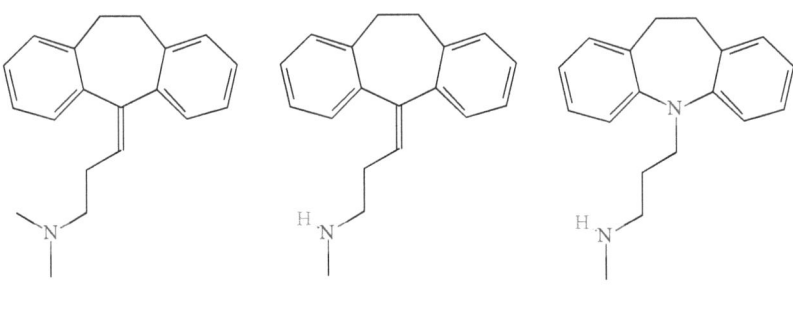

Amitripyline Nortriptyline Desipramine

Chemical Structure of Pain Medications

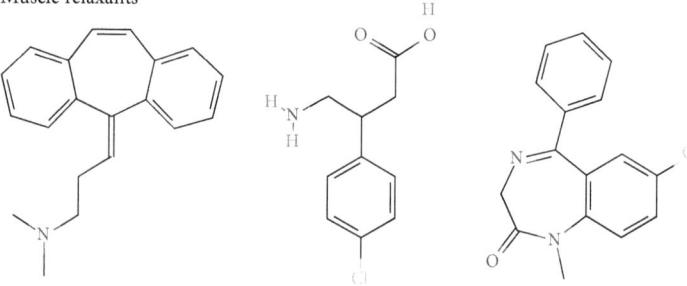

Venlafaxine

Duloxetine

Pain-active anticonvulsants

Carbamazepine

Oxcarbazepine

Topiramate

Muscle relaxants

Cyclobenzaprine

Baclofen

Diazepam

Chemical Structure of Pain Medications

Locally acting agents

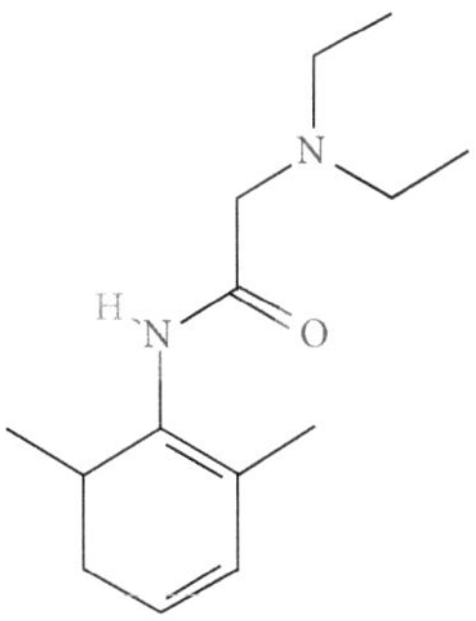

Lidocaine

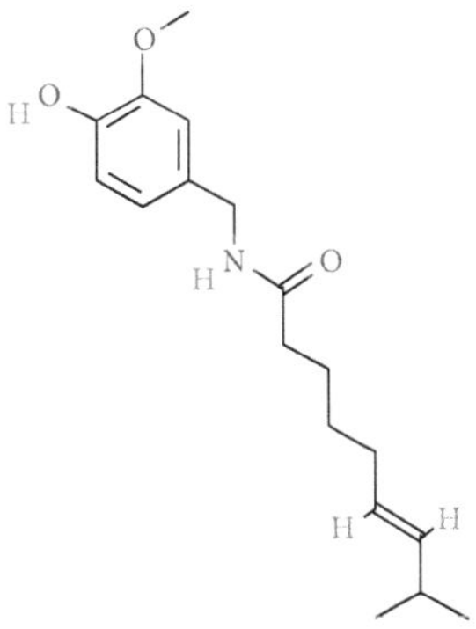

Capsaicin

Opioids

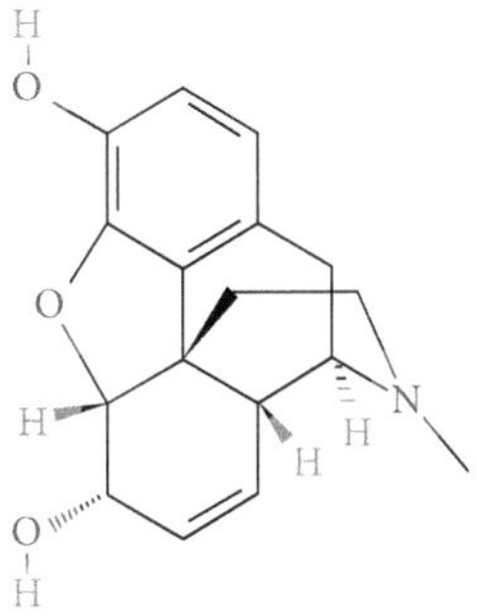

Morphine

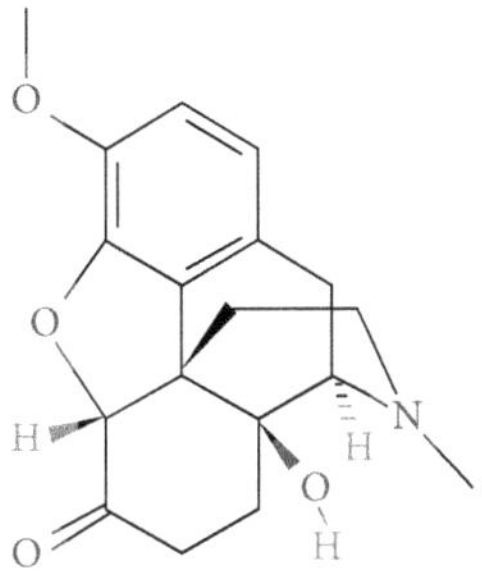

Oxycodone

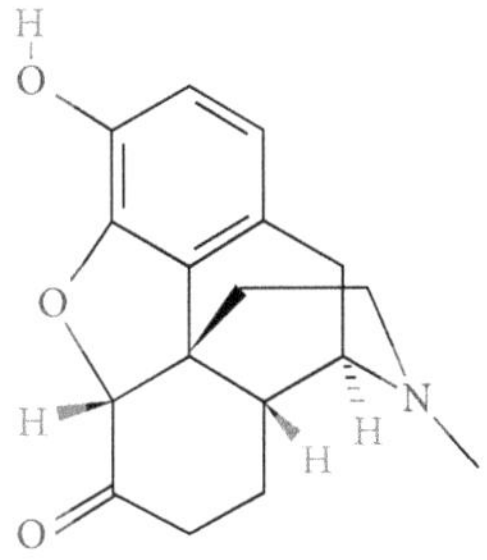

Hydromorphone

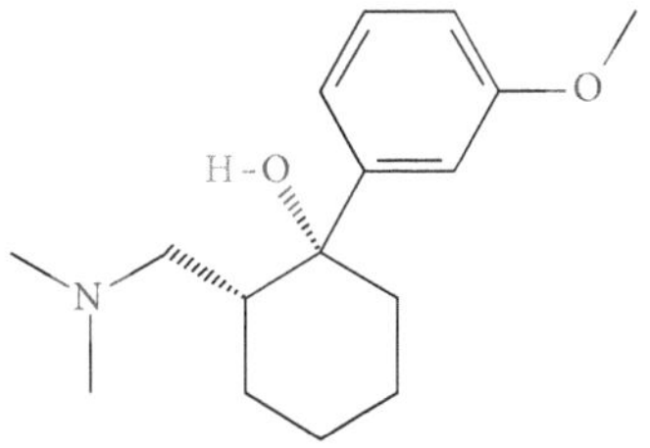

Tramadol

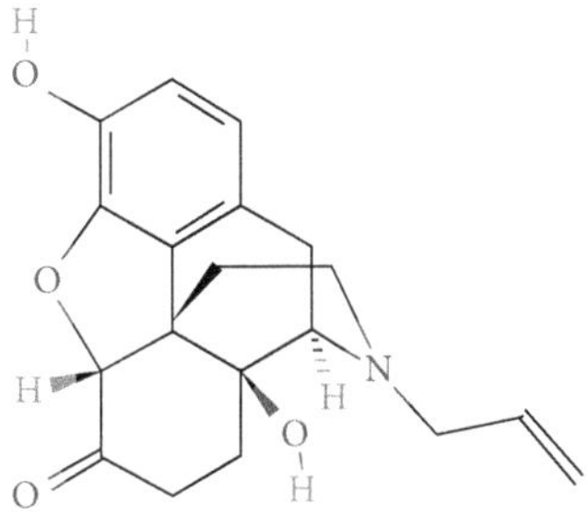

Naloxone

Selected neurotransmitters

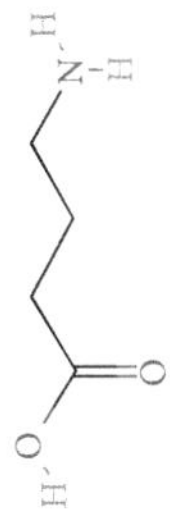

GABA

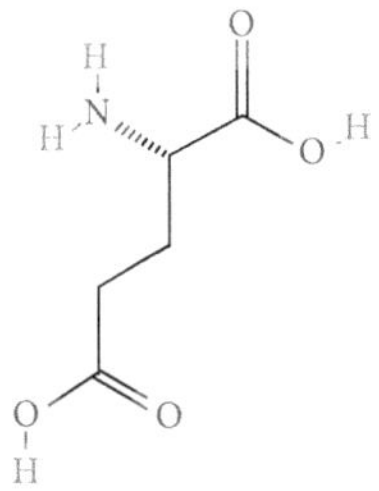

Glutamate

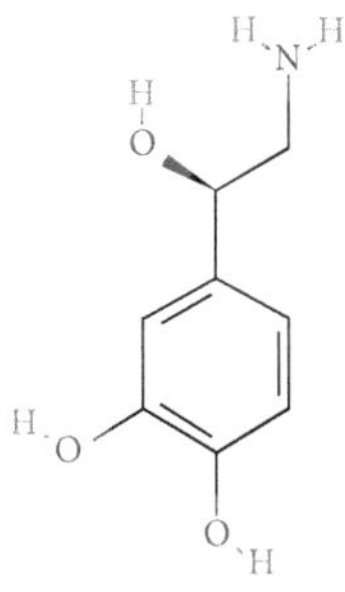

Norepinephrine

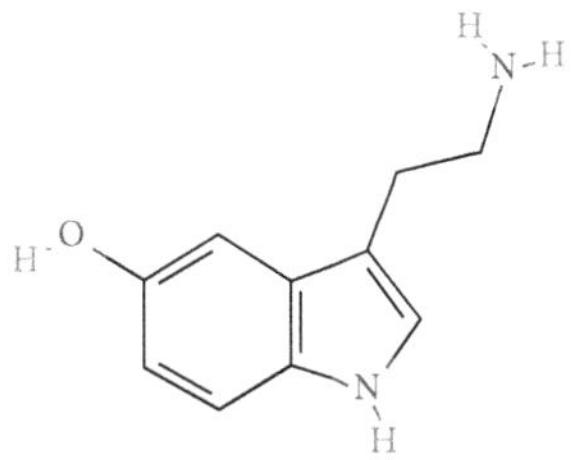

Serotonin

Appendix III
Comparison of Pain Treatments According to Pain Type

Pain Type	Specifics of mechanism	Conditions associated with pain mechanisms (examples)	Non-pharmacological treatments (examples)	Pharmacological treatments (examples)
Nociceptive	Activation of nociceptive afferents using ordinary mechanisms of sensing	pricks, burns, cuts, blows, breaks, crushes, chemical exposures	Cold or cooling Rubbing (counter irritant) Distraction	NSAIDs Local anesthetics Opioids (severe+acute/peri-procedural pain)
Inflammatory	Activation of afferents following modification in response to inflammatory mediators	arthritis, inflammation, infection	Warmth (heating pad, epsom salts), or cooling Gentle exercise, e.g., water-walking PT: Strengthening Stretching, bracing	NSAIDs Acetaminophen* (non anti-inflammatory) Disease modifying drugs Minimize opioid use
Neuropathic	Activation of nociceptive processing pathways due to disease or dysfunction of nervous system	Neuropathy, MS, transverse myelitis, Spinal cord injury, nerve damage	Distraction Self-management CBT/ACT PT, empathetic support	Pain-active antidepress. Pain-active anticonvuls. (e.g., gabapentinoids) Local anesthetics Minimize opioid use

Appendix IV
Adjustments in Treatment for Liver and Renal Failure

Metabolism and safety notes for selected medications used in common pain-associated conditions

Drug name	Dose range (normal)	Adjustments for Mild-mod. CKD	Adjustments for ESRD	Adjustments for mild hepatic compromise	Adjustments for hepatic impairment	Preg. Cat.	In breast-milk?
Acetaminophen	500–3,000 mg daily	Longer dose interval: q6h	Longer dose interval: q8h	Limit exposure	Avoid	B/B/B	Low, considered safe
Ibuprofen	400–2,400 mg daily	Avoid	Avoid	Caution	Avoid	C/C/D	Very low, analgesic of choice
Naproxen	250–1,000 mg daily	Avoid	Avoid	Caution	Avoid	C/C/D	Yes, low levels
Gabapentin	Max 3,600 mg total/day, taper up	Max 1,400 mg total/day	Max 300 mg total/day	No adjustment	No adjustment	C	Yes, low levels
Pregabalin	Max 300 mg total/day, taper up	Max 300 mg total/day	Max 75 mg total/day	No adjustment	No adjustment	C	Yes
Carbamazepine	400–800 mg daily, taper up slowly	No adjustment	Reduce dose by 25%	Caution	Avoid	D	Yes

Drug name	Dose range (normal)	Adjustments for Mild-mod. CKD	Adjustments for ESRD	Adjustments for mild hepatic compromise	Adjustments for hepatic impairment	Preg.Cat.	In breast-milk?
Amitriptyline	10 – 50 mg daily, taper up slowly	No adjustment	No adjustment	Caution: hepatotoxicity reported	Avoid: extensive hepatic metabolism	C	Yes, low levels
Nortriptyline	20-80 mg daily, taper up slowly	No adjustment	No adjustment	Caution: acute liver failure reported	Avoid: extensive hepatic metabolism	C	Yes, low levels
Venlafaxine	37.5 – 225 mg daily Taper up gradually	Reduce dose by 25-50%	Caution: reduce dose more than 50%	Reduce dose by 50%	Caution: reduce dose more than 50%	C	Yes
Duloxetine	30 – 60 mg daily Taper up gradually	Start low, reduce dose	Avoid: metabolites accumulate	Start low, reduce dose	Avoid: 5-fold increase in AUC	C	Yes
Tramadol	50-400 mg daily	Max 200 mg total/day	Avoid	Max 75 mg total/day	Avoid	C	Yes, low levels
Morphine	Variable	Reduce dose by 25%	Reduce dose 50%	Caution	Avoid	C	Yes* Oral: yes, IV: yes, Epidural: likely trivial
Oxycodone	Variable	Renal excretion: reduce dose	Renal excretion: avoid	Liver metabolism: reduce dose	Liver metabolism: avoid	C	Yes*

	Renal excretion: reduce dose	Renal excretion: avoid/caution	Liver metabolism: reduce dose	Liver metabolism: avoid		
Hydromorphone	Variable				C	Yes*
Fentanyl	Variable	Reduce dose 50%	Caution	Avoid	C	Yes*, See TOXNET

*The federal TOXNET notes that use of oral narcotics by breastfeeding mothers may result in infant death, alternatives should be used. See oxycodone reference below. NSAIDs, Ibuprofen and Naproxen are Category C for 1st and 2nd trimesters of pregnancy, but Category D for third trimester due to effects on ductus arteriosus.

Renal failure affects 44% of those over age 70.

CDC. Use of Prescribed NASAIDs but CKD stage definition and year. https://nccd.cdc.gov/ckd/detail.aspx?QNum=Q700

From DaVita: "Stage 1 with normal or high GFR (GFR > 90 mL/min) Stage 2 Mild CKD (GFR = 60-89 mL/min) Stage 3A Moderate CKD (GFR = 45-59 mL/min) Stage 3B Moderate CKD (GFR = 30-44 mL/min)"

Acetaminophen
https://online.epocrates.com/drugs/30601/acetaminophen/Adult-Dosing
http://toxnet.nlm.nih.gov/cgi-bin/sis/search2/r?dbs+lactmed:@term+@DOCNO+330

Ibuprofen
Servey J, Chang J. Over-the-Counter Medications in Pregnancy. Am Fam Physician. 2014 Oct 15;90(8):548-555. https://www.aafp.org/afp/2014/1015/p548.html
Choosing Wisely: Avoid nonsteroidal anti-inflammatory drugs (NSAIDs) in individuals with hypertension or heart failure or chronic kidney disease of all causes, including diabetes. American Family Physician. https://www.aafp.org/afp/recommendations/viewRecommendation.htm?recommendationId=36
http://toxnet.nlm.nih.gov/cgi-bin/sis/search2/r?dbs+lactmed:@term+@DOCNO+142

Naproxen
http://toxnet.nlm.nih.gov/cgi-bin/sis/search2/r?dbs+lactmed:@term+@DOCNO+195
https://online.epocrates.com/drugs/54/naproxen

Gabapentin
http://toxnet.nlm.nih.gov/cgi-bin/sis/search2/r?dbs+lactmed:@term+@DOCNO+358
https://globalrph.com/renal/gabapentin/
https://www.accessdata.fda.gov/drugsatfda_docs/label/2011/020235s036,020882s022,021129s022lbl.pdf

Pregabalin
http://toxnet.nlm.nih.gov/cgi-bin/sis/search2/r?dbs+lactmed:@term+@DOCNO+908
https://globalrph.com/renal/pregabalin/
https://www.accessdata.fda.gov/drugsatfda_docs/label/2012/021446s028lbl.pdf

Carbamazepine
http://toxnet.nlm.nih.gov/cgi-bin/sis/search2/r?dbs+lactmed:@term+@DOCNO+400
https://online.epocrates.com/drugs/165/carbamazepine
https://www.accessdata.fda.gov/drugsatfda_docs/label/2009/016608s101,018281s048lbl.pdf

Amitriptyline
https://toxnet.nlm.nih.gov/cgi-bin/sis/search2/r?dbs+lactmed:@or+%28@na+%22AMITRIPTYLINE%22+%29
https://online.epocrates.com/drugs/13501/amitriptyline/Adult-Dosing
https://livertox.nih.gov/Amitriptyline.htm

Nortriptyline
http://toxnet.nlm.nih.gov/cgi-bin/sis/search2/r?dbs+lactmed:@term+@DOCNO+314
https://livertox.nih.gov/Nortriptyline.htm
https://online.epocrates.com/drugs/1084/Pamelor

Venlafaxine
https://dailymed.nlm.nih.gov/dailymed/drugInfo.cfm?setid=9a30e1b5-272b-4109-ad6c-a3c9a895822f

Duloxetine
https://globalrph.com/renal/duloxetine/
https://dailymed.nlm.nih.gov/dailymed/drugInfo.cfm?setid=2f7d4d67-10c1-4bf4-a7f2-c185fbad64ba

Tramadol
https://globalrph.com/renal/tramadol/
https://toxnet.nlm.nih.gov/cgi-bin/sis/search2/r?dbs+lactmed:@term+@DOCNO+391
https://online.epocrates.com/drugs/1346/tramadol
https://www.accessdata.fda.gov/drugsatfda_docs/label/2009/020281s032s033lbl.pdf

Morphine
http://toxnet.nlm.nih.gov/cgi-bin/sis/search2/r?dbs+lactmed:@term+@DOCNO+370

Oxycodone
http://toxnet.nlm.nih.gov/cgi-bin/sis/search2/r?dbs+lactmed:@term+@DOCNO+378
https://www.accessdata.fda.gov/drugsatfda_docs/label/2015/022272s027lbl.pdf
https://dailymed.nlm.nih.gov/dailymed/drugInfo.cfm?setid=ae0de7f7-defe-41ec-8635-ee08948541f0#S12.3

Hydromorphone
http://toxnet.nlm.nih.gov/cgi-bin/sis/search2/r?dbs+lactmed:@term+@DOCNO+360

Fentanyl
http://toxnet.nlm.nih.gov/cgi-bin/sis/search2/r?dbs+lactmed:@term+@DOCNO+356
https://online.epocrates.com/drugs/1691/fentanyl

Appendix V
Back Pain Diagnosis Flow Diagram

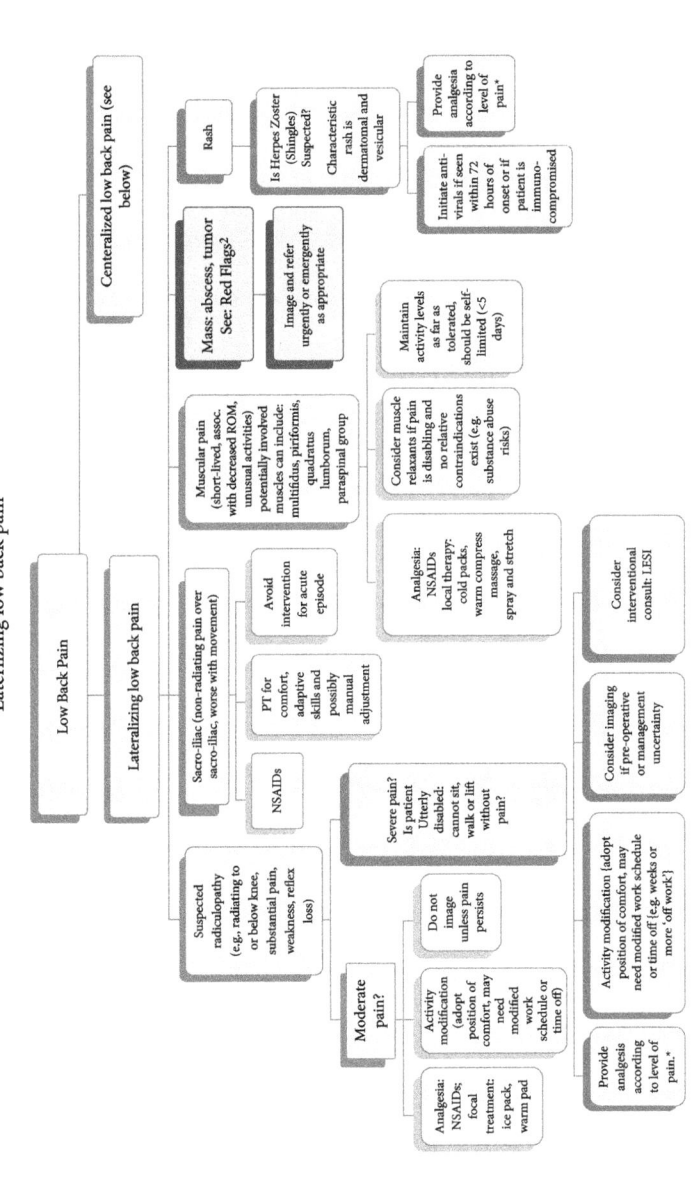

Centralized low back pain

Centralized Back Pain

Spinal cord injury or disease - myelopathy (e.g.: incontinence, bilateral weakness, reflex abberations) Red Flags: fever, chills, weight loss, known cancer[2]
- If new onset: image emergently
- Refer as appropriate

Vertebral fracture[1]
- Trauma: younger patients
- Atraumatic: older patients, osteoporosis, steroid exposure
- xray/CT
- xray, provide analgesia for pain

Ligamentous strain (poor posture, lack of ergonomic design)
- Ergonomic adaptation
- Physical therapy, conditioning, see chronic low back pain for details
- Exercise program - core strengthening

Centralized and Lateralized (See below)

Chronic low back pain
- Ergonomic adaptation
- Physical therapy and self-managed conservative care: conditioning exercise, cold packs, warm compress, trigger point massage, cold spray and stretch, iontophoresis, e-stim
- Exercise program - core strengthening and maintenance of activity
- Analgesia: NSAIDs, Acetaminophen or neuromodulating agents as appropriate

[1] Pain may be central and radiating (if nerve root compressed)

Centralized and Lateralized low back pain

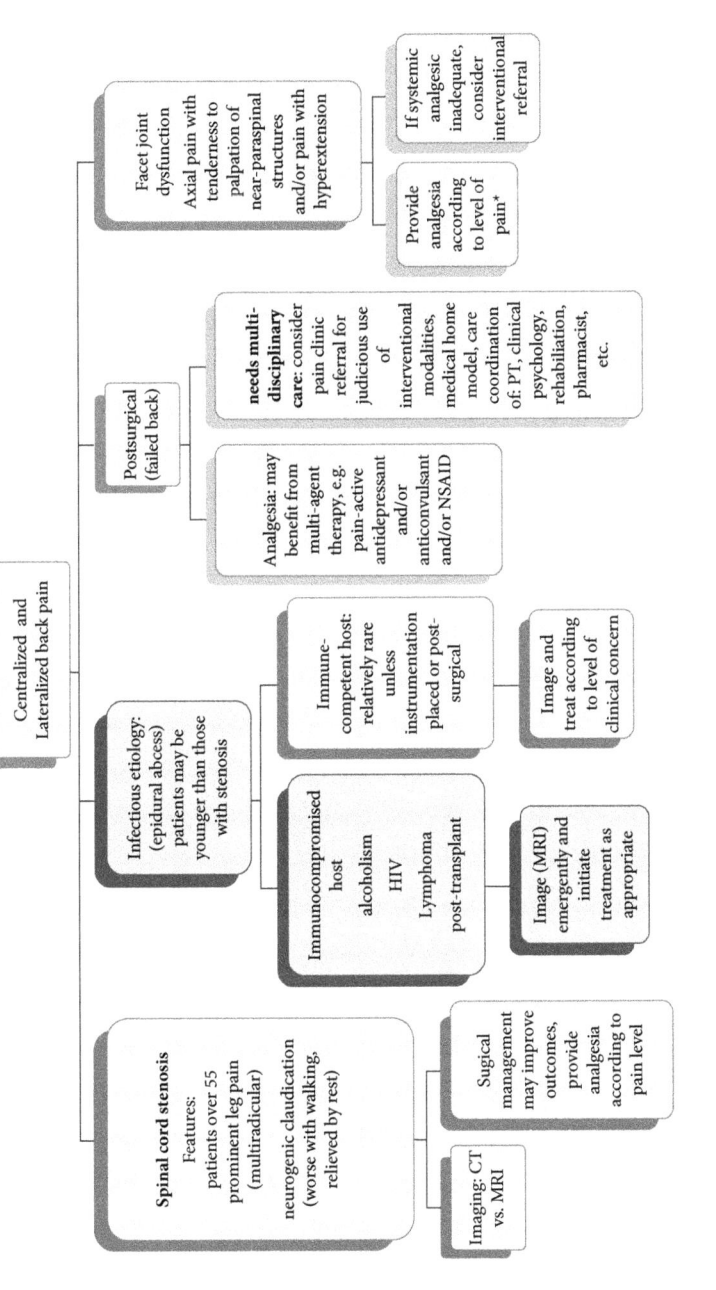

Appendix VI
Evidence-Based Basic Recommendations to Prevent or Reduce Chronic Pain*

7 DAILY ACTIVITIES TO HELP PREVENT CHRONIC PAIN (CAN BE USED AS A 'PRESCRIPTION')

- ☐ Walk for 20 minutes a day, outside when possible
  - ○ Stationary biking or swimming are good alternatives
  - ○ Yoga or tai chi may provide additional pain relief
- ☐ Drink 8 eight-ounce glasses of water
  - ○ Eliminate soda and fruit juice
  - ○ Limit alcohol to no more than 1 drink daily
- ☐ Eat 4 servings of vegetables and 2 servings of fruit
- ☐ Sit quietly and breathe deeply for three minutes at least once every day
  - ○ Mindfulness-based stress reduction decreases chronic pain
- ☐ Stretch Iliopsoas and pectoralis muscles
  - ○ Iliopsoas stretch: start with a gentle lunge, stand with one hand on countertop for stability
  - ○ Pectoralis stretch: with arms held straight out from body, bend elbows to 90 degrees, step into a corner or narrow doorframe to gently push arms back, feel stretch
- ☐ Strengthen quads and hip abductors
  - ○ Quad strengthening: lying on back, place pillow beneath one knee, press knee down into pillow and hold for 3 seconds, relax for 1 second. Repeat 30 times on each side.
  - ○ Hip abductor strengthening: lying on one side with legs straight, bend knees without flexing hips, feet will be behind you. Now raise the upper knee to 30 degrees, keeping the feet together, and hold for 3 seconds, relax. Repeat 20 times on each side.
- ☐ Set aside 8 hours a day for sleeping
  - ○ Remove TVs and computers from the bedroom permanently
  - ○ Stop using phone 1 hour before bedtime

* Patients with specific limitations or health conditions should consult with provider regarding details or modifications of these instructions.

NOTES REGARDING EVIDENCE FOR PAIN PREVENTION AND REDUCTION

Moderate daily exercise shows efficacy in multiple forms of chronic pain.[1]

Exposure to forest or 'green' environment has beneficial effects.[2]
Yoga and Tai Chi are beneficial against multiple forms of chronic pain.[3]

Adequate hydration is important for healthy function of kidneys, at risk with pain medication.[4]

Water consumption amounts may be adjusted for renal failure.
Avoidance of fruit juice and soda is associated with lower body weight.

Healthy diet recommendations should be followed for control of BMI, obesity is associated with multiple forms of chronic pain.

Meditative therapies, especially mindfulness-based stress reduction are just one form of evidence based cognitive strategies for the control of pain, detailed further in chapters 5 and 12.[3]

Stretching of iliopsoas and pectoralis muscles is associated with improved spinal alignment and lower levels of neck and low back pain.[5]

Strengthening of selected lower limb muscles is associated with reduced knee and hip pain; knee and hip osteoarthritis are among the most common causes of chronic pain.[6]

Sleep has a strong associated with pain; disrupted or limited sleep is associated with higher rates of chronic pain.[7]

REFERENCES

1. Geneen LJ, Moore RA, Clarke C, et al. Physical activity and exercise for chronic pain in adults: an overview of Cochrane Reviews. Cochrane Database Syst Rev. 2017 Apr 24;4:CD011279.
2. Park BJ1, Tsunetsugu Y, Kasetani T, Kagawa T, Miyazaki Y. The physiological effects of Shinrin-yoku (taking in the forest atmosphere or forest bathing): evidence from field experiments in 24 forests across Japan. Environ Health Prev Med. 2010 Jan;15(1):18–26.
3. Skelly AC, Chou R, Dettori JR, Turner JA, et al. Noninvasive Nonpharmacological Treatment for Chronic Pain: A Systematic Review. Rockville (MD): AHRQ (US); 2018 Jun.
4. U.S. Department of Health and Human Services and U.S. Department of Agriculture. 2015 – 2020 Dietary Guidelines for Americans. 8th Edition. December 2015. Available at https://health.gov/dietaryguidelines/2015/guidelines/. Accessed April 1, 2019.
5. Johnson, J. Treat Your Own Knees: Simple Exercises to Build Strength, Flexibility, Responsiveness and Endurance. 2003. Hunter House, Berkeley, CA.
6. Murinson, B. Take Back Your Back. 2011. Fair Winds Press.
7. Afolalu EF, Ramlee F, Tang NKY. Effects of sleep changes on pain-related health outcomes in the general population: A systematic review of longitudinal studies with exploratory meta-analysis. Sleep Med Rev. 2018 Jun;39:82–97.

Index

Tables, figures and boxes are indicated by *t*, f and *b* following the page number

For the benefit of digital users, indexed terms that span two pages (e.g., 52–53) may, on occasion, appear on only one of those pages.

ABC. *See* Addiction Behavior Checklist (ABC)
abdominal pain, 223
  case scenario, 259–60
  in children, 311
  emergencies, 226*t*
  and imaging, 223
aberrant drug behaviors, 341*b*
  prevalence of, 342
Aβ fibers, 9–11, 10–11*f*, 13*f*
abscess
  and atypical focal pain, 264–65
  brain, 228–29, 228*t*
  epidural, 250–51
    with epidural corticosteroid injection, 235–36
  spinal, 229
  soft tissue, 225
acceptance and commitment therapy (ACT), 16–17, 82*t*, 83, 112–14, 201–2, 203
  for older adults, 328
acetaminophen, 19*f*, 135, 245
  administration route, 246*t*
  adverse effects of, 136
  allergy to, 135
  and breastfeeding, 367
  dosage adjustments for kidney or liver disease, 367
  in older adults, 335
  dosage and administration of
    in adults, 135
    in children, 135
    by pediatric age group, 314*t*
  drug interactions with, 136
  formulations of, 135
  indications for, 135–36, 270*f*
  and liver disease, 135, 136
  mechanism of action of, 135, 246*t*
  for older adults, 330*t*
    risk-reduction strategies with, 335
  opioid-sparing effect, 315
  overdose, 136
  for pediatric fever, 135
  pharmacology of, 135
  precautions with, 246*t*
  pregnancy category, 367
  and renal impairment, 135
  side effects, 246*t*
  site of action, 244*f*
  trial of, for older adults unable to self-report, 325*t*
acetic acids, 137*t*
N-acetylcysteine, for acetaminophen overdose, 136
N-acetyl-*p*-benzoquinone imine (NAPQI), 136
acid-sensing ion channel (ASIC), 27–30
ACS. *See* acute compartment syndrome (ACS)
ACT. *See* acceptance and commitment therapy (ACT)
action potentials
  of off-cells, in pain modulation, 36–37, 37*f*
  of on-cells, in pain modulation, 36–37, 37*f*
  in pain signaling, 12, 21–22, 27–28, 30–31, 32*f*, 34–35*f*
active listening, 119–21, 121*b*
activities of daily living (ADLs), assessment of, in older adults, 322

acupressure
   for children, 312
   in pain treatment for older adults, 327
acupuncture, 206, 245
   auricular, 206
   "battlefield," 206
   for children, 312
   combined with other treatment modalities, 84–85
   for older adults, 327
acute compartment syndrome (ACS), 254
acute coronary syndrome, 223, 224t
acute pain
   behavioral manifestations of, 106–7
   case scenario, 241–42
   in children, 310
   in chronic opioid users, 255
   management of, 242, 244–51
   nonopioids for, 245, 246t
   nonpharmacologic therapies for, 245
   pharmacologic management of, 245
   poor management of, 27
   prevalence of, 45
addiction. *See also* opioid addiction
   iatrogenic, to opioids, 249
Addiction Behavior Checklist (ABC), 346, 348t
addiction specialist, referral to, 67–68
Aδ fibers, 9–11, 10–11f, 13f, 30, 244
adenosine triphosphate (ATP), 29–30
adherence toxicity, 329
adhesive capsulitis, 193
adjuvant (term), 134–35, 159
adjuvant analgesics, 134–35
ADLs. *See* activities of daily living (ADLs)
adolescent(s). *See also* pediatric pain assessment; pediatric pain management
   causes of pain in, 311
Adolescent Pediatric Pain Tool (APPT), 310
adrenergic receptors, dopamine binding to, and modulation of pain, 38
Advil Filmtabs, 137
affect, negative, and opioid misuse/addiction, 343–45
affective information, in pain-focused encounter, 106
aging. *See also* older adults
   and pain pathways, 23, 319–20
   and pain suppression pathways, 23

agitation, in older adults, 322
agoraphobia, SPS and, 303
alfentanil, 141t, 147
algogen (term), 58–59
algology, 58–59
allodynia, 55–56, 254–55
   causes of, 69
   with chronic migraine, 277f
   in complex regional pain syndrome, 297
   definition of, 69, 70t
   migraine and, 98–99, 277f, 278
   molecular machinery of, 29–30
   with postherpetic neuralgia, 295
   with ulnar neuropathy, 288–89
allostatic load, 76–77
alpha 2 (α2-) agonists, 19f
   site of action, 244f
amitriptyline, 165–66
   adverse effects of, 165–66
   and breastfeeding, 367
   dosage adjustments for kidney or liver disease, 367
   dosage and administration of, 165–66
   formulations of, 165–66
   indications for, 165–66
   mechanism of action of, 165–66
   pregnancy category, 367
   for shingles, 265
   therapy with, *case scenario,* 158–59
   topical, 173
AMPA receptor, in nociceptive transmission, 31–32, 32f, 33
analgesia. *See also* epidural analgesia; multimodal analgesia; neuraxial analgesia; patient-controlled analgesia (PCA)
   case scenario, 134, 154–56
   definition of, 70t
   mechanism of action of, neuroanatomy of, 18, 19f
   preventive, 255
analgesia (term), 58–59
analgesics. *See also* nonopioid analgesics; opioid(s); *specific analgesic*
   adjuvant, 134–35
   chemical structure of, 359
   combination of, 134
   standard systemic, 134

storage and disposal of, patient education about, 336
trial of, for older adults unable to self-report, 325t
variable responses to, 134
anchoring bias, 113b
anesthesia dolorosa, definition of, 70t
aneurysm(s)
aortic, rupture, 224t
intracranial, 227
anger, patient's, in clinical encounter, 92–93
angiotensin-converting enzyme inhibitors, and NSAIDs, interactions of, 140
ankle block, 252f
ankle fracture(s), 123–24
case scenario, 118
ankylosing spondylitis, NSAIDs for, 136–37
ankyrin 1, 28
anterior cingulate cortex, 16, 17f, 203
rostral, activation by painful stimuli, 106–7
antianxiety agents, for older adults, 330t
antibiotics, and statin-induced myopathy, 269
anticonvulsants, 161–65
for complex regional pain syndrome, 297–98
mechanism of action of, 159b
for migraine prophylaxis, 278–79
for older adults, 330t
in pain care, 159b, 159
side effects of, 278–79
antidepressants, 165–67. See also selective norepinephrine-serotonin reuptake inhibitors; selective serotonin reuptake inhibitors (SSRIs)
for complex regional pain syndrome, 297–98
newer, 167
for older adults, 330t
in pain care, 159, 270f
mechanism of action of, 160b
for painful peripheral neuropathy, 287–88
for postherpetic neuralgia, 295
side effects of, 278–79, 287–88
and statin-induced myopathy, 269

antifungals, and statin-induced myopathy, 269
anti-inflammatory drugs, site of action, 244f
antinuclear antibody (ANA), laboratory testing for, 110t
anxiety, 17–18. See also pain anxiety
in children, 313
chronic pain and, 78
in chronic pain patients, and opioid misuse/addiction, 343–44
disability caused by, 46
evaluation for, 78
interaction with other biopsychosocial variables, 79–80
mindfulness-based stress reduction for, 83–84
in older adults, 322, 324
opioid use and, 345
pain and, 43–44, 76, 78–79, 80–81
passive coping and, 81
and problematic opioid use, 351
anxiety disorders, in chronic pain patients, 340–42
aortic aneurysm rupture, 224t
APAP. See acetaminophen
appendicitis, 226t
appearance, patient's, assessment of, 355
APPT. See Adolescent Pediatric Pain Tool (APPT)
aquatic therapy, 201
arthritis
of knee, 201
in older adults, pharmacologic therapy for, 330t
arthritis pain
acetaminophen for, 135–36
disability caused by, 46
of knee, 194
in shoulder, 193
ascending pain pathways, 14, 15f, 27–30, 33, 244f
ASIC. See acid-sensing ion channel (ASIC)
aspirin, 137
dosage and administration of, 139t
for erythromelalgia, 301
half-life of, 139t
mechanism of action of, 138t
and Reye syndrome, 135

assessment, 245. *See also* clinical assessment; pain assessment
  of chest pain, 223
  in emergency department, 222
  perioperative, 243–44
  psychological, 77–80, 81
  in older adults, 322–24
assistive devices/orthotics
  in Ehlers-Danlos syndrome, 302
  in pain treatment for older adults, 327
astrocytes, 12–14
ATNB. *See* auriculotemporal nerve block (ATNB)
ATP. *See* adenosine triphosphate (ATP)
attention to pain, 15*f*, 16
aura, with migraine, 261
auriculotemporal nerve, 178
auriculotemporal nerve block (ATNB), 178–79
auriculotemporal neuralgia, 178
autogenic training, 203
autoimmune disorders
  and headache, 262
  and peripheral neuropathy, 286
autonomy, 48, 49, 124
availability bias, 113*b*
axial pain, chronic, 185, 186–87
axons, 21*f*, 21
  diameter of, and conduction velocity, 21–22
  myelination of, 21*f*, 21–22

back pain
  and cerebrospinal fluid analysis, 227, 228*t*
  diagnosis of, flow diagram for, 369–70
  and disability, 45
  disability caused by, 46
  economic burden of, 46
  mindfulness-based stress reduction for, 83–84
  palpation for, 99
  prevalence of, 45–46
  urgent, 266–68
baclofen, 171
  intrathecal, withdrawal, 237
  mechanism of action of, 171–72, 172*f*
  for SPS, 303
  topical, 173
  withdrawal, 237

Barton, Clara, 319
base-rate distortion, 113*b*
BDNF. *See* brain-derived neurotrophic factor (BDNF)
behavioral manifestations
  of acute pain, 106–7
  brain regions associated with, 14
  of chronic pain, 106–7
beneficence, 48, 124
benzodiazepines, 172–73. *See also* diazepam
  for SPS, 303
BFB. *See* biofeedback (BFB)
bias. See also *specific bias*
  affective distortions and, 113*b*
  cognitive distortions and, 113*b*
BIMS. *See* Brief Interview for Mental Status (BIMS)
biofeedback (BFB), 82*t*, 203
  for children, 313
  and cognitive-behavioral therapy, 84
  in pain treatment for older adults, 328
  and relaxation training, 84
biopsychosocial model, 77*f*, 77, 78*f*, 81, 118–22
  and safe pain care, 119
BK2 cell surface receptors, 29–30
bone metastases, in older adults, pharmacologic therapy for, 330*t*
bone morphogenetic protein
  BMP4, 21
  BMP7, 21
bone pain, NSAIDs for, 136–37
bone scan, 111*t*
Botox. *See* botulinum toxin
botulinum toxin injection, for migraine prophylaxis, 180
boundary issues, in clinical encounter, 92–93
BPI. *See* Brief Pain Inventory (BPI)
brachial plexus block, 252*f*, 252, 253*t*
bradykinin, 29–30
brain
  abscess, 228–29, 228*t*
  activation by painful stimuli, 106–7
  ascending nociceptive input to, 14, 15*f*, 27–30, 33
  cancer metastases to, 228
brain-derived neurotrophic factor (BDNF), in nociceptive transmission, 30–31, 32*f*, 32–33

brain tumor, 228
   and headache, 262, 263
breakthrough pain, 152
   in children, 315
breast milk, medications in, 144
Brief Interview for Mental Status
      (BIMS), 323
Brief Pain Inventory (BPI), 61, 64f, 322
Buddhists, 56–58
bupivacaine, dosage and administration
      of, 253–54
buprenorphine, 141t, 145
   dosage and administration of, 145
   formulations of, 145
   mechanism of action of, 247t
   for opioid use disorder, 351–52
   pharmacology of, 145
   prescribing of, 145
   trial of, for older adults unable to
      self-report, 325t
burnout
   prevention of, 124
   women and, 124
bursitis
   and hip pain, 283–84
   NSAIDs for, 136–37
   subacromial subdeltoid, 192
butorphanol, 141, 141t

Caesar, Julius, 41
CAGE-AID, 346, 348t
calcitonin gene-related peptide(s) (CGRP)
   and migraine, 261
   in nociceptive transmission, 30–31,
      32f, 32–33
calcium, in nociceptive transmission,
      30–31, 32f
calcium channel blockers
   for migraine prophylaxis, 278–79
   and statin-induced myopathy, 269
calcium channels, N-type, 168f, 168–69
CAM. See Confusion Assessment
      Measure (CAM)
cancer
   cerebral metastases, 228
   spinal metastases, 229
cancer pain, 45–46
   in children, opioids for, 315
   iatrogenic, 46
   multimodal treatment of, 206–7

neurophysiology of, 206–7
opioids for, 140–41
prehabilitation for, 206–7
prevalence of, 46
rehabilitation interventions for, 206–7
transmucosal immediate-release
      fentanyl for, 148
treatment of, 46
cannabinoids, for complex regional pain
      syndrome, 297–98
CAPA. See Clinically Aligned Pain
      Assessment (CAPA)
capsaicin, 9, 19f, 28–29, 169, 173, 270f
   contraindications to, 287–88, 295
   mechanism of action of, 169–70, 170f
carbamazepine, 163
   adverse effects of, 163
   and breastfeeding, 367
   dosage adjustments for kidney or liver
      disease, 367
   dosage and administration of, 163
   drug interactions with, 136, 163
   formulations of, 163
   indications for, 163
   pregnancy category, 367
   side effects of, 294
   for trigeminal neuralgia, 160, 163, 294
caregivers, 44–45
   of older adults
      evaluation of, 324
      and multimodal pain treatment, 324–27
   working with, in pain care, 214
carpal tunnel syndrome (CTS), 288–89
   testing for, 94
catastrophizing, 16–17, 44, 80, 82–83, 201–2
   in chronic pain patients, and opioid
      misuse/addiction, 343–44
   passive coping and, 81
cauda equina syndrome, 230, 231f
causalgia, definition of, 70t
CBT. See cognitive behavioral
      therapy (CBT)
celecoxib, 137
   administration route, 246t
   dosage and administration of, 139t
   half-life of, 139t
   mechanism of action of, 138t, 246t
   for older adults, 331
   precautions with, 246t
   side effects, 246t

celiac plexus block, 189
cellulitis, 225
central nervous system
　nociceptive transmission into, 12, 27
　pain processing in, 27
central neuropathic pain, definition of, 70t
central sensitization, 12–14, 13f, 16, 31–32, 254–55, 285–86
cerebrospinal fluid (CSF)
　analysis, in headache and back pain emergencies, 227, 228t
　leak, with intrathecal pump implantation, 236
cervical myelopathy, 279–80
C fibers, 9–11, 10–11f, 30, 244, 287
　as polymodal, 30
　stressed or dying back, detection of, 99–100
CGRP. *See* calcitonin gene-related peptide(s) (CGRP)
CGRP receptor-like receptor (CRLR), 32–33
change. *See* stages of change model
chaperone, for clinical encounter, 92–93
chemical copers, 344
chest pain, 223
　differential diagnosis, 223, 224t
chief complaint, 105
children. *See also* pediatric pain management
　acute versus chronic pain in, 310
　age 8 and older, pain assessment in, 310
　breakthrough pain in, 315
　causes pain of, 310–11
　comfort measures for, in stressful procedures, 312
　fever in, 135
　pain assessment in, 61–62, 62f, 63t, 307–10 (*see also* pediatric pain assessment)
　pain location in, determining, 309
　pain scales for, 310
　preschool, pain assessment in, 308t, 309
　school-age
　　causes of pain in, 311
　　pain assessment in, 308t, 309
Children's Hospital of Eastern Ontario Pain Scale (CHEOPS), 310
chiropractic, in pain treatment for older adults, 327

cholecystitis, 226t
cholecystokinin, and on-cell activity, 36–37
chronic hip pain, 283–84
　causes of, 283–84
chronic knee pain, 284–85
　management of, 284
　prevalence of, 284
chronic low back pain, 280–83
　causes of, 280
　centralizing, 281
　and disability, 280
　examination of patient with, 281–82
　key features of, 281
　lateralizing, 281
　management of, 282–83, 283f
　red flags for, 280–81
chronic migraine, 277–79
　allodynia with, 277f
　clinical features of, 278
　definition of, 278
　examination of patient with, 278
　management of, 278–79, 279f
chronic neck pain, 279–80
　causes of, 279–80
　management of, 279–80
chronic pain. *See also* persistent postsurgical pain
　and anxiety, 78
　assessment of, 202
　behavioral manifestations of, 106–7
　case scenario, 41–42, 273–74
　in children, 310
　and close social network, 44–45
　common conditions causing, 274–75
　definition of, 274
　development of, 27, 42
　dysfunctions caused by, 75–76, 77, 78f, 78
　early-life sexual abuse and, 92
　economic burden of, 46
　evidence-based management of, 274–75, 275f
　extremes of, 292
　impact of, 106–7
　individual impact of, 41–42, 43–44
　management of, 76, 274–75
　management with alcohol or illicit opioids, 47
　and mental health, 76, 78
　in neonates and infants, 311
　neuromodulating agents for, 160

in older adults, 275–76
prevalence of, 45–46, 274
prevention, evidence-based
  recommendations for, 38
and psychiatric disorders,
  comorbidity, 340–42
psychological interventions for, 202
reduction, evidence-based
  recommendations for, 38
risk factors for, 45–46
societal impact of, 41–42, 45–46
treatment of, 47–48
widespread, prevalence of, 45–46
chronic shoulder pain, 285–86
causes of, 285–86
management of, 285–86
chronic tension headache, 276–77
muscles and, 276–77, 277f
as musculoskeletal pain-related
  condition, 277
treatment of, 277
Churg-Strauss syndrome, and nerve
  vasculitis, 299
cingulate cortex/gyrus, 15–16, 22
classification, of pain, 54–56, 55f
clinical assessment
  case scenario, 90
  as critical skill, 90–91
  pain-focused, 92–93
Clinically Aligned Pain Assessment
  (CAPA), 321
clinical trials
  pain assessment tools as outcome
    measures for, 68
  of pain treatment, factors affecting,
    68, 69t
clonidine, 19f, 160b, 170
  administration route, 246t
  intrathecal, withdrawal, 237
  mechanism of action of, 246t
  precautions with, 246t
  side effects, 246t
  withdrawal, 237
codeine, 141t, 142–43
  administration route, 248t
  contraindications to, 143
    in adolescents, 315–16b
    in children younger than 12 years,
      315–16b
    in older adults, 334

equianalgesic dose, 248t
mechanism of action of, 247t
metabolism of, 143
onset and duration of action, 248t
cognitive behavioral therapy (CBT), 16–17,
  80, 81, 82, 82t, 83f, 201–2, 203, 204
  biofeedback and, 84
  for children, 312, 313
  combined with other treatment
    modalities, 84–85
  for older adults, 328, 330t
cognitive impairment
  in older adults, 322
    and pain assessment, 322, 325t
    and pain treatment plan, 329
  pain assessment tools used with, 62
  and pain treatment plan, 213–14
cognitive restructuring, 112–14
cognitive status, in older adults, assessment
  of, 322–23
cognitive therapy, 203
cold therapy, 245
  for erythromelalgia, 301
  in pain treatment for older adults, 327
collaboration, interprofessional, 112, 125
collagen, mutations of, 301
color scale, 61–62
COMFORT pain scale, 62
COMFORT Scale, 310
COMM. *See* Current Opioid Misuse
  Measure (COMM)
commission bias, 113b
commission error, 112–14
communication
  with colleagues, 126
  with patients, 126
communication about pain
  with pediatric patients, 61
  with special populations, 61
communication barriers, overcoming,
  122b, 201
comorbidity, and diagnostic
  evaluation, 112–14
compassion
  communication of, 119
  vs. empathy, 120–21
complementary and alternative
  modalities, 205–6
  active, 205
  passive, 206

complementary and alternative strategies, in pain treatment for older adults, 327
complex regional pain syndrome (CRPS), 181, 296–99
   case scenario, 291–92
   clinical features of, 297, 298*t*
   with evident nerve injury (CRPS II), 296
   and examination, 92–93
   mechanisms of, 297
   prevalence of, 296, 298*t*
   treatment of, 297, 298*t*
   without evident nerve injury (CRPS I), 296
computed tomography (CT), 110–11, 111*t*
   guidance, for interventions, 177
   head, 227
   spiral, 223–25
conduction velocity (CV), 9–11, 21–22
   and DRG neuron diameter, 9–11
   of primary afferent neurons, 9–11
Confusion Assessment Measure (CAM), 324
congenital insensitivity to pain, 292–93
   clinical features of, 293, 298*t*
   genetics of, 292, 293
   prevalence of, 292, 298*t*
   treatment of, 293, 298*t*
consent, for examination, 92–93
constipation
   in older adults, pharmacologic therapy for, 330*t*
   opioid-induced, 249
      in older adults, prevention of, 335
consultative assessments, 112
contingency management, 202
coordination, screening assessment of, 95
coping, passive vs. active, 81, 82–83
coping strategy(ies), 203
   in pain treatment for older adults, 328
corticosteroids, and NSAIDs, interactions of, 140
costochondritis, 224*t*
counterirritants, 270*f*
   for older adults, 331
cranial nerve(s), V, 178
cranial nerve testing, 95, 96, 355
craving. *See also* opioid craving
   definition of, 344
CRIES Pain Scale, 62, 63*t*, 64*f*

CRLR. *See* CGRP receptor-like receptor (CRLR)
CRPS. *See* complex regional pain syndrome (CRPS)
CT. *See* computed tomography (CT)
CTS. *See* carpal tunnel syndrome (CTS)
culture
   and experience and presentation of pain, 44, 45, 78–79
   and pain treatment for older adults, 328
Current Opioid Misuse Measure (COMM), 346, 348*t*
CV. *See* conduction velocity (CV)
cyclobenzaprine, for fibromyalgia, 300
cyclooxygenase (COX)
   COX-1, 137, 138*t*
   COX-2, 137, 138*t*
      inhibitors of, 137, 138–39
   COX-2 inhibitors, 246*t*
      for older adults, 331
   inhibitors, 160
   isoenzymes, 137
      NSAIDs selective for, 137, 138*t*
cytokines
   and inflammatory pain, 55–56
   proinflammatory, 29–30

Dalai Lama, 7
DeBakey, Michael, 221
decision-making. *See also* shared decision-making
   clinical
      diagnosis-centered approach to, 107*f*
      patient-centered approach to, 107*f*
deconditioning, pain and, 78, 81, 85
Defense and Veterans Pain Rating Scale (DVPRS), 325*t*
delirium, in older adults, 322, 324
dementia
   pain assessment tool used in, 62
   and pain treatment plan, 213–14
demyelination, in trigeminal neuralgia, 293–94
dental pain, ibuprofen-sodium for, 137
depression, 17–18
   in children, 313
   in chronic pain patients, and opioid misuse/addiction, 343–44
   disability caused by, 46
   evaluation for, 78

interaction with other biopsychosocial
    variables, 79–80
mindfulness-based stress reduction
    for, 83–84
in older adults, 322, 323
opioid use and, 345
pain and, 43–44, 76, 78–79, 81, 160b
dermatomes, 97
    of lower torso and limbs, 97f
dermatomyositis, 268–69
Descartes, René, 56–58, 58f
descending modulation of pain,
    33–38, 34–35f
descending pain pathways, 17f, 17,
    160f, 244f
desipramine, 166–67
development, of pain system, 18–23
dexmedetomidine
    administration route, 246t
    mechanism of action of, 246t
    precautions with, 246t
    side effects, 246t
diabetes, 23
    SPS and, 303
diabetic amyotrophy, 265, 266f
diabetic neuropathy, 11, 110t, 286. *See
    also* painful diabetic peripheral
    neuropathy (PDPN)
    in older adults, pharmacologic therapy
        for, 330t
diagnosis/diagnoses, 104
    collaborative, 112
    multiple possible, 112–14
    precision of, 104
    process of, 104
Diagnosis, Intractability, Risk, and Efficacy
    (DIRE) scale, 345–46, 347t
diagnostic momentum, 113b
diagnostic reasoning, 104
    awareness of, 112
    errors in, avoiding, 112–15
    foundational elements of, 105–8
    and headache, 103–4
    key characteristics of pain in, 105, 106t
diagnostic testing, 109
diaphragmatic breathing, 84
    for children, 312
diarylheterocyclics, 137t
diazepam
    adverse effects of, 172–73

drug interactions with, 172–73
    mechanism of action of, 172f, 172–73
diclofenac, 138–39
    dosage and administration of, 139t
    half-life of, 139t
    hepatic injury with, 139–40
    mechanism of action of, 138t
    for older adults, 331
diet, in pain treatment for older adults, 329
differential diagnosis, 108–9, 119–20
    development of, 109
    physical examination and, 108
    process of, 104
    rare (catastrophic) entities in, 109
diffuse noxious inhibitory control
    (DNIC), 17–18
diflunisal
    dosage and administration of, 139t
    half-life of, 139t
    mechanism of action of, 138t
diphenoxylate, 141t, 147
diphenylheptanes, 141, 141t, 148
DIRE. *See* Diagnosis, Intractability, Risk,
    and Efficacy (DIRE) scale
disability
    definition of, 207
    determination of, 208
        by Social Security Administration,
        pain and, 207
    and legal action, 208
    related to pain, determination of, 207–8
disability system
    healthcare provider and, 208, 209f
    patient and, 208, 209f
distal symmetric polyneuropathy
    (DSPN), 286–88
    evaluation of, 286–87
    treatment of, 287–88, 288f
distraction, 15f, 16, 204
    for children, 312
    in pain treatment for older adults, 328
DNIC. *See* diffuse noxious inhibitory
    control (DNIC)
dopamine
    antinociceptive effect of, 38
    pronociceptive effect of, 38
    in reward system, 345
dorsal root ganglion (DRG), 8–9, 12, 17f, 31f
    aberrant sympathetic sprouts into, 170, 171f
    development of, 20f, 20–21

DRG. *See* dorsal root ganglion (DRG)
Drug Abuse Screening Test (DAST-10), 346, 348*t*
drug-seeker(s)/drug-seeking, 45, 48, 49, 66, 79
drug toxicity, in older adults, pharmacologic therapy for, 330*t*
Drug Use Disorders Identification Test (DUDIT), 346, 348*t*
dry needling, 201, 206
DSPN. *See* distal symmetric polyneuropathy (DSPN)
duloxetine, 167
 and breastfeeding, 367
 dosage adjustments for kidney or liver disease, 367
 for painful peripheral neuropathy, 287–88
 pregnancy category, 367
duodenal ulcers, NSAID-related, 138
DVPRS. *See* Defense and Veterans Pain Rating Scale (DVPRS)
dynorphins, opioid receptor binding, 140–41
dysesthesia, definition of, 70*t*

ectopic pregnancy, 225–27
 ruptured, 226*t*
education
 interprofessional, 125
 patient-provider, 121*f*
Ehlers-Danlos syndrome, 298*t*, 301–2
elderly, pain assessment tools for, 62
electrical stimulation, 201, 206–7
electromagnetic therapies, in pain treatment for older adults, 328–29
emergency(ies). *See also* pain emergency(ies)
 associated with pain, 222–31
 complications of pain treatment as, 222–38
emergency department, pain in, 221–22
emotional support, of patient, 119–20
empathy, 124
 communication of, 119
 vs. compassion, 120–21
 usefulness of, 120–21
encephalitis, 228–29, 228*t*
 fungal, 228*t*
 tuberculous, 228*t*
 viral, 228–29, 228*t*

endometriosis, 303–4
endorphins, opioid receptor binding, 140–41
energy field therapies, in pain treatment for older adults, 328–29
enkephalin, 17–18
 opioid receptor binding, 140–41
enolic acids, 137*t*
enteric neurons, 20–21
environmental factors
 with low back pain, 282–83, 283*f*
 in pain self-management, 212, 275*f*
ephaptic transmission, in trigeminal neuralgia, 293–94
Epicureans, 56–58
Epicurus, 241
epididymitis, 225–27
epidural analgesia, 250*f*, 250, 252*f*
 contraindications to, 250–51
 indications for, 250–51
 monitoring during, 250–51
 in obstetrics, 251–52
 side effects of, 250–51
epidural space, 250*f*
epidural steroid injection(s) (ESIs), 183
 complications of, 233
 interlaminar approach for, 183–84
 risks of, 185
 technique for, 183, 185*f*
 transforaminal approach for, 184–85
equianalgesic doses, of opioids, 150, 151*t*, 154–56
ERK. *See* extracellular signal-regulated kinases (ERK)
error(s)
 affective, 112–14, 113*b*
 cognitive, 112–14, 113*b*
 in diagnostic reasoning, 112–15
 disclosure of, 114
 prevention of, 112–15
 reducing, through effective clinical reasoning, 115*b*, 115
erythromelalgia, 292, 298–99*b*, 300–1
 clinical features of, 298*t*, 301
 genetics of, 293
 mechanisms of, 301
 prevalence of, 298*t*, 300
 treatment of, 298*t*, 301
ESIs. *See* epidural steroid injection(s) (ESIs)

ethics
    and pain alleviation, 58
    of pain alleviation, 42
    in pain practice, 124
    of pain treatment, 48–49
ethnicity, and experience and presentation of pain, 44
etodolac
    dosage and administration of, 139t
    half-life of, 139t
    mechanism of action of, 138t
etoricoxib, mechanism of action of, 138t
evoked potentials, 22
exercise, 201. *See also* strengthening exercises
    for fibromyalgia, 300
    for low back pain, 282–83, 283f
    in pain self-management, 210, 275f
    in pain treatment for older adults, 327
    for prevention or reduction of chronic pain, 373–74
    therapeutic, 205
expectancy, 213, 213t
extracellular signal-regulated kinases (ERK), in nociceptive transmission, 31–33
extremes of pain, 292
    case scenario, 291–92
    clinical features of, 298t, 304
    prevalence of, 298t, 304
    treatment pearls for, 298t, 304
eye(s), shingles and, 265
eye movement testing, 95

face, nerves of, 178, 179f
Face, Legs, Arms, Cry, Consolability Scale (FLACC), 310
Faces Pain Scale (FPS), 61–62, 309–10
Faces Pain Scale-Revised (FPS-R), 62, 64f, 309f, 310, 325t
facet joint cysts, 185–86
facet joint dysfunction, detection of, 100
facet joint injection, intra-articular, 185, 186f
facial pain
    and cranial nerve testing, 95
    new-onset, 264
    sinusitis and, 264
factitious disorder, 269–70
fascia iliaca block, 253t

fear, specific to pain, 80–81
fear avoidance, 43–44, 80–81
Federal Pain Research Strategy, 49
female(s), and pain risk, 78
femoral nerve, diabetic amyotrophy, 265, 266f
femoral nerve block, 252f, 252, 253t
fenamic acids, 137t
fenoprofen
    dosage and administration of, 139t
    half-life of, 139t
    mechanism of action of, 138t
fentanyl, 141, 147, 148. *See also* transmucosal immediate-release fentanyl (TIRF)
    administration route, 248t
    and breastfeeding, 367
    dosage adjustments for kidney or liver disease, 367
    dosage and administration of, 148
    drug interactions with, 148
    equianalgesic dose, 248t
    equianalgesic doses of, 150, 151t
    formulations of, 148
    mechanism of action of, 247t
    onset and duration of action, 248t
    pharmacology of, 148
    pregnancy category, 367
    transdermal, 148
fever, in children, 135
FFT. *See* Fortin finger test (FFT)
fibromyalgia, 17–18, 300
    clinical features of, 300
    mechanisms of, 300
    mindfulness-based stress reduction for, 83–84
    in older adults, pharmacologic therapy for, 330t
    prevalence of, 300
    sex distribution of, 300
    treatment of, 300
finger-to-nose test, 95
FLACC tool, 62, 63t, 64f
flu, and headache, 263
fluoroscopy, 177
flurbiprofen
    dosage and administration of, 139t
    half-life of, 139t
    mechanism of action of, 138t
focal pain, atypical, 264–65

foreign language speakers, pain assessment tools for, 62
Fortin finger test (FFT), 100
FPS. *See* Faces Pain Scale (FPS)
FPS-R. *See* Faces Pain Scale-Revised (FPS-R)
fracture(s)
  ankle, 123–24
    case scenario, 118
  hip, pain management for, 252
  in older adults, pharmacologic therapy for, 330*t*
  rib, 187–88
    pain management for, 243, 252
  vertebral, 229
frequency bias, 113*b*
frozen shoulder, 193
Functional Pain Scale, 325*t*
fundamental attribution bias, 113*b*

GABA, 17–18, 161
  diazepam and, 172*f*, 172–73
  GABA-A, benzodiazepines and, 172–73
  GABA-B, baclofen and, 171–72, 172*f*
  and nociceptive modulation in spinal dorsal horn, 38
  in pain modulation, 35, 36–37
  in periaqueductal gray, 35
  production of, impairment of, 302
  in rostral ventromedial medulla, 36–37
gabapentin, 19*f*, 26–27, 161, 245
  administration route, 246*t*
  adverse effects of, 162
    in older adults, 162
  and breastfeeding, 367
  for complex regional pain syndrome, 297–98
  dosage adjustments for kidney or liver disease, 367
  dosage and administration of, 161–62
  efficacy of, 161
  formulations of, 161–62
  half-life of, 161–62
  indications for, 161
  mechanism of action of, 38, 159*b*, 161, 162*f*, 246*t*
  for painful peripheral neuropathy, 287–88
  pharmacology of, 161, 162
  precautions with, 246*t*
  pregnancy category, 367
  side effects, 246*t*, 287–88
  topical, 173
gabapentinoids. *See also* gabapentin; pregabalin
  mechanism of action of, 38
  for phantom limb pain, 300
  for postherpetic neuralgia, 295
GAD-7. *See* Generalized Anxiety Disorder-7 (GAD-7)
GAD65 antibodies, 302
GAI. *See* Geriatric Anxiety Inventory (GAI)
gait
  assessment of, 95, 96, 263, 276–77, 281–82
  in older adults, 327
  in cauda equina syndrome, 230
  in multiple sclerosis, 263
  normal-pressure hydrocephalus and, 264
  optimization, with diabetic neuropathy, 287–88
gambler's fallacy, 113*b*
gamma-aminobutyric acid. *See* GABA
gangrene, 225
garlic, 28–29
gastric ulcers, NSAID-related, 138
gastroesophageal reflux disease, 224*t*
gastrointestinal system, nociception in, 11
gate control theory, 76–77, 203
  psychoeducation about, 81–82
Gawande, Atul, 26
GDS. *See* Geriatric Depression Scale (GDS)
gender, and pain, 17–18, 78
Generalized Anxiety Disorder-7 (GAD-7), 78, 85
genitofemoral nerve block, 188
Geriatric Anxiety Inventory (GAI), 324, 325*t*
Geriatric Depression Scale (GDS), 323, 325*t*
geriatric patients. *See* aging; elderly
GiA. *See* nucleus reticularis gigantocellularis pars alpha (GiA)
giant cell arteritis. *See* temporal arteritis
glaucoma, 262, 263
glenohumeral joint injection, 192
glia, 8–9
  spinal, 13*f*

glioblastoma multiforme, 228
global burden of illness, 46
glutamate, in nociceptive transmission, 30–32, 32f, 33, 35, 160f
gluteus/hip external rotation exercise, 284
glycine, and nociceptive modulation in spinal dorsal horn, 38
GONB. *See* greater occipital nerve block (GONB)
gout, NSAIDs for, 136–37
graded motor imagery, 203
graphic rating scale (GRS), 222
gravity-reducing treadmill, 201
gray matter, changes linked to persistent pain, 43
greater occipital nerve(s), 178
  compression, tenderness associated with, 277f
greater occipital nerve block (GONB), 179
guided imagery, in pain treatment for older adults, 328
Guillain-Barré syndrome, 228t, 230

hamstring strain, 112
hamstring stretch, 285
handicap, definition of, 207
HbA1$_c$, laboratory testing for, 110t
headache, 227. *See also* migraine; tension headache
  autoimmune disorders and, 262
  benign, 260
  brain tumor and, 262, 263
  brain tumor (neoplasm) and, 228
  caffeine-withdrawal, 103–4, 105, 106t
  case scenario, 103–4
  causes of, 260
  and cerebrospinal fluid analysis, 227, 228t
  in children, 311
  chronic daily, 276
  and cranial nerve testing, 95
  diagnostic reasoning and, 103–4
  as emergency, 227
  examination of patient with, 276–77, 277f
  infection and, 263
  laboratory testing and, 110t
  neurologic deficits with, 261, 276b
  new or worsening, 260–64
  nonbenign, 262

obstructive sleep apnea and, 261
in older adults, 264, 276b
palpation for, 98
postdural puncture, 236
screening neurologic exam for, 263, 276–77
sinusitis and, 264
thunderclap, 227
with visual impairment, 262–60
headache diary, 278–79
healthcare professionals, impact of pain on, 46–48
heat therapy, in pain treatment for older adults, 327
Helsinki declaration, 58
hematoma
  epidural, 234, 235, 250–51
  wound, with intrathecal drug delivery system implantation, 235
hemicrania, 121–22
Hemingway, Ernest, 291
hepatitis, and nerve vasculitis, 299
hepatitis C, 263
  laboratory testing for, 110t
hip abductor strengthening, 284, 373
hip fracture(s), pain management for, 252
hip joint replacement, 283–84
hip pain. *See also* chronic hip pain
  osteoarthritis and, 283–84
Hippocrates, 56–58
historical perspective, on pain, pain terminology, and pain assessment, 56–59
history, and diagnosis, 104
history of present illness (HPI), 91. *See also* illness narrative
history-taking, 91. *See also* illness narrative
HIV, 263
  pain-associated conditions with, 110t
  peripheral neuropathy, lamotrigine for, 163–64
Hogans tapping test (HTT), 99–100
home exercise programs, 112–14
homeostasis, 76–77
Horowitz's Impact of Event Scale, 324
5HT. *See* serotonin
HTT. *See* Hogans tapping test (HTT)
hydration, for prevention or reduction of chronic pain, 373–74

hydrocodone, 141t, 142–43, 144
  with acetaminophen (Vicodin), 247t
  dosage and administration of, 144
  equianalgesic doses of, 150, 151t
  formulations of, 144
  mechanism of action of, 247t
  and other analgesics, combined, 144
  pharmacology of, 144
hydrogen ions, 29–30
hydromorphone, 141t, 142–43
  administration route, 248t
  adverse effects of, 143
  and breastfeeding, 367
  dosage adjustments for kidney or liver disease, 367
  dosage and administration of, 143
  equianalgesic dose, 248t
  equianalgesic doses of, 150, 151t
  formulations of, 143
  mechanism of action of, 247t
  onset and duration of action, 248t
  pharmacology of, 143
  pregnancy category, 367
5-hydroxytryptamine (5-HT) receptors
  excitatory vs. inhibitory, 38
  subtypes, 38
hyperalgesia, 254–55. See also wind-up
  causes of, 69
  chronic opioid use and, 142
  definition of, 69, 70t
  detection of, 99–100
  molecular machinery of, 29–30
  PANos-mediated, 16
  with postherpetic neuralgia, 295
  with ulnar neuropathy, 288–89
hyperesthesia, definition of, 70t
hyperpathia, definition of, 70t
hyperpolarization, of cell membrane, and modulation of nociception, 38
hypertension, 23
hypervigilance, 15f, 16–17
hypnosis, 84, 203, 245
  for children, 312
  in pain treatment for older adults, 328
hypoalgesia, definition of, 70t
hypoesthesia, definition of, 70t
hypotension, with epidural analgesia, 250–51
hypothalamic-pituitary-adrenal (HPA) axis dysregulation, 76–77

IASP. See International Association for the Study of Pain (IASP)
IBS. See irritable bowel syndrome (IBS)
ibuprofen, 245
  administration route, 246t
  and breastfeeding, 367
  dosage adjustments for kidney or liver disease, 367
  dosage and administration of, 139t
    by pediatric age group, 314t
  formulations of, 137
  half-life of, 139t
  intravenous, 136–37
  mechanism of action of, 138t, 246t
  for migraine, 261
  for older adults, risk-reduction strategies with, 335
  opioid-sparing effect, 315
  pregnancy category, 367
  side effects, 246t
ibuprofen-sodium, 137
idiopathic intracranial hypertension (IIH), 262
IIH. See idiopathic intracranial hypertension (IIH)
ileus, opioid-induced, 249
iliohypogastric nerve block, 188, 189, 252f
ilioinguinal nerve block, 188, 189, 252f
iliopsoas stretch, 373, 285
iliotibial band syndrome, 112
  and hip pain, 283–84
illness narrative
  and diagnosis, 104, 109
  with multiple pain-associated conditions, 105, 106t
  obtaining, 105
  pain-focused, 91–92
  professional's role in, 119–20
imaging, 110, 111t
  and abdominal pain, 223
  guidance, for interventions, 177
  and low back pain, 110–11
IMMPACT Consortium, recommendations for pain assessment, 308t, 309
immune response
  opioids and, 249
  postoperative pain and, 243
impairment
  definition of, 207
  determination of, 208

and legal action, 208
support for patients with, 207, 208
impulsivity, in pain patients with negative affect, and risk of opioid misuse/addiction, 344
indomethacin
  dosage and administration of, 139t
  half-life of, 139t
  mechanism of action of, 138t
infant(s). *See also* pediatric pain management
  acute pain in, 311
  causes of pain in, 311
  chronic pain in, 311
  pain assessment in, 307
    tools for, 62, 63t
  pain prophylaxis in, 22
  response to pain, 18–19
infection(s)
  headache caused by, 228–29, 228t, 263
  with intrathecal drug delivery system implantation, 235
  spine pain caused by, 229
inflammation
  neurogenic, 33
  and nociception in small intestine, 11
inflammatory mediators, 29–30, 55–56
inflammatory pain, 54, 55f, 55
  etiology of, 57t
  pharmacologic treatment of, 270f
  treatment of, 57t, 363
inflammatory soup, 28–30
information gathering, from patient, 119–20, 120f, 121f
Initiative on Methods, Measurement and Pain Assessment in Clinical Trials. *See* IMMPACT Consortium
inspection, 97
  abnormalities seen on, 94
insufficient information bias, 113b
insula, 15f, 15–16, 203
integrative therapies, 275f
  for complex regional pain syndrome, 297–98
  for low back pain, 282–83, 283f
intercostal nerve block, 187, 252f
interdisciplinary programs, for pediatric pain management, 312, 313

interleukin(s) (IL)
  IL-6, 29–30
  IL-1β, 29–30
interleukin receptor(s) (IL-R)
  IL-1R, 29–30
  IL-6R, 29–30
International Association for the Study of Pain (IASP)
  definition of pain, 53–54, 70t
  lexicon and taxonomy of pain, 69, 70t
interneurons, 13f, 160f
  inhibitory, 12–14, 17–18
interprofessional competencies, core, related to pain, 46–47
interprofessional practice, 208–10
interventional pain management, 177
  case scenario, 176–77
  CT guidance, 177
  fluoroscopy for, 177
  head and face procedures, 178–81
  landmark technique, 177
  large joint procedures, 192–95
  neck procedures, 181–83
  neuraxial procedures, 183–87
  pelvic procedures, 190–92
  trunk procedures, 187–90
  ultrasound guidance, 177
intervertebral disk(s). *See* spinal disk
interview
  affective information in, 106, 119–20
  as critical skill, 90–91
  open-ended questions in, 92, 105, 120–21
  three-function model of, 120f
  updated three-function model of, 121f
intracranial hemorrhage (ICH), 227
intrathecal drug delivery, 196
  and baclofen withdrawal, 237
  bleeding complications with, 235
  candidates for, 196
  and cerebrospinal fluid leak, 236
  and clonidine withdrawal, 237
  complications of, 234
  devices for, 234f, 234
  indications for, 196, 234
  infectious complications with, 235
  and meningitis after pump implantation, 235
  and opioid effects, 236
  and opioid withdrawal, 237

intrathecal drug delivery (cont.)
    and postdural puncture headache, 236
    postimplantation complications
        with, 235
    refill complications, 238
    risks of, 197
    systems for, 196
    technique for, 196
intravenous immunoglobulin(s) (IVIG),
        for SPS, 303
ion channel-selective agents, 168–70
    in pain care, 159
Iowa Pain Thermometer (IPT), 325t
irritable bowel syndrome (IBS), 268
    case scenario, 259–60
isoniazid, drug interactions with, 136
itching. See pruritus
IVIG. See intravenous
        immunoglobulin(s) (IVIG)

Joint Commission, pain assessment and
        management standards, 66, 242
joint position testing, 99–100
joint replacement, in older adults, 283–84
justice, ethical principle of, 48, 124
juvenile idiopathic arthritis, 311
juvenile rheumatoid arthritis, 311

KA. See kainite (KA) receptor
Kahlo, Frida, 273
kainite (KA) receptor, in nociceptive
        transmission, 31–32, 33
Katz Index of Independence in ADLs, 322
Keele, Kenneth, 59
ketamine, 19f, 169, 245
    administration route, 246t
    mechanism of action of, 16, 169f,
        169, 246t
    for phantom limb pain, 300
    precautions with, 246t
    side effects, 246t
    site of action, 244f
    topical, 173
ketoprofen
    dosage and administration of, 139t
    half-life of, 139t
    mechanism of action of, 138t
    topical, 173
ketorolac
    administration route, 246t

    dosage and administration of, 139t
    half-life of, 139t
    intranasal, 136–37
    mechanism of action of, 138t, 246t
    parenteral, 136–37
    side effects, 246t
key characteristics of pain, 91, 105b, 105
    in diagnostic reasoning, 105, 106t
kidney disease
    medication dosage adjustments for, 144
    NSAIDs and, 139–40
kinesiology taping, 201
King, Stephen, 117
knee, arthritis of, 201
knee intra-articular joint injection, 194
knee pain. See also chronic knee pain
    management of, 284–85
    prevention of, exercises for, 284

laboratory testing, 110, 110t
lamotrigine, 163
    adverse effects of, 164
    dosage and administration of, 164
    drug interactions with, 164
    formulations of, 164
    mechanism of action of, 163–64, 164f
large-fiber testing, 99–100
laser, 201
LAST. See local anesthetic systemic
        toxicity (LAST)
Lawton Instrumental ADLs, 322
LEADERS LEAD (mnemonic), 115b
learned helplessness, 43–44
legitimation, 120–21
lesser occipital nerve(s), 178
lesser occipital nerve block (LONB), 179
Lessing, Doris, 117
levorphanol, 141t, 150
lidocaine, 19f, 168, 173, 270f
    dosage and administration of, 253–54
    mechanism of action of, 168f, 168
    for painful peripheral
        neuropathy, 287–88
    pharmacology of, 168
    precautions with, 295
    trial of, for older adults unable to
        self-report, 325t
lifestyle change, positive, 123
limb pain, 225
lipid emulsion (Intralipid), 253–54

listening. *See also* active listening
  to illness narrative, 91, 92
lithium, and NSAIDs, interactions of, 140
litigation, and pain resolution, 208
liver disease
  medication dosage adjustments for, 144
  NSAIDs and, 139–40
local anesthetics
  dosage and administration of, 253–54
  in epidural analgesia, 250
  mechanism of action of, 168*f*, 168
  site of action, 244*f*
  toxicity of, 250–51
local anesthetic systemic toxicity
    (LAST), 253–54
locus ceruleus, 17*f*, 17–18, 35
LONB. *See* lesser occipital nerve
    block (LONB)
loperamide, 141*t*, 147
low back pain. *See also* chronic low
    back pain
  and clinical assessment, 90–91
  collaborative care for, 112
  diffuse, in Guillain-Barré syndrome, 230
  and disability, 45, 46
  with disk injury, 267–68
  emergent causes of, 268
  evaluation of, 99, 280
  imaging and, 110–11
  management of, 282–83, 283*f*
  physical therapy for, 112
  prevalence of, 90–91
  provocative maneuvers for, 94
  red flags for, 280–81
LPGi. *See* nucleus paragigantocellularis
    lateralis (LPGi)
lumbar puncture (LP), 227
lumiracoxib, mechanism of action of, 138*t*
lupus cerebritis, laboratory testing and, 110*t*
Lyme disease, 228–29, 263, 264
  laboratory testing and, 110*t*
  peripheral neuropathy in, 286

magnetic resonance imaging (MRI),
    110–11, 111*t*
  of brain, in headache patient, 263
  of neck, 279–80
Maimonides, 56–58
malignancy. *See also* cancer; tumor(s)
  in children, 311

malingering, 269–70
manipulation, 94
manual therapy, 201
Marley, Bob, 199
massage, in pain treatment for older
    adults, 327
MBBs. *See* medial branch block(s) (MBBs)
MBSR. *See* mindfulness-based stress
    reduction (MBSR)
McGill Pain Questionnaire (MPQ), 59, 61, 64*f*
mechanic's hands, 268–69
meclofenamate
  dosage and administration of, 139*t*
  half-life of, 139*t*
  mechanism of action of, 138*t*
medial branch block(s) (MBBs), 186
medial branch radiofrequency ablation, 186
medical history, of older adults, 320–21
medication safety
  with low back pain, 282–83, 283*f*
  in pain self-management, 211, 275*f*
meditation, 211, 245
  for children and adolescents, 312
  guided, 84
meditation-oriented recovery
    enhancement, 211
melastatin 8, 28
meloxicam
  dosage and administration of, 139*t*
  half-life of, 139*t*
  mechanism of action of, 138*t*
Melzack, Ron, 59
Memorial Pain Assessment Card (MPAC), 61
meningitis, 228–29, 228*t*
  with intrathecal drug delivery system
      implantation, 235
menorrhagia, NSAIDs for, 136–37
mental health
  in older adults, assessment of, 322–24
  pain and, 76, 78–79
mental preparation, in pain
    self-management, 211
mental status, assessment of, 94–95,
    96, 355
menthol, 28–29
meperidine, 141*t*, 147
  adverse effects of, 147
  formulations of, 147
  mechanism of action of, 147
  neurotoxicity of, 147

meralgia paresthetica, 70t, 265, 266f
metabolic neuropathy, 286
metabotropic glutamate receptor (mGluR), in nociceptive transmission, 31–32, 33
methadone, 141t, 149
　administration route, 248t
　adverse effects of, 149
　deaths caused by, 149
　dosage and administration of, 149
　equianalgesic dose, 248t
　formulations of, 149
　half-life of, 149
　mechanism of action of, 149, 247t
　for older adults, 331
　onset and duration of action, 248t
　for opioid use disorder, 351–52
　pharmacology of, 149
N-methyl-D-aspartate. See NMDA
methylnaltrexone bromide, 335
mGluR. See metabotropic glutamate receptor (mGluR)
microglia, 12–14
migraine, 105, 106t, 121–22, 260. See also chronic migraine
　and allodynia, 98–99, 277f, 278
　botulinum toxin injection for, 180
　case scenario, 103–4
　chronic, allodynia with, 277f
　clinical features of, 261, 278
　and differential diagnosis, 109
　disability caused by, 46
　neurologic deficits with, 261, 277–78
　NSAIDs for, 136–37
　in older adults, 264
　pathophysiology of, 261
　prevalence of, 261, 277–78
　prophylaxis, 278–79
　treatment of, 136–37, 261
milnacipran, 167
mind–body connection, 76
mind–body therapies
　for low back pain, 282–83, 283f
　in pain self-management, 211
mindfulness, 211
　for children and adolescents, 312
　clinicians', 125–26
mindfulness-based stress reduction (MBSR), 81, 82t, 83–84, 211
　for prevention or reduction of chronic pain, 373

mindfulness strategies, 83
Mini-Cog, 323
Mini-Mental Status Exam (MMSE), 325t
mirror pain, with postherpetic neuralgia, 295
mirror visual feedback, 203
MMSE. See Mini-Mental Status Exam (MMSE)
MOBID-2 pain scale, 62
Modified Caregiver Strain Index, 324
modulation of pain, 9, 15f, 16–18
　descending, 33–38, 34–35f
　negative pathways, 17
　neurocognitive, in rehabilitation, 202–4
　positive pathways, 16
　supraspinal, 16–17
monoamine oxidase inhibitors, 160b
mononeuropathy, definition of, 70t
mononeuropathy multiplex, definition of, 70t
mood
　assessment of, 355
　and problematic opioid use, 351
mood disorders, in chronic pain patients, 340–42
morphine, 134, 141t, 142–43
　administration route, 248t
　and breastfeeding, 367
　and cardiovascular outcomes, 223
　dosage adjustments for kidney or liver disease, 367
　dosage and administration of, 143
　　by pediatric age group, 314t
　elimination half-life of, 143
　equianalgesic dose, 248t
　equianalgesic doses of, 150, 151t
　extended-release (ER), 134
　formulations of, 143
　immediate-release (IR), 134
　mechanism of action of, 247t
　onset and duration of action, 248t
　in pediatric pain management, 314t, 315
　pharmacology of, 143
　pregnancy category, 367
　and renal impairment, 143
　trial of, for older adults unable to self-report, 325t
morphine sulfate equivalent dose, 332
Morton neuroma, 100
motivational interviewing, 203

motor examination, screening, 95, 96
motor weakness, 99–100
MPAC. *See* Memorial Pain Assessment Card (MPAC)
MPQ. *See* McGill Pain Questionnaire (MPQ)
MRI. *See* magnetic resonance imaging (MRI)
MS. *See* multiple sclerosis (MS)
multimodal analgesia, 245. *See also* pain care: multimodal approach for
  case scenario, 8
  preventive, 255
multiple sclerosis (MS), 262, 263
  and atypical focal pain, 264–65
  and facial pain, 264
muscle, knots in, palpation for, 99
muscle spasm, 99
muscle tone, assessment for, 99
musculoskeletal pain
  in children, 311
  disability caused by, 46
  prevalence of, 45–46
music therapy, 245
  in pain treatment for older adults, 328
mustard, 28–29
myalgia, 268–69
  statin-associated, 268–69
myelination, 18–19
  central, 22
  peripheral, 21*f*, 21, 22
  of primary afferent neurons, 9–11, 10–11*f*
myelopathy, cervical, 279–80
myofascial pain syndrome, in older adults, pharmacologic therapy for, 330*t*
myopathy, statin-associated, 268–69
myositis, 268–69

nabumetone
  dosage and administration of, 139*t*
  half-life of, 139*t*
  mechanism of action of, 138*t*
nalbuphine, 141*t*
  mechanism of action of, 247*t*
naloxegol, 335
naloxone, 141–42, 141*t*, 146
  dosage and administration of, 146, 147*t*, 248*b*
  formulations of, 146
  and long-acting opioids, 248*b*

  for opioid overdose, 146, 147*t*, 232
naltrexone, 141*t*, 146
  elimination half-life of, 146
  formulations of, 146
  pharmacology of, 146
NAPQI. *See* N-acetyl-*p*-benzoquinone imine (NAPQI)
naproxen
  administration route, 246*t*
  and breastfeeding, 367
  dosage adjustments for kidney or liver disease, 367
  dosage and administration of, 139*t*
  half-life of, 139*t*
  mechanism of action of, 138*t*, 246*t*
  pregnancy category, 367
  side effects, 246*t*
  and sumatriptan, combined, 136–37
narcotics, oral, and breastfeeding, 367
narrative. *See* illness narrative; pain narrative
National Pain Strategy (2016), 49
natural/herbal therapies, in pain treatment for older adults, 329
nausea and vomiting, opioid-induced, 249
neck, nerves of, 178, 179*f*
neck pain. *See also* chronic neck pain
  and disability, 45
  disability caused by, 46
  palpation for, 99
  urgent, 266–68
neck stiffness, 228–29
neonate(s). *See also* pediatric pain management
  acute pain in, 311
  causes of pain in, 311
  chronic pain in, 311
  pain assessment in, 307
neospinothalamic tract, 14, 15*f*, 15–16
nerve block(s). *See also* peripheral nerve block(s); regional anesthesia; *specific nerve*
  diagnostic, 177
  for older adults, 334
nerve endings, nociceptive, 9–11
nerve growth factor, 11, 29–30
  and inflammatory pain, 55–56
nerve injury
  with epidural analgesia, 250–51
  persistent pain after, 254–56
nerve root compression, cervical, 279–80

nerve root levels, 97
neural crest, 20f, 20–21
    slug expression, 20f, 21
neural fold, 20f, 20–21
neuralgia, definition of, 70t
neural groove, 20f, 20–21
neural tube, 20–21
    closure of, 20–21
neuraxial analgesia, 183–87, 250–51,
        334. See also epidural steroid
        injection(s) (ESIs); regional
        anesthesia
    complications of, 233
    and epidural hematoma, 234
    morphine for, 143
    with opioids, adverse effects and safety
        issues, 248, 249, 250–51, 252
    oxycodone for, 144–45
neuregulin 1, 21–22
neuritis, definition of, 70t
neuroablation, 177
neurocognitive modulation of pain, in
        rehabilitation, 202–4
neurofeedback, 203
neurogenesis, 20
neurogenic claudication, 267
neuroinflammation, 12, 13f
neurokinin 1 (NK1) receptor, in
        nociceptive transmission,
        32f, 32–33
neurologic examination, screening, 94, 263
neuroma
    definition of, 100
    intercostal, 187–88
    Morton, 100
    proximal limb (stump), pain from,
        versus phantom limb pain, 295, 296
neuroma testing, 100
neuromatrix theory of pain, 76–77
neuromodulating agents, 134–35. See also
        specific agent
    for chronic pain, 160
    classes of, 159, 160–61
    definition of, 159
    efficacy of, 160–61
    indications for, 270f
    mechanisms of action of, and multidrug
        combinations, 160
    multiple, combined, 160
    for neuropathic pain, 160

for older adults, 331
    therapy with, case scenario, 158–59
    topical, 173
neuromodulation, 18, 177, 195. See also
    spinal cord stimulation
neuropathic pain, 12–14, 13f, 54, 55f, 56,
    269–70. See also distal symmetric
    polyneuropathy (DSPN);
    painful diabetic peripheral
    neuropathy (PDPN)
    case scenario, 158–59
    definition of, 70t
    etiology of, 57t
    IASP definition of, 56
    laboratory testing and, 110t
    management of, 38
    neuromodulating agents for, 160
    in older adults, pharmacologic therapy
        for, 330t, 334, 336
    pharmacologic treatment of, 270f
    prevalence of, 45–46
    research-oriented revised
        definition of, 56
    suspected, in older adults unable to
        self-report, 325t
    treatment of, 57t, 363
neuropathy, 55f
    definition of, 70t
neurostimulators, for older adults, 334
Neurotip, 99–100
neurotransmitter receptors
    in descending modulation of
        pain, 34–35f
    in nociceptive transmission, 30–33, 32f
neurotransmitters, 26–27
    in descending modulation of
        pain, 34–35f
    and nociceptive modulation in spinal
        dorsal horn, 38, 160f
    in nociceptive transmission, 30–33, 32f
    opioid use and, 345
neurotrophins, 20–21
newborn
    pain control in, 18–23
    pain exposure, effects on brain
        development, 43
    pain prophylaxis in, 22
    pain system development in, 18–23
    response to pain, 18–19, 20
NGF. See nerve growth factor

NK1. *See* neurokinin 1 (NK1) receptor
NMDA antagonists, 16, 169f, 169, 247t
NMDA receptor, in nociceptive
    transmission, 31–32, 32f, 33
nocebo effect, 213t
nociception
    chemically induced, 28–29, 29t
    definition of, 70t
    mechanical, 27–28
    molecular machinery of, 27
    thermal, 28
nociception (term), 58–59
nociceptive (term), 58–59
nociceptive neuron, definition of, 70t
nociceptive pain, 54, 55f
    definition of, 70t
    etiology of, 57t
    in older adults, pharmacologic therapy for, 330t, 334
    opioids for, 140–41
    pharmacologic treatment of, 270f
    suspected, in older adults unable to self-report, 325t
    treatment of, 57t, 363
nociceptive processing
    case scenario, 26–27
    cortical and subcortical, 15f, 15
nociceptive stimulus, definition of, 70t
nociceptive transmission, 244f, 244
    anterograde, 33
    ascending, 14, 15f, 27–30, 33 (*see also* ascending pain pathways)
    bidirectional modulation of, 36–38
    into central nervous system, 12, 27
    postsynaptic descending facilitation of, 33–35, 34–35f
    postsynaptic descending inhibition of, 33–35, 34–35f
    presynaptic descending facilitation of, 33–35, 34–35f
    presynaptic descending inhibition of, 33–35, 34–35f
    retrograde, 33
nociceptor(s), 8–9, 10–11f
    activation of, 54–55
    classification of, 9
    definition of, 70t
    mechanical, 27–28
    peripheral, 244
    polymodal, 9–11

somatic, 9
visceral, 11
nociceptor (term), 58–59
nocifensive (term), 58–59
nocifensive withdrawal reflex, 26, 36–37
nonmaleficence, 48, 124
nonopioid analgesics, 135–36. See also
    specific analgesic
    for acute pain, 245, 246t
    combinations of, 245
nonsteroidal anti-inflammatory drugs
    (NSAIDs), 19f, 136–40, 245
    administration route, 246t
    adverse effects of, 138
    cardiovascular effects of, 138–39
    chemical classes of, 137, 137t
    clinical applications of, 136–37
    contraindications to, 138–39
        in older adults, 335
    dosage and administration of, 139t
    drug interactions with, 140
    efficacy, interpatient variability of, 138
    formulations of, 136–37
    gastrointestinal protection with, in older adults, 335
    and gastroprotective agents, combined, 136–37
    half-life of, 139t
    hepatic effects of, 139–40
    hepatic injury with, 139–40
    indications for, 270f
    mechanism of action of, 246t
    nanoformulated, 136–37
    for older adults, 330t, 331
        risk-reduction strategies with, 335
    and other analgesics, combined, 136–37
    for pediatric fever, 135
    precautions with, 246t
    renal effects of, 139–40
    side effects, 246t
    topical, 136–37
        for older adults, 331
    trial of, for older adults unable to self-report, 325t
nonverbal patients, pain scale for, 62
norepinephrine, 17f, 17–18
    reuptake inhibition, 160b
normal-pressure hydrocephalus, 264

nortriptyline, 166
   and breastfeeding, 367
   dosage adjustments for kidney or liver disease, 367
   pregnancy category, 367
notochord, 20*f*, 20–21
noxious stimulus, 9
   definition of, 70*t*
NRM. *See* nucleus raphe magnus (NRM)
NRS. *See* numeric rating scale (NRS)
NSAIDs. *See* nonsteroidal anti-inflammatory drugs (NSAIDs)
Nubian. *See* nalbuphine
nucleus paragigantocellularis lateralis (LPGi), 36*f*, 36
nucleus raphe magnus (NRM), 17*f*, 17–18, 36*f*, 36
nucleus reticularis gigantocellularis pars alpha (GiA), 36*f*, 36
numeric rating scale (NRS), 59, 60*f*, 60, 64*f*, 68, 222, 243–44, 325. *See also* Brief Pain Inventory (BPI)
Nuremberg code, 58
nutrition, for prevention or reduction of chronic pain, 373–74

obsessive-compulsive disorder (OCD), pain and, 43–44
obstetric pain
   anatomic sources of, 251*f*, 251
   case scenario, 241–42
   epidural analgesia for, 251–52
obstructive sleep apnea (OSA), 261
OCC. *See* Opioid Compliance Checklist (OCC)
occipital neuralgia, 105, 106*t*, 178, 277*f*, 278
occupational therapy, for children, 313
off-cells, in pain modulation, 36–37, 37*f*, 38
older adults
   adherence toxicity in, 329
   age-related physiologic changes in, 334
   agitation in, 322
   anxiety in, 322, 324
   caregivers
      evaluation of, 324
      and multimodal pain treatment, 324–27
   chronic pain in, 275–76
   cognitive impairment in, 322
      and pain assessment, 322, 325*t*
      and pain treatment plan, 329
   cognitive status in
      assessment of, 322–23
      and pain treatment plan, 329
   delayed treatment of pain in, 324–27
   delirium in, 322, 324
   depression in, 322, 323
   drug dosage and administration in, 334
   drug prescribing for
      principle of, 334
      recommendations for, 334
   drug toxicity in, risk factors for, 329, 334
   falls in, 322
   function, assessment of, 322
   gabapentin side effects in, 162
   joint replacement in, 283–84
   medical history of, 320–21
   medication adverse effects in, reduction/prevention of, 334
   medication safety in, 334
   medication tolerance in, 329
   mental health in, assessment of, 322–24
   mild pain in, pharmacologic therapy for, 336
   mixed/undetermined pain in, pharmacologic therapy for, 330*t*, 334
   moderate pain in, pharmacologic therapy for, 336
   multimodal pain treatment for, 324–36, 325*t*, 328*f*
      complementary and alternative strategies in, 327
      medications in, 329, 330*t*
   neuropathic pain in, pharmacologic therapy for, 330*t*, 334, 336
   with new or worsening headache, 264, 276*b*
   nociceptive pain in, pharmacologic therapy for, 330*t*, 334
   opioid abuse/misuse by, 335–36
   opioids for, 332–33
   opiophobia in, 329
   pain assessment in, 320–24
      comprehensive, 320, 321*f*
      focused, 320, 324, 325*t*
   pain in
      deleterious consequences of, 320
      prevalence of, 319–20

pain interference with function, and pain management, 334
pain management in, *case scenario,* 319
pain narrative of, 321–22
pain severity in, and pain management, 334
pain type in, and pain management, 330*t*, 334
persistent pain in, analgesic management of, 330
pharmacodynamics in, 334
pharmacogenetics in, 334
pharmacokinetics in, 334
physical abilities of, and pain treatment plan, 329
polypharmacy in, 329
post-traumatic stress disorder in, 322, 324
psychological assessment in, 322–24
severe pain in, pharmacologic therapy for, 336
somatic pain in, pharmacologic therapy for, 330*t*
subgroups at increased risk for pain, 320
suicidal ideation in, 322
undertreatment of pain in, 324–27
visceral pain in, pharmacologic therapy for, 330*t*
weight of, and drug treatment, 334
oligodendrocytes, 22
omission bias, 113*b*
on-cells, in pain modulation, 36–37, 37*f*, 38
operant conditioning, 202
opioid(s), 19*f*, 48, 134, 140–52. See also *specific opioid*
  aberrant drug behaviors and, 341*b*
  abuse of, 142, 340 (see also opioid addiction)
    definition of, 341*b*
    by older adults, 335–36
    prevalence of, 340–42
  for acute pain, 245
  administration routes for, 140–41, 245
  adverse effects and safety issues, 231*t*, 232, 245–49
  adverse effects of, 141–42, 142*t*
  around-the-clock dosing of, 150
  chronic users, acute pain in, 255
  class effects of, 141
  classification of, 141, 141*t*
  clinical applications of, 140–41

for complex regional pain syndrome, 297–98
contraindications to, 300, 303
  in older adults, 331
conversions between, 150, 154–56
deaths caused by, 47, 119, 140
discontinuation of, 351–52
dosage and administration of, by pediatric age group, 314*t*
dose conversions, 134
drug interactions with, 141–42
for dying patients, 47
endogenous, 17*f*, 17–18
  in periaqueductal gray, 35
equianalgesic doses of, 150, 151*t*, 154–56, 248*t*
extended-release (ER), 150
  for older adults, 331
iatrogenic addiction to, 249
illicit, 47
and immune modulation, 249
incomplete cross-tolerance, 151–52
intoxication, 141–42
intrathecal, adverse effects and safety issues, 236
long-acting, 150
  naloxone and, 248*b*
  for older adults, 331
mechanism of action of, 38, 245, 247*t*
misuse of, 142, 340. See also opioid addiction
  in chronic pain patients, management of, 351–52
  clinician-based measures, 346, 348*t*
  definition of, 341*b*
  generic instruments for identifying, 346–50, 348*t*
  identification of patients at risk for, 345–46
  management of patients at risk for, 350–51
  neurobiological factors affecting, 345
  by older adults, 335–36
  opioid-specific instruments for identifying, 346–50, 348*t*
  over course of therapy, identification of patients, 346–50, 348*t*
  risk factors for, 342–44
  self-report questionnaires on, 346, 348*t*
  urine toxicology screening for, 346

opioid(s) (*cont.*)
  naturally occurring, 142–43
  and nociceptive modulation in spinal dorsal horn, 38
  for older adults, 330*t*, 331
    risk-reduction strategies with, 335
  and orthopedic surgery, 204–5
  overdose (*see* opioid overdose)
  in patient-controlled analgesia, 249
  for pediatric pain management, 313, 315
  physical dependence on, 142, 339, 351–52
  policy changes related to, 47
  precautions with, 247*t*
  prescribed, 47, 119
  prescription guidelines for, 140, 350–51
  rapid-acting, for older adults, 331
  risk–benefit with, 153
  rotation, in pediatric pain management, 315
  short-acting, for older adults, 331
  site of action, 244*f*
  and stigma, 45
  storage and disposal of, patient education about, 336
  subcutaneous injection near intrathecal device, 238
  synthetic, 147
  tolerance, 142, 151–52, 255, 341*b*
    in older adults, 329
  use, early life trauma and, 92
  for vaso-occlusive pain crises in sickle cell disease, 230–31
  withdrawal, 142, 146, 237
opioid abuse-deterrent drugs, for older adults, 333
opioid addiction, 339. *See also* opioid use disorder (OUD)
  case scenario, 340
  in chronic pain patients, 340–42
    demographic and background factors affecting, 342
    management of, 351–52
    psychological factors affecting, 343, 344–45, 351
    risk factors for, 342–44
  diagnosis of, 350
  identification of patients at risk for, 345–46
  management of patients at risk for, 350–51
  neurobiological factors affecting, 345
  prevalence of, 340–42
  risk factors for, 342–44
opioid agonist(s), 141, 141*t*, 142*t*, 247*t*
opioid alternatives, 47
opioid antagonist(s), 141, 141*t*, 247*t*
  in opioid abuse-deterrent drugs, 333
Opioid Compliance Checklist (OCC), 346, 348*t*
opioid craving, in pain patients with negative affect, and risk of opioid misuse/addiction, 344
opioid crisis, 47, 49, 140
  economic burden of, 46
opioid detoxification, 352
opioid overdose, 47, 119, 140, 141–42, 146, 232
  naloxone for, 146, 147*t*, 232
  treatment of, 232
opioid receptors, 140–41
  and adverse effects of opioids, 141, 142*t*
  in periaqueductal gray, 35
  in rostral ventromedial medulla, 36–37
opioid risk assessment, 345–46
Opioid Risk Tool (ORT), 335–36, 345–46, 347*t*
opioid-sparing effect, 245, 315
opioid treatment agreement, 350–52
opioid use disorder (OUD), 47, 49. *See also* opioid addiction
  buprenorphine for, 145
  definition of, 341*b*
  DSM-V diagnostic criteria for, 341*b*, 342, 350
  methadone for, 149
  naltrexone for, 146
opiophobia, 329
opium poppy, 142–43
optic neuritis, 263
oral pain, with dental caries, 311
ORT. *See* Opioid Risk Tool (ORT)
orthotics. *See* assistive devices/orthotics
Orwell, George, 259
Osler, William, 103
osteoarthritis
  and hip pain, 283–84
  of knee, 194
  pain of, 55*f*
    NSAIDs for, 136–37

OTC. *See* over-the-counter (OTC) pain relievers
Oucher—Numeric Rating Scale, 310
Oucher—Photographic, 310
outcome bias, 112–14, 113*b*
overconfidence bias, 112–14, 113*b*
over-the-counter (OTC) pain relievers, hazards of, 274–76
oxaprozin
   dosage and administration of, 139*t*
   half-life of, 139*t*
oxcarbazepine, 163
   for trigeminal neuralgia, 160
oxycodone, 141*t*, 142–43, 144
   with acetaminophen (Percocet), 247*t*
   administration route, 248*t*
   and breastfeeding, 367
   dosage adjustments for kidney or liver disease, 367
   dosage and administration of, 144
      by pediatric age group, 314*t*
   equianalgesic dose, 248*t*
   equianalgesic doses of, 150, 151*t*
   extended-release (ER), 134
   formulations of, 144
   immediate-release (IR), 134
   mechanism of action of, 247*t*
   onset and duration of action, 248*t*
   pharmacology of, 144
   pregnancy category, 367
oxymorphone, 141*t*, 142–43, 144
   elimination half-life of, 144
   equianalgesic doses of, 150, 151*t*
   extended-release (ER), 144
   formulations of, 144
   pharmacology of, 144

pacing, 204
PACSLAC-II. *See* Pain Assessment Checklist for Seniors with Limited Ability to Communicate (PACSLAC-II)
PADT. *See* Pain Assessment and Documentation Tool (PADT)
PAG. *See* periaqueductal gray (PAG)
pain
   affective component of, 106, 119–20
   classes of, overlap and interaction of, 54, 55*f*
   classification of, 54–56, 55*f*
   definition of, 242
   historical perspective on, 56–58
   IASP definition of, 53–54, 70*t*
   impact on healthcare professionals, 46–48
   impact on social network, 44–45
   individual variation in, 65*f*, 65–66
   as intersubjective, 106–7
   mixed/undetermined
      in older adults, pharmacologic therapy for, 330*t*, 334
      suspected, in older adults unable to self-report, 325*t*
   as not "subjective," 106–7
   subjective features of, 121–22
   of undetermined pathology, 269–70
Pain, Enjoyment, and General Activity (PEG) Scale, 322
PAIN-AD, 62
PAINAD. *See* Pain Assessment in Advanced Dementia Scale (PAINAD)
pain anxiety, 80, 82–83. *See also* anxiety
   affective component of, 106
Pain Anxiety Symptoms Scale (PASS), 80–81
pain assessment
   accepting patient's self-report in, 65–66
   case scenario, 52–53
   challenges and difficulty of, 53
   of chest pain, 223
   in children, 61–62, 62*f*, 307–10 (*see also* pediatric pain assessment)
   clinician's responsibilities in, 65–68
   contingency-based approach to, 67*f*, 67–68
   in emergency department, 222
   historical perspective on, 59
   IMMPACT Consortium recommendations for, 308*t*, 309
   in older adults, 320–24
      comprehensive, 320, 321*f*
      focused, 320, 324, 325*t*
   patient's responsibilities in, 65, 68
   perioperative, 243–44
   principles of, 62
   and reassessment, 68
   standard clinical approach (QRSTUVW), 308*t*
   supportive environment for, 68

Pain Assessment and Documentation Tool (PADT), 346, 348t
Pain Assessment Checklist for Seniors with Limited Ability to Communicate (PACSLAC-II), 325t
Pain Assessment in Advanced Dementia Scale (PAINAD), 325t
pain assessment tools, 59–68
  behavioral, 62
  key characteristics of, 65
  multidimensional, 59, 61
  as outcome measures for clinical trials, 68
  unidimensional, 59
pain-associated condition(s)
  with manifestations in multiple areas, 105
  multiple
    appraising, 105, 106t
    prioritzing, 105
pain care. *See also* pain management
  cognitive impairment and, 213–14
  coordinated evidence-based approach for, 208–10, 210f
  cultural considerations in, 44
  dementia and, 213–14
  disparities in, 44, 45
  liguistic competence and, 44
  multimodal approach for, 47–48, 126–27, 127f, 201, 208–10, 210f, 274–75, 275f (*see also* multimodal analgesia)
  in older adults, 324–36, 325t, 328f
  professional conduct in, 118–22
  psychological factors in, 201
  safe, biopsychosocial model and, 119
  and working with caregivers, 214
pain catastrophizing. *See* catastrophizing
Pain Catastrophizing Scale (PCS), 80, 85
pain control, early, 18–23
pain emergency(ies), *case scenario,* 221–22
pain-exaggerating patients, 66–68
painful diabetic peripheral neuropathy (PDPN), 286–88
  treatment of, 287–88, 288f
pain intensity, measurement of, 59
pain management. *See also* pain care
  and accreditation, 242
  combined approaches for, 84–85
  in emergency department, 223
  historical perspective on, 58

pain medication(s)
  chemical structure of, 359
  dosage adjustments for kidney or liver disease, 144
  pregnancy categories of, 144
Pain Medication Questionnaire (PMQ), 346, 348t
pain medicine specialist, referral to, 67–68
pain narrative. *See also* illness narrative
  of older adults, 321–22
pain pathway(s), 8, 244f, 244
  aging and, 23, 319–20
  ascending, 14, 15f, 27–30, 33, 244f
  central, 15f
  descending, 17f, 17, 160f, 244f
  multidimensional experience of, 76–77
  in peripheral nervous system, 8–9, 244
pain prevention plan, 212
pain psychology
  case scenario, 75–76, 78f, 78, 85
  concepts of, 80–81
  interventions, 81–85, 82t
  and response to treatment, 85
pain reassessment, 68
pain scales, 59
  for children, 310
  for pediatric patients, 61–62, 62f, 63t
  selection of, based on patient characteristics, 62, 64f
pain sensation
  decreased, 11, 292, 293
  increased, 293 (*see also* allodynia; hyperalgesia)
pain sensitivity
  aging and, 319–20
  interpersonal relationships and, 44
pain summation, temporal and spatial, 12–14, 13f
pain suppression pathways, aging and, 23
pain terminology, 69
  historical perspective on, 58–59
pain threshold, 9
  definition of, 70t
  reduced, chronic opioid use and, 142
pain tolerance level
  definition of, 70t
  reduced, chronic opioid use and, 142
pain underestimation, 66f, 66
paleospinothalamic tract (PSTT), 14, 15f

palpation, 94, 96–97
  for headache, 98
  for neck and back pain, 99
pancreatitis, 226t
PANos. *See* primary afferent nociceptors (PANos)
PANs. *See* primary afferent neurons (PANs)
papaverine, 142–43
Papaver somniferum, 142–43
parabrachial nucleus, 15f
paracetamol. *See* acetaminophen
parallel pathway model, for treatment and diagnosis, 108f
paravertebral block, 252f, 252, 253t
paresthesia, definition of, 70t
PASS. *See* Pain Anxiety Symptoms Scale (PASS)
patellofemoral pai, 201
paternalism, 48, 49
patient-centered care, 122–23
  providers' role in, 123
patient-controlled analgesia (PCA), 249
  for older adults, 334
patient feedback, and clinician ratings, 128
Patient Health Questionnaire (PHQ), 325t
  PHQ-2, 323
  PHQ-9, 78, 85, 323
patient narrative. *See* illness narrative
PCS. *See* Pain Catastrophizing Scale (PCS)
PDPN. *See* painful diabetic peripheral neuropathy (PDPN)
PDUQ-p. *See* Prescription Drug Use Questionnaire—Patient version (PDUQ-p)
pectoralis stretch, 285, 373
pediatric pain assessment
  in children age 8 and older, 310
  in infants, 307
  in neonates, 307
  observational measures for, 310
  pain quality tools for, 310
  pain scales for, 310
  in preschool children, 308t, 309
  in school-age children, 308t, 309
  self-report pain intensity measures for, 310
pediatric pain management, 311–16
  acetaminophen for, 135, 313, 315
    dosage and administration by age group, 314t

case scenario, 306–7
challenges of, 307
ibuprofen for, 313, 315
  dosage and administration by age group, 314t
interdisciplinary programs for, 312, 313
key concepts of, 311
morphine in, 314t, 315
  dosage and administration by age group, 314t
nonpharmacologic strategies, 312
NSAIDs for, 135, 313
opioid rotation in, 315
opioids for, 313, 315
  dosage and administration by age group, 314t
oxycodone in, dosage and administration by age group, 314t
pharmacologic approaches, 313
pediatric pain specialist, 313
PEG Scale. *See* Pain, Enjoyment, and General Activity (PEG) Scale
pelvic inflammatory disease, 225–27
pelvic pain, 225, 264–65
  with endometriosis, 303–4
perception of pain, 9, 15–16
  exaggeration of, 15f
Percocet, 247t
periaqueductal gray (PAG), 16, 17f, 17–18
  in descending modulation of nociception, 35
  structure of, 36f
pericarditis, NSAIDs for, 136–37
perioperative pain, acetaminophen for, 135–36
peripheral nerve(s)
  development of, 21f, 21
  structure of, 58f
peripheral nerve block(s), 16, 252–54
  clinical applications of, 252, 253t
  complications of, 253–54, 253t
  contraindications to, 254
  of head and face, 178
  ultrasound guidance of, 253f, 253
peripheral nerve vasculitis, 299
  clinical features of, 299
  diagnosis of, 299
  mechanisms of, 299
  treatment of, 299

peripheral nervous system (PNS), in pain transmission, 27
peripheral neuropathic pain, definition of, 70t
peripheral neuropathy. *See also* distal symmetric polyneuropathy (DSPN); painful diabetic peripheral neuropathy (PDPN)
　lamotrigine for, 163–64
　treatment of, 287–88, 288f
peripheral neuropathy testing, 99
peripheral sensitization, 16, 33
permission(s), patient's, during examination, 92–93, 94
persistent postsurgical pain, 254–56
personality disorders, in chronic pain patients, 340–42
　and opioid misuse/addiction, 343–44
personality traits, in pain patients with negative affect, and risk of opioid misuse/addiction, 344
personalized treatment plan, 42
phantom limb pain, 295–96, 298–99b
　clinical features of, 296, 298t
　versus comcomitant pain from other factors, 295, 296
　mechanisms of, 295
　in older adults, pharmacologic therapy for, 330t
　prevalence of, 295, 298t
　treatment of, 296, 298t
　use in psychoeducation, 81–82
pharmacodynamics, age-related changes in, 334
pharmacogenetics, in older adults, 334
pharmacokinetics, age-related changes in, 334
phenanthrenes, 141, 141t, 142
　antagonists, 141t, 146
　full agonists, 141t, 143
　mixed agonist-antagonists, 145
　mixed/partial agonists, 141t
phenylacetic acids, 137t
phenylpiperidines, 141, 141t, 147
phenytoin, 165
　adverse effects of, 165
　mechanism of action of, 159b
PHN. *See* postherpetic neuralgia (PHN)
phonophobia, with migraine, 278

phospholipase C (PLC), in nociceptive transmission, 31–32
photophobia, 228–29
　with migraine, 278
PHQ. *See* Patient Health Questionnaire (PHQ)
physical activity, in pain self-management, 210, 275f
physical examination
　chaperone for, 92–93
　consent for, 92–93
　information from, and diagnostic reasoning, 108
　pain caused by, 93
　pain-focused, 93–98
　permission from patient during, 92–93, 94
　special maneuvers in, 98
physical therapy, 112–14, 275f
　for children, 312, 313
　combined with other treatment modalities, 84–85
　for low back pain, 112
　for older adults, 330t
　in pain treatment for older adults, 327
　psychologically informed, 201
　in rehabilitation setting, 201–2
Pieces of Hurt tool, 310
pinched nerve, pain of, 55f
PIPT. *See* psychologically informed physical therapy (PIPT)
piriformis injection, 192
piriformis syndrome, 55f, 112, 192
　and examination, 92–93
piriformis testing, 111
piroxicam
　dosage and administration of, 139t
　half-life of, 139t
　mechanism of action of, 138t
Pittsburgh Sleep Quality Index (PSQI), 322, 325t
PKA. *See* protein kinase A (PKA)
PKC. *See* protein kinase C (PKC)
placebo effects, 68, 69t, 213, 213t
plasmapheresis, for SPS, 303
PLC. *See* phospholipase C (PLC)
PMQ. *See* Pain Medication Questionnaire (PMQ)
pneumonia, 224t

polyarteritis nodosa, and nerve vasculitis, 299
polymodal nociceptor(s), 9–11
polymyositis, 268–69
polyneuropathy, definition of, 70t
polypharmacy, in older adults, 329
positioning, in pain treatment for older adults, 327
positron emission tomography, 111t
postdural puncture headache, 236, 250–51
postherpetic neuralgia (PHN), 265, 294–95
  clinical features of, 295
  epidemiology of, 294
  mechanisms of, 294
  in older adults, pharmacologic therapy for, 330t
  treatment of, 295
postoperative pain, 55. See also persistent postsurgical pain
  breast cancer surgery and, 206–7
  cardiac effects of, 242–43
  endocrine effects of, 243
  gastrointestinal effects of, 243
  immune system effects of, 243
  musculoskeletal effects of, 243
  nervous system effects of, 243
  in older adults, pharmacologic therapy for, 330t
  opioids for, 140–41
  in orthopedic surgery, 204–5
  physiologic impact of, 242–43
  prevalence of, 45
  pulmonary effects of, 243
poststroke syndrome, in older adults, pharmacologic therapy for, 330t
post-traumatic stress disorder (PTSD)
  assessment tool for, 324
  in older adults, 322, 324
  pain and, 43–44, 76, 78
potassium channels, 27–28
prednisone, 171
  in pain care, indications for, 171
  topical, 173
prefrontal cortex, 16, 203
pregabalin, 19f, 162
  administration route, 246t
  adverse effects of, 163
  and breastfeeding, 367
  dosage adjustments for kidney or liver disease, 367

dosage and administration of, 162–63
formulations of, 162–63
half-life of, 162–63
indications for, 162
mechanism of action of, 246t
for painful peripheral neuropathy, 287–88
precautions with, 246t
pregnancy category, 367
side effects, 246t, 287–88
trial of, for older adults unable to self-report, 325t
pregnancy. See also ectopic pregnancy
  and abdominal imaging, 223–25
  and pelvic pain, 225–27
pregnancy category(ies), of common pain medications, 144
prehabilitation, 204
  for cancer pain, 206–7
  definition of, 204
  individualized trimodal approach to, 205
  interventions used in, 204, 205
  to support pain control, 204–5
prehabilitation program, implementation of, 205
Preparedness for Caregiving Scale, 324
Prescription Drug Use Questionnaire—Patient version (PDUQ-p), 346, 348t
prevention
  case scenario, 8
  primary, 49
  secondary, 49
  tertiary, 49
primary afferent neurons (PANs), 12, 16, 160f, 171f
  structural and functional features of, 9–11, 10–11f
primary afferent nociceptors (PANos), 8–9, 12, 16
  activation of, 9
  classification of, 9–11
  decreased, 11
  dynamic regulation of, 11
  structural and functional features of, 9–11
problem list, 108–9
  creation of, 109

Procedure Behavior Check List
(PBCL), 310
Procedure Behavior Rating Scale—Revised
(PBRS-R), 310
professionalism
 case scenario, 118
 patient feedback about, 128
progressive muscle relaxation, 84
propionic acids, 137t
propoxyphene, 141t, 148
prostaglandin(s)
 and inflammatory pain, 55–56
 NSAIDs and, 137, 139–40
 PGE2, 29–30
prostanoid receptor E2 (EP2), 29–30
protein kinase A (PKA), in nociceptive
 transmission, 32–33
protein kinase C (PKC), in nociceptive
 transmission, 31–33
protons, 29–30
providers
 motivations of, 124
 role of, 123–27
provocative maneuvers, 94, 111
pruritus
 with epidural analgesia, 250–51
 opioid-induced, 249
pseudoaddiction, 230–31, 341b
PSQI. See Pittsburgh Sleep Quality
 Index (PSQI)
PSTT. See paleospinothalamic tract (PSTT)
psychiatric disorders
 in chronic pain patients, 340–42
  and opioid addiction/misuse, 343
  and problematic opioid use, 343, 351
  neurobiological factors affecting, 345
psychoeducation, 81
psychological intervention(s), 81–85, 275f
 for children, 312, 313
 combined with other treatment
  modalities, 84–85
 for complex regional pain
  syndrome, 297–98
 evidence-based, 82t
 for low back pain, 282–83, 283f
 for older adults, 330t
 for pain, 202
 for problematic opioid use, 351
 in rehabilitation, 202
 and response to treatment, 85

psychologically informed physical therapy
 (PIPT), 201
PT. See physical therapy
PTSD. See post-traumatic stress
 disorder (PTSD)
public health approach, to pain care, 49
pudendal nerve block, 191
pudendal neuralgia, 191
pudendal neuropathy, 225–27, 293–94
pulmonary embolus, 224t
pupillary light reflex, 95
Putuhepa, Queen, 158
P2X3 receptor, 29–30

qi gong, 205, 211
QRST characteristics of pain, 91,
 105b, 308t
QRSTUVW pain assessment, 308t
quad strengthening, 284, 373
question(s), open-ended, 92, 105, 120–21

radicular compression syndromes, 267
radicular pain, epidural steroid injections
 for, 183
radiculopathy, 266
 epidural steroid injections for, 183
 and low back pain, 281–82
 in older adults, pharmacologic therapy
  for, 330t
radiofrequency ablation (RFA), 177
 of medial branches of spinal nerves, 186
radiography, 110–11, 111t
Ramachandran, V. S., 75
RAMP1. See receptor activity–modifying
 protein 1 (RAMP1)
range of motion
 active, 94
 assessment of, 97, 98
 passive, 94
rapport, building, 120f, 120–22, 121f
rash, lamotrigine-induced, 164
Rathmell, James P., 176
receptor activity–modifying protein
 1 (RAMP1), in nociceptive
 transmission, 32–33
referral(s), 67–68, 92, 112
 for atypical focal pain, 264–65
 for motor weakness, 99–100
referred pain
 palpation for, 94

visceral, 12*t*
reflection, 120–21
reflective practice, 124
reflexes, 22
reflex testing, 96, 99–100
regional anesthesia, 250
rehabilitation
   behavioral interventions in, 202
   for cancer-related pain, 206–7
   case scenario, 200
   for children, 312, 313
   interventions for, 201
   neurocognitive modulation of pain
      in, 202–4
   in outpatient clinical practice, 208
   pain management and, 201
   physical therapy in, 201–2
   principles of, 200–1
   psychological interventions in, 202
      central neurophysiologic
         models, 203
      cognitive and coping models, 203
      operant model, 202
      peripheral physiologic models, 203
relationship-centered care, providers' role
   in, 123
relaxation training, 84, 203, 245
   biofeedback and, 84
remifentanil, 147
reminiscence therapy, in pain treatment for
   older adults, 328
REMs. *See* Risk Evaluation and Mitigation
   Strategies (REMs)
renal colic, in older adults, pharmacologic
   therapy for, 330*t*
renal stone, 226*t*
rescue, 275*f*
research
   IMMPACT Consortium
      recommendations for, 308*t*, 309
   on pain management, 49
respiratory arrest, opioid-induced, 232
respiratory depression
   with epidural analgesia, 250–51
   opioid-induced, 232, 236, 248
reticulospinothalamic tract. *See*
   paleospinothalamic tract (PSTT)
reward system
   dopaminergic, 345
   and opioid misuse, 345

Rexed lamina/laminae
   I, 12–14, 13*f*, 17–18, 30, 31*f*
   II, 12–14, 13*f*, 30, 31*f*
   V, 12–14, 13*f*, 15*f*, 17–18, 30
Reye syndrome, 135
rheumatoid arthritis, 262
   juvenile, 311
   and nerve vasculitis, 299
   pain of, NSAIDs for, 136–37
rheumatoid factor, laboratory testing
   for, 110*t*
rib fracture, 187–88
   pain management for, 243, 252
rippling effect of pain, 42, 43*f*
Risk Evaluation and Mitigation Strategies
   (REMs), 335–36
rituximab, for SPS, 303
rofecoxib, mechanism of action of, 138*t*
rostral ventromedial medulla (RVM),
   17*f*, 17–18
   bidirectional modulation of pain, 36–38
   in descending modulation of
      nociception, 35, 36, 37*f*
   structure of, 36*f*
Rumi, 89
RVM. *See* rostral ventromedial
   medulla (RVM)

sacroiliac joint
   anatomy of, 190–91
   dysfunction, 112, 225–27
      testing for, 100
   injection, nerve block, and
      radiofrequency ablation, 190
sacroiliac stress maneuvers, 111
safety factor, 21–22
salicylates, 137*t*, 270*f*
   nonacetylated, for older adults, 330
satellite glia cells (SGCs), 10–11*f*, 12
scalp
   nerves of, 178, 179*f*
   peripheral nerve blocks of, 178
Schwann cells, 20–22, 21*f*
   satellite, 20*f*, 171*f*
Schweitzer, Albert, 306
sciatica, 192
   and hip pain, 283–84
sciatic nerve, 192
sciatic nerve block, 252*f*, 252, 253*t*
SCN9A gene mutations, 293, 301

scotomas, 261
Screener and Opioid Assessment for Patients With Pain–Revised (SOAPP-R), 345–46, 347t
Screening Instrument for Substance Abuse Potential (SISAP), 345–46, 347t
SCS. *See* spinal cord stimulator (SCS)
search satisfying bias, 113b
second-order neurons, 12–14, 13f, 16, 17–18, 31–32, 33
sedation
  drugs causing, 232
  opioid-induced, 232, 248
    in older adults, prevention of, 335
selective serotonin/norepinephrine reuptake inhibitors, 17–18, 19f, 167
  for fibromyalgia, 300
  mechanism of action of, 38
  for older adults, 330t
  in pain care, mechanism of action of, 160b
selective serotonin reuptake inhibitors (SSRIs), 160b, 167
self-efficacy, 112–14
  low, in chronic pain patients, and opioid misuse/addiction, 343–44
self-management of pain, 112–14, 126, 127f, 274–75
  active strategies, 112–14, 275f
  comprehensive approach for, 208–10, 274–75, 275f
  coordination with provider-directed management, 126, 127f
self-management plan(s)
  coordinated multimodal, 210f, 210, 275f
  environmental factors in, 212, 275f
  medication safety in, 211, 275f
  mental preparation in, 211
  mind–body therapies in, 211
  pain prevention plan in, 212
  physical activity in, 210, 275f
  sleep optimization in, 211, 275f, 373
self-medication, in pain patients with negative affect, and risk of opioid misuse/addiction, 344
self-report, of pain, 65–66
sensation seeking, in pain patients with negative affect, and risk of opioid misuse/addiction, 344
sensitization. *See also* central sensitization
  definition of, 70t

sensory discrimination training, 203
sensory ganglion/ganglia, 10–11f, 12
sensory loss
  in distal symmetric polyneuropathy, 287
  in painful diabetic peripheral neuropathy, 287
sensory nerve(s), ablation, 177
sensory neurons, 8–9
sensory testing
  for peripheral neuropathy, 99–100
  screening, 95, 96
seroma, with intrathecal drug delivery system implantation, 235
serotonergic agents, and NSAIDs, interactions of, 140
serotonin, 17f, 17–18
  antinociceptive effect of, 38
  and nociception, 38
serotonin syndrome, 147, 232
  causes of, 232–33
  diagnostic criteria for, 232–33
  differential diagnosis, 232–33
  signs of, 232–33
  treatment of, 233
sexual abuse, early-life, as risk factor, 92
SF-MPQ, 64f
SGCs. *See* satellite glia cells (SGCs)
shared decision-making, 120f, 122
Sherrington, 58–59
shingles, 230, 265. *See also* postherpetic neuralgia (PHN)
  ophthalmic involvement in, 265
  treatment of, 265
  vaccination against, 294
shoulder, anatomy of, 193f, 285–86
shoulder injections, 192
shoulder pain, 192. *See also* chronic shoulder pain
sickle cell disease, 311
  opioids for, 315
  vaso-occlusive pain crises in, 230
Simons, David and Lois, 89
sinusitis, 264
  chronic, 264
SISAP. *See* Screening Instrument for Substance Abuse Potential (SISAP)
sleep
  in older adults, assessment of, 322
  optimization

in pain self-management, 211, 275f, 282–83, 283f, 330
in pain treatment for older adults, 327
slipping rib syndrome, 187–88
SLR. *See* straight leg raise (SLR)
small-fiber testing, 99–100
small intestine, nociception in, 11
SMART goals, 125–26, 126t
SNRIs. *See* selective serotonin/norepinephrine reuptake inhibitors
SOAPP-R. *See* Screener and Opioid Assessment for Patients With Pain–Revised (SOAPP-R)
social factors, and pain, 78
social isolation, 78
social network, impact of pain on, 44–45
Social Security Administration, disability determination process, pain and, 207
social support, 44, 67–68, 77f, 77–78, 324
somatic pain
 focal and neuropathic, 264–65
 in older adults, pharmacologic therapy for, 330t
somatization, in chronic pain patients, and opioid misuse/addiction, 343–44
somatoform pain disorders, in older adults, pharmacologic therapy for, 330t
somatosensory cortex (SI), 15f, 15–16
SONB. *See* supraorbital nerve block (SONB)
sonic hedgehog (Shh), 20f, 21
spinal column
 anatomy of, 184f
 stabilization of, 229
spinal cord, stroke, 230
spinal cord stimulation, 195f, 195. *See also* neuromodulation
spinal cord stimulator (SCS), 195
spinal disk herniation, 266
 in older adults, pharmacologic therapy for, 330t
spinal disk injury, 266, 267–68
spinal dorsal horn, 12–14, 13f, 16, 35, 160f
 in ascending transmission, 30–33, 31f
 bidirectional modulation by rostral ventromedial medulla, 36–38
 in descending modulation of pain, 33–38, 34–35f, 160f
 sites of drug action in, 174f

spinal pain, 229, 267–68
spinal stenosis, 267
 central, 279–80
 cervical, 279–80
 lateral, 279–80
 pain of, 55f
spine
 age-related changes in, 267
 degeneration of, 281–82, 282f
 metastatic involvement of, 229
spine pain, evaluation of, 99
spinothalamic tract (STT), 15f
 in nociceptive signaling, 14, 244
spirituality, 43
spiritual strategy(ies), in pain treatment for older adults, 328–29
spondylosis, 185, 186–87, 279–80
SPS. *See* stiff-person syndrome (SPS)
stages of change model, 125, 125t
statins
 drug interactions with, and risk of myopathy, 268–69
 myalgias associated with, 268–69
stellate ganglion block, 181, 182f
sternocleidomastoid muscle, palpation, precautions with, 276–77, 277f
steroids. *See also* epidural steroid injection(s) (ESIs); prednisone
 annual dose of, 233
 injection of, 177
 long-term use, effects of, 171
 in pain care, 171
Stevens-Johnson syndrome, 162
stiff-person syndrome (SPS), 302–3
stigma, 45, 49, 79
stimulus–response curve, nociceptive, 54–55
Stoics, 56–58
straight leg raise (SLR), 94, 97, 99, 111
 seated, 99
strengthening exercises
 for prevention of hip and knee pain, 284
 for prevention or reduction of chronic pain, 373
strength testing, 94, 95
 pain caused by, 93
stress, 79
stretching, for prevention or reduction of chronic pain, 285, 373

stroke, 227, 264
    and atypical focal pain, 264–65
    spinal cord, 230
STT. See spinothalamic tract (STT)
subacromial subdeltoid bursa
        injection, 192
subarachnoid hemorrhage (SAH), 227
subjective complaint, 91. See also illness
        narrative
subjective phenomena, clinician's
        understanding of, 121
"subjectivity," of pain, 106–7
substance abuse
    early-life sexual abuse and, 92
    pain and, 78
substance P, in nociceptive transmission,
        30–31, 32f, 32–33, 35
Subutex. See buprenorphine
sufentanil, 141t, 147
suicidal ideation, in older adults, 322
suicidality, 43–44
    tricyclic antidepressants and, 165
sulfones, 137t
sulindac
    dosage and administration of, 139t
    half-life of, 139t
    mechanism of action of, 138t
sunburn, pain of, 16, 55f
supraorbital nerve, 178
    neuralgia, 178
supraorbital nerve block (SONB), 178
supratrochlear nerve, 178
surgical pain management, 177, 195–97
Sutton's slip, 113b
sympathetic sprouts, abnormal, into dorsal
        root ganglion, 170, 171f
symphysis pubis, anterior, laxity of, 225–27
synaptic pruning, 18–19
synaptogenesis, 18–19
syphilis, 228–29, 263, 264
    laboratory testing and, 110t
systemic lupus erythematosus, 262
    laboratory testing and, 110t
    and nerve vasculitis, 299

tai chi, 205
tapentadol, 141t, 149
tapping test. See also Hogans tapping
        test (HTT)
    for distal symmetric polyneuropathy, 287

taut bands, palpation for, 96–97, 99, 111
TCAs. See tricyclic antidepressants
        (TCAs)
temporal arteritis, 262
temporomandibular joint (TMJ)
        disorder, 264
tenderness, palpation for, 96–97
tendonitis, NSAIDs for, 136–37
tension headache, 105, 106t, 121–22, 260.
        See also chronic tension headache
    acetaminophen for, 135–36
    and differential diagnosis, 109
    examination of patient with,
        276–77, 277f
    muscles and, 276–77, 277f
    as musculoskeletal pain-related
        condition, 277
    in older adults, pharmacologic therapy
        for, 330t
    treatment of, 277
terminology. See pain terminology
TG. See trigeminal ganglion (TG)
thalamus, 15f, 16, 244
    ventral posterior lateral (VPL), 14,
        15f, 15–16
thebaine, 142–43
therapeutic alliance, building, 120–21, 122
third-order neurons, 33
Tinel sign, 94
TIRF. See transmucosal immediate-release
        fentanyl (TIRF)
tolmetin
    dosage and administration of, 139t
    half-life of, 139t
    mechanism of action of, 138t
topical treatment, 173f, 173
    for complex regional pain
        syndrome, 297–98
    for erythromelalgia, 301
    indications for, 270f
    for older adults, 330t, 331
    for painful peripheral
        neuropathy, 287–88
    for postherpetic neuralgia, 295
topiramate, 164
    adverse effects of, 165
    dosage and administration of, 165
    drug interactions with, 165
    formulations of, 165
    indications for, 164–65

mechanism of action of, 159b, 164f, 164–65
tramadol, 141t, 150
  and breastfeeding, 367
  contraindications to
    in adolescents, 315–16b
    in children younger than 12 years, 315–16b
  dosage adjustments for kidney or liver disease, 367
  pregnancy category, 367
transcutaneous electrical nerve stimulation, 201, 245
  for older adults, 327
transdermal on-body injectors, for older adults, 334
transduction, 8–9
  of mechanical stimuli, 27–28
  of pain stimuli, 9–11
transient receptor potential (TRP), 27–29
  TRPV1, agonist, 169–70, 170f
transmission of pain, 9, 12–14
transmucosal immediate-release fentanyl (TIRF), 148
transverse myelitis, 229
transversus abdominis plane block, 252f, 252, 253t
trauma
  acute pain associated with
    imaging and, 110–11
    opioids for, 140–41
  assessment of, 225
  early-life, 92
  persistent pain after, 254–56
Travell, Janet, 89
treatment. *See also* clinical trials; pain care
  active approaches to, 123
  case scenario, 8
  comprehensive, 127f
  contingency-based approach to, 67f, 67–68
  development of, 18
  emerging trends in, 18
  ethics of, 48–49
  unpredictable responses to, 42
  variable responses to, 42
triage cueing bias, 113b
tricyclic antidepressants (TCAs), 165
  adverse effects of, 165
  contraindications to, 303
  for fibromyalgia, 300

mechanism of action of, 165, 166f
  for migraine prophylaxis, 278–79
  for older adults, 330t
  in pain care, 165
    mechanism of action of, 160b
  for shingles, 265
trigeminal ganglion (TG), 8–9, 12
trigeminal nerve, 178
  branches, blocks of, 180
trigeminal nerve block, 180
trigeminal neuralgia, 264, 293–94
  clinical features of, 294, 298t
  diagnostic nerve block for, 180
  mechanism for, 293
  in older adults, pharmacologic therapy for, 330t
  prevalence of, 298t
  therapeutic nerve block for, 180
  treatment of, 160, 163, 294, 298t
trigger points, 94, 98–99, 111, 269–70
  palpation for, 276–77, 277f
  and tension headache, 260–61
TrkB. *See* tropomyosin receptor kinase B (TrkB)
tropomyosin receptor kinase A (TrkA), 29–30
tropomyosin receptor kinase B (TrkB), in nociceptive transmission, 32f, 32–33
TRP. *See* transient receptor potential (TRP)
tumor(s). *See also* brain tumor
  and atypical focal pain, 264–65
  in children, 311
tumor necrosis factor (TNF)
  receptors, 29–30
  TNF-α, 29–30

ulcer(s), NSAID-related, 138
ulnar neuropathy, 288–89
ultrasound, 110–11, 111t
  abdominal, 223–25
  guidance, for interventions, 177
  guidance of peripheral nerve block, 253f, 253
  of soft tissue abnormalities, 264–65
  vascular, 225
universal precautions, 211–12
urinary retention
  with epidural analgesia, 250–51
  opioid-induced, 236–37, 249

urinary tract infection, 225–27
urine toxicology screening (UTS), for opioid misuse, 346
UTS. See urine toxicology screening (UTS)
UVW characteristics of pain, 91, 105b, 308t

valdecoxib, mechanism of action of, 138t
valproic acid, 165
　adverse effects of, 165
Vane, John Robert, 133
vanilloid 1 and 2, 28
VAS. See visual analog scale (VAS)
vasculitis, 262, 299
VDS. See Verbal Descriptor Scale (VDS)
venlafaxine, 167
　and breastfeeding, 367
　dosage adjustments for kidney or liver disease, 367
　pregnancy category, 367
veracity, 48
verbal descriptor rating scale (VRS), 60f, 60–61, 64f
Verbal Descriptor Scale (VDS), 325t
vertebral fractures, 229
VGCCs. See voltage-gated calcium channel(s) (VGCCs)
vibration testing, 99–100
Vicodin, 247t
viscera
　nociceptive-type innervation in, 11
　referred pain patterns of, 12t
visceral bias, 113b
visceral pain
　case scenario, 259–60
　in older adults, pharmacologic therapy for, 330t
vision impairment, headache with, 262
visual analog scale (VAS), 60f, 60, 64f, 310.
　See also Memorial Pain Assessment Card (MPAC)
　for children 8 years old and older, 310

visual testing, 95
vitamin B12 deficiency, 99–100
vitamin deficiencies, and peripheral neuropathy, 286
Volkow, Nora, 339
voltage-gated calcium channel(s) (VGCCs), 30–31, 32f
voltage-gated potassium channels, 30
voltage-gated sodium channels, 30
VRS. See verbal descriptor rating scale (VRS)

warfarin
　drug interactions with, 136
　and NSAIDs, interactions of, 140
WDR. See wide dynamic range (WDR) neurons
Wegener syndrome, and nerve vasculitis, 299
weight loss, 201
　in pain treatment for older adults, 329
Weir Mitchell, Silas, 296–97, 298–99b, 300–1
West Nile virus, 228–29
wide dynamic range (WDR) neurons, 12–14, 13f, 16
wind-up, 13f, 22, 99–100, 287
Wong-Baker FACES Pain Rating Scale, 62f, 62, 310
Woolf, Virginia, 52

yoga, 205–6, 211
　for children, 312
　for prevention or reduction of chronic pain, 373

ziconotide, 168
　mechanism of action of, 168f, 168–69
zygapophyseal joint
　dysfunction, detection of, 100–1
　osteoarthritis, detection of, 100–1

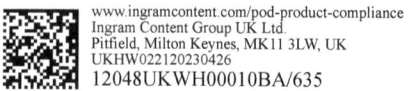